ROUTLEDGE INTERNATIONAL HANDBOOK OF MEDICAL EDUCATION

Twenty-first-century medical schools, postgraduate bodies and other medical education organisations are responding to rapid advances in medicine, healthcare delivery, educational approaches and technology, and globalisation. Differences in geography, culture, history and resources demand diversity amongst educational systems. This important volume is designed to help medical educators working in today's challenging circumstances by providing an overview of best practices and research in medical education.

The *Routledge International Handbook of Medical Education* provides a practical guide to and theoretical support for the major education challenges facing teachers, managers and policy makers around the world. Highlighting how resources can be used to provide effective and sustainable responses to the key issues facing medical educators, the handbook offers a truly international perspective of best practices with contributing editors and authors from around the globe.

The *Routledge International Handbook of Medical Education* recognises the need to maintain established best practices when appropriate and to respond adaptively to cultural differences and local conditions facing medical education. This topical book deals with the key challenges facing medical education by the different stakeholders, including:

- selection and admission of students to study medicine;
- competences necessary for graduates to enable them to recognise and address emerging health issues and policies;
- teaching and learning processes that are necessary to meet tomorrow's challenges;
- approaches to assessment, including the integration of assessment and learning;
- design and management of complex curricula that provide educational strategies to meet regional and global problems.

A unique, diverse and illustrative resource of best practices in medical education, the handbook is stimulating reading for all educators of present and future healthcare professionals.

Khalid A. Bin Abdulrahman, MD, Professor of Family Medicine & Medical Education; Vice Rector for Planning, Development and Quality; Professor Chair, Dr AlKholi Chair for Developing Medical Education in Saudi Arabia, Al Imam Mohammad Ibn Saud Islamic University (IMSIU), Saudi Arabia.

Stewart Mennin, BS, MS, PhD, Principal, Mennin Consulting and Associates; Professor Emeritus, Department of Cell Biology and Physiology; Assistant Dean Emeritus, Educational Development and Research, University of New Mexico School of Medicine, Albuquerque, New Mexico, USA.

Ronald M. Harden, OBE, MD, FRCP(GLAS.), FRCS(ED.), FRCPC, Professor Emeritus Medical Education, University of Dundee, General Secretary Association for Medical Education in Europe (AMEE), Editor, Medical Teacher, UK.

Catherine Kennedy, MA(Hons), MSc, PhD, Education Officer, Association for Medical Education in Europe (AMEE), Dundee, UK.

ROUTLEDGE INTERNATIONAL HANDBOOK OF MEDICAL EDUCATION

*Edited by Khalid A. Bin Abdulrahman,
Stewart Mennin, Ronald M. Harden
and Catherine Kennedy*

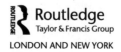

LONDON AND NEW YORK

First published 2016
by Routledge
2 Park Square, Milton Park, Abingdon, Oxon OX14 4RN

and by Routledge
711 Third Avenue, New York, NY 10017

Routledge is an imprint of the Taylor & Francis Group, an informa business

© 2016 K.A. Bin Abdulrahman, S. Mennin, R.M. Harden and C. Kennedy

The right of K.A. Bin Abdulrahman, S. Mennin, R.M. Harden and C. Kennedy to be identified as the authors of the editorial material, and of the authors for their individual chapters, has been asserted in accordance with sections 77 and 78 of the Copyright, Designs and Patents Act 1988.

All rights reserved. No part of this book may be reprinted or reproduced or utilised in any form or by any electronic, mechanical, or other means, now known or hereafter invented, including photocopying and recording, or in any information storage or retrieval system, without permission in writing from the publishers.

Trademark notice: Product or corporate names may be trademarks or registered trademarks, and are used only for identification and explanation without intent to infringe.

British Library Cataloguing-in-Publication Data
A catalogue record for this book is available from the British Library

Library of Congress Cataloging in Publication Data
The Routledge handbook of medical education / edited by Khalid A. Bin Abdulrahman, Ronald M. Harden, and Stewart Mennin.
  p. ; cm.
Handbook of medical education
Includes bibliographical references and index.
I. Abdulrahman, Khalid A. Bin, editor. II. Harden, Ronald M., editor.
III. Mennin, Stewart, editor. IV. Title: Handbook of medical education.
 [DNLM: 1. Education, Medical. W 18]
 R834
 610.71—dc23
 2015004353

ISBN: 978-0-415-81573-4 (hbk)
ISBN: 978-0-203-06620-1 (ebk)

Typeset in Bembo
by Swales & Willis Ltd, Exeter, Devon, UK

Printed and bound in the United States of America by Edwards Brothers Malloy on sustainably sourced paper.

CONTENTS

Notes on contributors xvi
Preface xxx
Acknowledgements xxxiii
List of abbreviations xxxiv

PART 1
The mission of the medical school 1

1 Rethinking the mission of the medical school 3
  Trevor Gibbs

  Case study 1.1: The new mission of the Faculty of Medicine of
    Tunis, Tunisia, Africa 4
  Ahmed Maherzi

  Case study 1.2: James Cook University School of Medicine, Australia 5
  *Sarah Larkins, Richard Murray, Tarun Sen Gupta, Simone Ross
  and Robyn Preston*

  Case study 1.3: Northern Ontario School of Medicine, Canada 7
  Roger Strasser

  Case study 1.4: The Ateneo de Zamboanga University-School of Medicine
    (ADZU-SOM), Philippines 8
  Fortunato L. Cristobal

  Case study 1.5: Lessons from eight medical schools in South Africa –
    the CHEER collaboration 9
  Stephen Reid

Contents

2   The role of the doctor and the competencies expected from the doctor of the future   18
Stefan Lindgren and David Gordon

     Case study 2.1: Easing the transition to clinical work – the role of an internship orientation programme in India   20
Rita Sood

3   Why outcome-based education (OBE) is an important development in medical education   27
Ronald M. Harden

     Case study 3.1: An integrated and community-oriented curriculum at the University of Geneva Faculty of Medicine, Switzerland   28
Anne Baroffio, Nu Viet Vu and Mathieu Nendaz

     Case study 3.2: Implementing an outcome- or competency-based approach in practice in Indonesia   31
Nancy Margarita Rehatta and Adrianta Surjadhana

     Case study 3.3: Sharing learning outcomes across health disciplines in Australia   32
Maree O'Keefe and Amanda Henderson

     Case study 3.4: Towards a competency-based curriculum – the focus of undergraduate medical education curriculum renewal at the Université de Sherbrooke, Canada   33
Marianne Xhignesse, Denis Bédard, Ann Graillon, Sharon Hatcher, Frédéric Bernier, Sylvie Houde, Daniel Gladu, Paul Chiasson and Ève-Reine Gagné

     Case study 3.5: Assessment of paediatric residents based on ACGME competencies in the USA   35
J. Lindsey Lane, Jennifer Soep and M. Douglas Jones, Jr

     Case study 3.6: Basic science integration into the whole curriculum at the Faculty of Medicine, King Abdulaziz University, Saudi Arabia   39
Abdulmonem Al-Hayani

4   How many medical students? Matching the number and types of students to a country's needs   43
Victor Lim, Abu Bakar Suleiman and Mei Ling Young

     Case study 4.1: Malaysia   47
Kok Leong Tan, Ankur Barua, Sami Abdo Radman Al-Dubai, Hematram Yadav and John Arokiasamy

     Case study 4.2: The Netherlands   48
Kok Leong Tan, Ankur Barua, Sami Abdo Radman Al-Dubai, Hematram Yadav and John Arokiasamy

Case study 4.3: South Africa 49
Kok Leong Tan, Ankur Barua, Sami Abdo Radman Al-Dubai, Hematram Yadav and John Arokiasamy

Case study 4.4: Saudi Arabia 50
Mohammad Yahya Al-Shehri

PART 2
The student 55

5 Should students be admitted to medical school directly from high school or as university graduates? 57
Trudie Roberts and Tadahiko Kozu

Case study 5.1: Catering for the school-leaver, Bond University, Gold Coast, Australia 58
Michelle McLean

Case study 5.2: Supporting transition to university study, Austral University, Argentina 60
Angel Centeno

Case study 5.3: A 30-year history of graduate-entry medical education programmes in Japan 61
Tadahiko Kozu

Case study 5.4: The experience of graduate entry into a medical programme – the case of College of Medicine, King Saud Ben Abdul-Aziz University for Health Sciences, Riyadh, Saudi Arabia 62
Ali I. Al Haqwi and Ibrahim A. Al Alwan

Case study 5.5: Graduate entry – the St George's experience, London, UK 63
Peter McCrorie

Case study 5.6: External influence in medical education, South Korea 65
Ducksun Ahn

6 How do we select students with the necessary abilities? 72
Jon Dowell

Case study 6.1: Selecting students with the necessary abilities, Aga Khan University, Pakistan 73
Rukhsana W. Zuberi and Laila Akbarali

Case study 6.2: Assessing non-academic attributes for medical and dental school admissions using a situational judgement test, United Kingdom 75
Fiona Patterson, Emma Rowett, Máire Kerrin and Stuart Martin

Contents

  Case study 6.3: The true fairy tale of the Multiple Mini-Interview,
   McMaster University, Canada   78
  Harold I. Reiter and Kevin W. Eva

  Case study 6.4: Consequences of 'selecting out' in the Netherlands   82
  Fred Tromp and Margit I. Vermeulen

7 The secret ingredient: the students' role and how they can be
  engaged with the curriculum   86
  Khalid A. Bin Abdulrahman and Catherine Kennedy

  Case study 7.1: Student engagement at the Faculty of Medicine
   in Helsinki   91
  Minna Kaila, Anna T. Heino, Kari Heinonen and Anne Pitkäranta

  Case study 7.2: Student involvement – from scratch, over self-sustainability,
   to the future, University of Maribor, Slovenia   94
  Marko Zdravkovic, Kristijan Jejcic and Ivan Krajnc

  Case study 7.3: Student mini-projects – celebrating World Health Day,
   United Arab Emirates   97
  Venkatramana Manda, Ishtiyaq A. Shaafie and Kadayam G. Gomathi

  Case study 7.4: Engaging students to take a global view of healthcare
   through the global determinants of health and development course
   in Trinity College Dublin   98
  Katherine T. Gavin and Orla Hanratty

8 Student mobility: a problem and an opportunity   101
  Athol Kent and Chivaugn Gordon

  Case study 8.1: Humanity in the workplace – Department of Obstetrics
   and Gynaecology, University of Cape Town, South Africa   103
  Veronica Mitchell, Alexandra Muller and Chivaugn Gordon

  Case study 8.2: The Cuban controversy – training South African medical
   students in Cuba   105
  Chivaugn Gordon

PART 3
The curriculum   111

9 Curriculum planning in the 21st century   113
  Ronald M. Harden

  Case study 9.1: The University of Dundee curriculum,
   United Kingdom   114
  Gary Mires and Claire MacRae

Case study 9.2: Training competent doctors for sub-Saharan Africa – experiences from an innovative curriculum in Mozambique   116
Janneke Frambach and Erik Driessen

Case study 9.3: Outcome-based curriculum in a new medical school in Peru   118
Graciela Risco de Domínguez

10   Authentic learning in health professions education: problem-based learning, team-based learning, task-based learning, case-based learning and the blend   128
Hossam Hamdy

Case study 10.1: Implementation of computer-assisted PBL sessions to medical students at Faculty of Medicine, Suez Canal University, Egypt   132
Somaya Hosny and Yasser El-Wazir

Case study 10.2: Integrated assessment in problem-based learning promotes integrated learning   134
Raja C. Bandaranayake

Case study 10.3: Authentic learning via problem-based learning – reflections from a Malaysian medical school   135
William K. Lim

Case study 10.4: The effect of team-based learning on students' learning in a basic science course at the Universidad Peruana de Ciencias Aplicadas Medical School   137
Denisse Champin

Case study 10.5: Teaching and learning basic medical sciences in the clinical environment using a task-based learning approach at the University of Sharjah, United Arab Emirates   138
Hossam Hamdy

Case study 10.6: Improving students' decision-making skills on the surgical rotation   139
Jonas Nordquist

11   Introducing early clinical experience in the curriculum   144
Ruy Souza and Antonio Sansevero

Case study 11.1: The challenges of integrating early clinical experience into the curriculum – Bond University, Australia   145
Richard Hays

Case study 11.2: Integrating early clinical experience in the curriculum – experience from a teaching hospital in United Arab Emirates   146
Manda Venkatramana and Pankaj Lamba

Case study 11.3: Early clinical exposure in graduate-entry medicine at Swansea University – Learning Opportunities in the Clinical Setting (LOCS)   148
Paul Kneath Jones and Judy McKimm

Case study 11.4: Integrating early clinical experience in the curriculum of the pre-clinical years at the Faculty of Medicine, Suez Canal University, Egypt   150
Somaya Hosny and Mirella Youssef Tawfik

Case study 11.5: Student-run clinics provide authentic patient care roles and activities for early learners, University of California, San Francisco, USA   152
H. Carrie Chen

12   Benefits and challenges associated with introducing, managing, integrating and sustaining community-based medical education   157
Regina Helena Petroni Mennin

Case study 12.1: Flinders University Parallel Rural Community Curriculum   158
Jennene Greenhill

Case study 12.2: Community-oriented education, Faculty of Medicine, University of Airlangga, Indonesia   160
Nancy Margarita Rehatta and Adrianta Surjadhana

Case study 12.3: The Selectives Programme for undergraduate medical students, Nelson R. Mandela School of Medicine, University of KwaZulu-Natal, KwaZulu-Natal, South Africa   163
Stephen Knight and Jacqueline van Wyk

Case study 12.4: '... and my patient died happy and cured', an experience in Brazil   166
Ruy Souza

Case study 12.5: Beyond the hospital, Brazil, South America   167
Regina Helena Petroni Mennin

13   Integration of the sciences basic to medicine and the whole of the curriculum   171
Stewart Mennin

Case study 13.1: Integration of simulation-based clinical correlation pedagogy within an anatomy curriculum, Kuala Lumpur, Malaysia   176
Nicole Shilkofski and Carmen Coombs

Case study 13.2: Clinical odontologists teaching basic sciences for health, integrating basic/clinic, different methodologies and disciplines in Argentina at the National University of Rio Negro Dental School – why it works   178
Elena I. Barragán

Case study 13.3: Basic science integration into the whole curriculum at the Faculty of Medicine, King Abdulaziz University, Saudi Arabia 179
Abdulmonem Al-Hayani

14 Implementing interprofessional education: what have we learned from experience? 188
Dawn Forman and Betsy VanLeit

Case study 14.1: Weaving interprofessional education into the medical curriculum at the University of Notre Dame, in Western Australia 191
Carole Steketee and Donna B. Mak

Case study 14.2: Developing community-engaged interprofessional education in the Philippines 193
Elizabeth R. Paterno, Louricha A. Opina-Tan and Dawn Forman

Case study 14.3: COBES at Moi University, Faculty of Health Sciences, Eldoret, Kenya 195
Simeon Mining and Dawn Forman

Case study 14.4: Interprofessional education in a rural clinical setting – a quick-start innovation for final-year health professional students, University of Otago, New Zealand 197
Sue Pullon, Eileen McKinlay, Peter Gallagher, Lesley Gray, Margot Skinner and Patrick McHugh

Case study 14.5: Applying interprofessional education in primary care facilities for fourth-year students at the Faculty of Medicine, Suez Canal University, Egypt 198
Somaya Hosny and Mohamed H. Shehata

Case study 14.6: Interprofessional education to prepare health professionals for rural practice in underserved New Mexico communities, USA 199
Betsy VanLeit

PART 4
Teaching and learning 205

15 How can learning be made more effective in medical education? 207
Stewart Mennin

Case study 15.1: The Primary Care Curriculum at the University of New Mexico School of Medicine 211
S. Scott Obenshain

Case study 15.2: Jack's dead and the boys have gone 213
Sweeney (2006: 3–4)

Case study 15.3: Addressing the educational needs for the 21st century – the Duke-National University of Singapore experience ... 215
Sandy Cook and Robert Kamei

16 New technologies can contribute to a successful educational programme ... 221
John Sandars

Case study 16.1: Digital story telling (DST) to enhance reflection on service learning, University of Pretoria, South Africa ... 222
Jannie Hugo

Case study 16.2: Using blogs to engage students and teaching staff in a medical school, University of Dundee, UK ... 223
Natalie Lafferty

Case study 16.3: Two models of decentralised medical education, United States ... 225
Ruth Ballweg, David Talford and Jared Papa

Case study 16.4: Using communication technology for surgical skills teaching in Uganda – a pilot study among intern doctors at Mulago National Referral and Teaching Hospital ... 227
Josaphat Byamugisha, Yosam Nsubuga, Mark Muyingo, Amy Autry, Sharon Knight, Felicia Lester, Gerald Dubowitz and Abner Korn

Case study 16.5: An online hyperlinked radiology case repository to facilitate postgraduate training in diagnostic radiology, National University of Singapore ... 228
Goh Poh Sun

Case study 16.6: Mobile devices for learning and assessment in clinical settings, University of Leeds, UK ... 230
Gareth Frith

PART 5
Assessment ... 235

17 How to implement a meaningful assessment programme ... 237
Lambert Schuwirth

Case study 17.1: Assessment in family medicine rotation, College of Medicine, King Saud University, Saudi Arabia ... 238
Eiad AlFaris, Hussain Saad Amin and Naghma Naeem

Case study 17.2: Implementing a meaningful assessment programme, Medical University of Vienna, Austria ... 239
Michael Schmidts and Michaela Wagner-Menghin

Case study 17.3: Implementing a meaningful assessment programme, St George's University of London, UK 242
Jonathan Round

18 Written and computer-based approaches are valuable tools to assess a learner's competence 247
Reg Dennick

Case study 18.1: Computer-based testing – a paradigm shift in student assessment in India 259
Bipin Batra

19 More attention is now paid to assessment of clinical competence and on-the-job assessment 263
Vanessa C. Burch

Case study 19.1: The use of workplace-based assessment in the UK Foundation Programme 265
Steve Capey and Richard Hays

Case study 19.2: Role of feedback for inference clarification during a mini-CEX encounter at the Instituto Cardiovascular de Buenos Aires, Argentina 268
Alberto Alves de Lima

Case study 19.3: Organising and running a simulation training workshop for core surgical trainees in the United Kingdom 270
T. James Royle and Steve B. Pandey

Case study 19.4: How to assess trainees' clinical competence performing endoscopies in a postgraduate residency programme at the Pontificia Universidad Católica de Chile 271
Arnoldo Riquelme

Case study 19.5: Introducing workplace-based assessment in a reformed, undergraduate curriculum at King Saud University, Saudi Arabia 274
Hamza Abdulghani and Gominda Ponnamperuma

PART 6
The medical school 279

20 International and transnational models for delivering medical education: the future for medical education 281
John Hamilton and Shajahan Yasin

Case study 20.1: Establishment of a branch campus medical
  school – Newcastle University Medicine Malaysia   283
Philip Bradley

Case study 20.2: Establishment of Monash University's Jeffrey Cheah
  School of Medicine and Health Sciences, Malaysia   284
Shajahan Yasin

Case study 20.3: The International Medical University, Kuala Lumpur,
  Malaysia   289
Victor Lim

Case study 20.4: Transnational medical education between Australia
  and the United States of America   290
David Wilkinson

21 Creating and sustaining medical schools for the 21st century   294
David Wilkinson

Case study 21.1: Mandatory versus curricular objective. Do we mean it
  when we say it? Southern Illinois University School of Medicine   295
Debra L. Klamen

Case study 21.2: A tale of two medical schools in Australia   297
Ian Wilson

Case study 21.3: Developing a distributed model of medical education
  to help meet the healthcare needs of the population of British
  Columbia, Canada   299
David Snadden

22 Recognising leadership and management within the medical school   304
Khalid A. Bin Abdulrahman and Trevor Gibbs

Case study 22.1: Recognising leadership, management and other
  responsibilities within the medical school – an example from Pakistan   308
Rukhsana W. Zuberi and Farhat Abbas

Case study 22.2: Starting a new medical school in Southern Africa –
  University of Namibia Medical School   311
Jonas Nordquist

Case study 22.3: Steps towards establishing a new medical college in
  Saudi Arabia – an insight into medical education in the Kingdom   313
Khalid A. Bin Abdulrahman and Farid Saleh

23 How teaching expertise and scholarship can be developed, recognised
  and rewarded   318
Deborah Simpson, Maryellen E. Gusic and M. Brownell Anderson

Case study 23.1: Dr Lasz Lo – clinician teacher (teaching
   activity category) 321
Deborah Simpson, Hina Mahboob, Richard J. Battiola and John R. Brill

Case study 23.2: Supporting the continuum of faculty development
   through a department for educational development, Aga Khan
   University, Pakistan 323
*Rukhsana W. Zuberi, Syeda K. Ali, Sheilla K. Pinjani, Shazia Sadaf and
Naveed Yousuf*

Case study 23.3: Institution(alising) education in a healthcare system,
   Singapore 325
Sandy Cook, Robert Kamei and Koo Wen Hsin

Case study 23.4: Aligning academic promotion with medical school
   missions and faculty roles, Eastern Virginia Medical School,
   United States 325
Elza Mylona, Aaron I. Vinik and Christine C. Matson

24 Accreditation and programme evaluation: ensuring the quality of
    educational programmes 330
    Dan Hunt, Ducksun Ahn, Barbara Barzansky and Donna Waechter

Case study 24.1: Accreditation standards as a tool to drive organisational
   culture change, The University of California, Davis, United States 331
Mark Servis and Claire Pomeroy

Case study 24.2: Using medical education accreditation standards as the
   foundation for creating Canada's first new medical school in 30 years,
   Northern Ontario School of Medicine, Canada 334
Joel H. Lanphear and Marie Matte

Case study 24.3: Overhauling the accreditation standards of the Taiwan
   Medical Accreditation Council 336
Chi-Wan Lai, Keh-Min Liu, Yan-Di Chang and Chyi-Her Lin

Case study 24.4: Developing an accreditation system from South Korea ... 338
Ducksun Ahn

Case study 24.5: Establishing a quality assurance system of medical
   education in Indonesia 340
Puti Marzoeki

PART 7
The future of medical education   353

25 Looking toward the future of medical education: fit for purpose 355
    Stewart Mennin

Index   361

CONTRIBUTORS

Farhat Abbas, MD, FCPS, FRCS, FRCSEd, FEBU, FACS. The Hussein Cumber Professor of Surgery (Urology), Department of Surgery, Dean Medical College, Aga Khan University, Pakistan

Sami Abdo Radman Al-Dubai, MBBS, MPH, DrPH, Senior Lecturer in Community Medicine, International Medical University, Kuala Lumpur, Malaysia

Hamza Abdulghani, DPHC, ABFM, FRCGP, MMEd, Professor of Medical Education and Family Medicine, Head of the Assessment and Evaluation Unit, Department of Medical Education, College of Medicine, King Saud University, Riyadh, Saudi Arabia

Ducksun Ahn, MB, MA(Art), MA(Ethics), FRCSC, Professor of Plastic Surgery and Medical Humanities, College of Medicine, Korea University

Laila Akbarali, MBA, MA(Educational Management), EdD, Senior Associate Registrar, Aga Khan University, Pakistan

Ibrahim A. Al Alwan, MRCP(UK), FAAP, FRCPC, Professor of Pediatrics and Dean, College of Medicine, King Saud bin Abdulaziz University for Health Sciences, Consultant, Pediatric Endocrinology, Ministry of NGHA, Riyadh, Saudi Arabia

Eiad AlFaris, MBBS, MSc, MRCGP, MMed, Professor of Family Medicine and Medical Education, Supervisor of the King Saud University Chair for the Development of Medical Education, Head of Family Medicine, King Saud University, Saudi Arabia

Ali I. Al Haqwi, MD, MRCGP(UK), ABFM, MHPE, PhD(Med Edu), Associate Professor/Consultant, Family Medicine, King Abdulaziz Medical City, National Guard Health Affairs, Chairman, Department of Medical Education, College of Medicine, King Saud bin Abdulaziz University for Health Sciences, Riyadh, Saudi Arabia

Contributors

Abdulmonem Al-Hayani, MBBS, DipFMS, PhD, LIFBA, Dean Students Affairs, Professor, Faculty of Medicine, King Abdul Aziz University, Jeddah, Saudi Arabia

Syeda K. Ali, MBBS, MHPE, PhD, Associate Professor, Department for Educational Development, Faculty of Health Sciences, Medical College, Aga Khan University, Karachi, Pakistan

Mohammad Yahya Al-Shehri, MBBS, FACS, D Med Ed., Professor of Surgery, King Saud University, Riyadh, Saudi Arabia

Alberto Alves de Lima, MD, MHPE, PhD, Professor of Cardiology; Director, Educational and Research Department, Instituto Cardiovascular de Buenos Aires, Affiliated to the School of Medicine, University of Buenos Aires, Argentina

Hussain Saad Amin, Assistant Professor and Consultant, Course Organizer COMM 421 (Males), Family and Community Medicine Department, College of Medicine, King Saud University, Saudi Arabia

M. Brownell Anderson, MEd, Vice President, International Programs, National Board of Medical Examiners, Philadelphia, Pennsylvania, USA

John Arokiasamy, MBBS, MSc, MPH, Professor in Community Medicine, International Medical University, Kuala Lumpur, Malaysia

Amy Autry, MD, Professor, Department of Obstetrics, Gynecology, and Reproductive Sciences, University of California, San Francisco, California, USA

Ruth Ballweg, MPA, PA-C, Professor and Senior Advisor on Advocacy, Health Policy and PA Global Development, MEDEX Northwest PA Section, Department of Family Medicine, School of Medicine, University of Washington, Seattle, Washington, USA

Raja C. Bandaranayake, MBBS, PhD, MSEd, FRACS, Consultant and Visiting Professor in Medical Education, Gulf Medical University, Ajman, United Arab Emirates

Anne Baroffio, PhD, Senior Lecturer in Medical Education, University of Geneva Faculty of Medicine, Geneva, Switzerland

Elena I. Barragán, MD, MHPE, PhD, Full Professor, Odontology School, University of Rio Negro, and Professor at the Biomedical Department, Faculty of Medical Sciences, National University of Comahue, Patagonia, Argentina

Ankur Barua, MBBS, MD, FRIPH, FRAS, Senior Lecturer in Community Medicine, International Medical University, Kuala Lumpur, Malaysia

Barbara Barzansky, PhD, MHPE, LCME Co-Secretary, Director, Undergraduate Medical Education, American Medical Association, Chicago, Illinois, USA

Contributors

Bipin Batra, MBBS, DMRD, DNB, PGDHHM, Professor and Executive Director, National Board of Examinations, India

Richard J. Battiola, MD, Director Internal Medicine Residency Program, Aurora Health Care and Associate Professor, Medicine (Clinical Adjunct), University of Wisconsin School of Medicine and Public Health, Milwaukee, Wisconsin, USA

Denis Bédard, PhD, Professor of Higher Education Teaching and Learning, Faculty of Education, Université de Sherbrooke, Sherbrooke, Quebec, Canada

Frédéric Bernier, MD, MHA, FRCPC, Associate Professor of Medicine (Endocrinology), Faculty of Medicine and Health Sciences, Université de Sherbrooke, Sherbrooke, Quebec, Canada

Khalid A. Bin Abdulrahman, MD, Professor of Family Medicine & Medical Education; Vice Rector for Planning, Development and Quality; Professor Chair, Dr AlKholi Chair for Developing Medical Education in Saudi Arabia, Al Imam Mohammad Ibn Saud Islamic University (IMSIU), Saudi Arabia

Philip Bradley, PhD, BSc(Hons), Professor of Medical Education Development and Head of School of Medical Education, Faculty of Medical Sciences, Newcastle University, Newcastle upon Tyne, UK

John R. Brill, MD, MPH, Director Clinical Student Education, Aurora Health Care, Professor, Family Medicine (Clinical Adjunct), University of Wisconsin School of Medicine and Public Health, and Medical College of Wisconsin, Milwaukee, Wisconsin, USA

Vanessa C. Burch, Professor and Chair of Clinical Medicine, Department of Medicine, Faculty of Health Sciences, University of Cape Town, Cape Town, South Africa

Josaphat Byamugisha, MBChB, DipObs, MMed, PhD, Chair, Department of Gynaecology and Obstetrics, School of Medicine, Makerere University College of Health Sciences, Makerere University College of Health Sciences, Kampala, Uganda

Steve Capey, Director of Assessment, College of Medicine, Swansea University, Swansea, UK

Angel Centeno, MD, PhD, FACP, FAcadMedEd, Chair, Department of Medical Education, Faculty of Biomedical Sciences, Austral University, Buenos Aires, Argentina

Denisse Champin, MD, FACP, MA Higher Education, Director, School of Medicine Universidad Peruana de Ciencias Aplicadas, Lima, Perú

Yan-Di Chang, MD, EdM, Former Program Manager, Medical Educators for Humanities Program, Taipei, Taiwan

H. Carrie Chen, MD, MSEd, Director, Health Professions Education Pathway, Director, Pediatric Core Clerkship, Professor of Clinical Pediatrics, Department of Pediatrics, University of California, San Francisco, UCSF Benioff Children's Hospital, USA

Contributors

Paul Chiasson, MD, CMFC, Centre de Formation Médicale du Nouveau-Brunswick, Professor, Department of Family and Emergency Medicine, Faculty of Medicine and Health Sciences, Université de Sherbrooke, Sherbrooke, Quebec, Canada

Sandy Cook, PhD, Associate Professor and Senior Associate Dean, Education, Duke-NUS Graduate Medical School Singapore, Singapore

Carmen Coombs, MD Emergency Medicine, Clinical Assistant Professor, Seattle Children's Hospital, Seattle, Washington, USA

Fortunato L. Cristobal, MD, MPH, MHPEd, FPPS, Dean, Ateneo de Zamboanga University School of Medicine, Zamboanga City, Philippines

Reg Dennick, BSc, PhD, MEd, FHEA, Professor of Medical Education, Assistant Director of Medical Education, School of Medicine, University of Nottingham, Nottingham, UK

Graciela Risco de Domínguez, MD, Doctor in Medicine (PhD), Dean of the School of Health Sciences, Universidad Peruana de Ciencias Aplicadas (UPC), Lima, Peru

Jon Dowell, BMSc, BMBS, MD, MRCGP, FHEA, Professor of General Practice and Admissions Convenor Dundee Medical School, Dundee, Scotland, UK

Erik Driessen, MA, PhD, Associate Professor, School of Health Professions Education and Chair, Department of Educational Development and Research, Faculty of Health, Medicine and Life Sciences, Maastricht University, Maastricht, Netherlands

Gerald Dubowitz, MD, Associate Professor, Department of Anesthesia and Perioperative Care, University of California, San Francisco, California, USA

Yasser El-Wazir, Professor and Head of Physiology Department, Faculty of Medicine, Suez Canal University, Ismailia, Egypt. Director of the Quality Assurance Center, Suez Canal University, Egypt

Kevin W. Eva, PhD, Hon FAcadMEd, Associate Director and Senior Scientist, Centre for Health Education Scholarship; Professor and Director of Education Research and Scholarship, Department of Medicine, University of British Columbia, Vancouver, Canada

Dawn Forman, PhD MBA, Visiting Professor University of Derby, UK, and University of Chichester, UK, Adjunct Professor Curtin University, Australia, and Auckland University of Technology, New Zealand

Janneke Frambach, MA(Hons), MSc(Hons), PhD, Assistant Professor, School of Health Professions Education, Faculty of Health, Medicine and Life Sciences, Maastricht University, Maastricht, Netherlands

Gareth Frith, BA, Technology Enhanced Learning Manager, Leeds Institute of Medical Education, School of Medicine, University of Leeds, Leeds, UK

Contributors

Ève-Reine Gagné, MD, FRCPC, Vice-Dean, Undergraduate Medical Education, Faculty of Medicine and Health Sciences, Université de Sherbrooke, Sherbrooke, Quebec, Canada

Peter Gallagher, RN, MA, PhD, Medical Education Advisor University of Otago, Wellington, New Zealand

Katherine T. Gavin, MB BCh BAO, BSc, MBA, PhD, Healthcare Management Consultant, formerly Clinical Lecturer in Medical Education, Trinity College Dublin, Ireland

Trevor Gibbs, MD, DA, MMedSci, FRCGP, SFHEA, FAcadMED, Consultant in Medical Education, Primary Care and Adolescent Health and the Development Officer for the Association for Medical Education in Europe (AMEE)

Daniel Gladu, Dipl. Ed., 3rd cycle, CHRP, Education Design Specialist, Office of Undergraduate Medical Education, Faculty of Medicine and Health Sciences, Université de Sherbrooke, Sherbrooke, Quebec, Canada

Kadayam G. Gomathi, PhD, GradDipHPE, Professor of Biochemistry, College of Medicine, Gulf Medical University, Ajman, United Arab Emirates

Chivaugn Gordon, MBChB, Dip HIV Man. Dip. Mental Health, Lecturer and Head of Undergraduate Obstetrics and Gynaecology Education, Faculty of Health Sciences, University of Cape Town, Cape Town, South Africa

David Gordon, FRCP, FMedSci, President, World Federation for Medical Education, Ferney-Voltaire, France

Ann Graillon, MD, MHA, FRCPC, Professor, Department of Pediatrics, Centre de Pédagogie des Sciences de la Santé (CPSS), Faculty of Medicine and Health Sciences, Université de Sherbrooke, Sherbrooke, Quebec, Canada

Lesley Gray, FFPH, MPH, MSc, Senior Lecturer, Department of Primary Health Care and General Practice, University of Otago, Wellington, New Zealand

Jennene Greenhill, RN, BA, MSPD, PhD, Professor and Associate Dean, Flinders University Rural Clinical School, Coordinator Masters of Clinical Education, Renmark, Australia

Tarun Sen Gupta, MBBS, PhD, FACRRM, FRACGP, Professor of Health Professional Education and Director of Medical Education, College of Medicine and Dentistry, James Cook University, Townsville, Australia

Maryellen E. Gusic, MD, Chief Medical Education Officer, Association of American Medical Colleges, Washington, District of Columbia, USA

Hossam Hamdy, MBChB, MCh, FRCS, FACS, PhD(Edu), Professor of Surgery and Medical Education, Vice Chancellor for Medical and Health Sciences Colleges; Dean, College of Medicine, University of Sharjah, Sharjah, United Arab Emirates

Contributors

John Hamilton, BA, DipEd, MEd(TESOL), Lecturer/Educational Developer, Department of Academic Support and Development, College of Health and Biomedicine, Victoria University, Melbourne, Australia

Orla Hanratty, BEd, MSc, Lecturer in Education in the School of Education, Trinity College Dublin and Learning Development Officer in Dublin Institute of Technology. Formerly Curriculum Advisor and Lecturer in Medical Education in the School of Medicine, Trinity College Dublin, Ireland

Ronald M. Harden, OBE, MD, FRCP(GLAS.), FRCS(ED.), FRCPC, Professor Emeritus Medical Education University of Dundee, General Secretary, Editor, Medical Teacher Association for Medical Education in Europe (AMEE), UK

Sharon Hatcher, MD, FCFP, Saguenay Medical Program Director, Associate Dean, Faculty of Medicine and Health Sciences, Université de Sherbrooke, Sherbrooke, Quebec, Canada

Richard Hays, MBBS PhD MD FRACGP, Professor of Medical Education (Dean of Medicine) at the University of Tasmania, Hobart, Australia

Anna T. Heino, Medical Student, University of Helsinki, Finland

Kari Heinonen, MD (medical student during the writing of the manuscript), University of Helsinki, Finland

Amanda Henderson, RN, RM, PhD, Nursing Director (Education), Queensland Health Research Fellow, ALTC Discipline Scholar (Health), Australian Learning and Teaching Fellow, Professor, Griffith Health, Griffith University, Princess Alexandra Hospital, Queensland, Australia

Somaya Hosny, MD, PhD, MHPE, Professor, Dean, Faculty of Medicine, Suez Canal University, Egypt

Sylvie Houde, PhD, Educational Developer, Centre de Pédagogie des Sciences de la Santé (CPSS), Faculty of Medicine and Health Sciences, Université de Sherbrooke, Sherbrooke, Quebec, Canada

Koo Wen Hsin, MBBS(S'pore), FRCP(Edin), Associate Professor, Duke-NUS Graduate Medical School Singapore, Group Director, Education, Singhealth, Singapore

Jannie Hugo, MB, ChB, M Fam Med, Professor and Head, Department of Family Medicine, University of Pretoria, South Africa

Dan Hunt, MD, MBA, LCME Co-Secretary, Senior Director for Accreditation Services, Association of American Medical Colleges, Washington, DC, USA

Kristijan Jejcic, MD, Resident of Psychiatry, University Medical Centre Maribor, Slovenia; formerly Vice-Dean for Student Affairs, Faculty of Medicine, University of Maribor, Slovenia

Contributors

M. Douglas Jones Jr, MD, Professor, Department of Pediatrics, University of Colorado School of Medicine, Aurora, Colorado, USA

Paul Kneath Jones, RGN, BSc, Honorary Associate Professor and Programme Director, Swansea College of Medicine, Swansea, UK

Minna Kaila, MD, PhD, Special Competence in Medical Education, Professor, Faculty of Medicine, University of Helsinki; President, Association for Medical Education in Finland, Helsinki, Finland

Robert Kamei, MD, Professor and Vice Dean, Education, Duke-NUS Graduate Medical School Singapore, Singapore; Professor of Pediatrics, Duke University School of Medicine, Durham NC, USA

Catherine Kennedy, MA(Hons), MSc, PhD, Education Officer, Association for Medical Education in Europe (AMEE), Dundee, UK

Athol Kent, MBChB, MPhil, FRCOG, FCOG(SA) Ad Eundem, Emeritus Associate Professor, Department of Obstetrics and Gynaecology, Faculty of Health Sciences, University of Cape Town, South Africa

Máire Kerrin, BSc, MSc, PhD, CPsychol, Director at the Work Psychology Group, UK

Debra L. Klamen, MD, MHPE, Professor and Chair, Department of Medical Education, Associate Dean for Education and Curriculum, Southern Illinois University School of Medicine, Springfield, Illinois, USA

Sharon Knight, MD, Associate Professor, Department of Obstetrics, Gynecology and Reproductive Sciences, University of California, San Francisco, California, USA

Stephen Knight, BSc(Med), MBBCh(Wits), DTM&H, DPHC(Ed), FCPHM(SA), Public Health Medicine Physician, School of Nursing and Public Health, College of Health Sciences, University of KwaZulu-Natal, Durban, South Africa

Abner Korn, MD, Professor , Department of Obstetrics, Gynecology, and Reproductive Sciences, University of California, San Francisco, California, USA

Tadahiko Kozu, MD, Professor Emeritus, formerly Professor of Gastroenterology and Chairman of Department of Medical Education, Tokyo Women's Medical University, Tokyo, Japan

Ivan Krajnc, MD, PhD, Professor of Internal Medicine and Dean, Faculty of Medicine, University of Maribor, Slovenia

Natalie Lafferty BSc(Hons), Director Technology in Learning, Technology and Innovation in Learning Team, College of Medicine, Nursing and Dentistry, University of Dundee, Dundee, UK

Contributors

Chi-Wan Lai, MD, Chairman, Taiwan Medical Accreditation Council, Taipei, Taiwan

Pankaj Lamba, MBBS, DO(Gold Medalist), DNB FRCS(Glasg), GradDipHPE, Clinical Assistant Professor in Ophthalmology, Gulf Medical University, Specialist in Ophthalmology, GMC Hospital and Research Center, Ajman, United Arab Emirates

J. Lindsey Lane, BMBCh, Professor and Vice Chair of Education, Department of Pediatrics, University of Colorado School of Medicine, Aurora, Colorado, USA

Joel H. Lanphear, PhD, Interim Senior Associate Dean for Academic Affairs, Central Michigan University College of Medicine, Mount Pleasant Michigan, USA

Sarah Larkins, MBBS, MPH&TM, BMedSci PhD, FRACGP, FARGP, Professor and Associate Dean of Research, College of Medicine and Dentistry, Co-Director, Anton Breinl Research Centre for Health Systems Strengthening, James Cook University, Townsville, Australia

Felicia Lester, MD, MPH, Assistant Professor, Department of Obstetrics, Gynecology, and Reproductive Sciences, University of California, San Francisco, California, USA

Victor Lim, MB, MSc, FRCPath, Vice President (Education) and Professor of Pathology, International Medical University, Kuala Lumpur, Malaysia

William K. Lim, BPharm, FSHP(Aust), MS, PhD, Associate Professor, Faculty of Medicine and Health Sciences, Universiti Malaysia Sarawak, Sarawak, Malaysia

Chyi-Her Lin, MD, Professor of Pediatrics, College of Medicine, National Cheng-Kung University, Tainan, Taiwan

Stefan Lindgren, MD, PhD, FACP, FRCP, Professor in Medicine, Senior Consultant in Gastroenterology, Past President World Federation for Medical Education, Lund University, University Hospital Skane, Sweden

Keh-Min Liu, DDS, PhD, Professor of Anatomy, School of Medicine; Chair, Center of Medical Education Research, College of Medicine, Kaohsiung Medical University, Kaohsiung, Taiwan

Claire MacRae, BMSc(Hons) PGCE, Staff Development Officer at University of Dundee, Dundee, Scotland, UK

Hina Mahboob, MD, Associate Director Internal Medicine Residency Program, Aurora Health Care and Assistant Professor, Medicine (Clinical Adjunct), University of Wisconsin School of Medicine and Public Health, Milwaukee, Wisconsin, USA

Ahmed Maherzi, MD, Professor of Paediatrics and Dean of Tunis Medical School, University of Tunis El Manar, Tunisia

Contributors

Donna B. Mak, MBBS, MPH, Chair, Population and Preventive Health Domain, School of Medicine, University of Notre Dame, Fremantle, Australia

Venkatramana Manda, MBBS, MS, FRCSEd, GradDipHPE, Clinical Professor of Surgery and Dean, College of Medicine, Consultant Surgeon, GMC Hospital and Research, Center, Gulf Medical University, Ajman, United Arab Emirates

Stuart Martin, BSc, MSc, CPsychol, Senior Psychologist at the Work Psychology Group, UK

Puti Marzoeki, MD, MPH, Senior Health Specialist, World Bank, Jakarta, Indonesia

Christine C. Matson MD, Glenn Mitchell Chair in Generalist Medicine, Chair, Department of Family and Community Medicine, Eastern Virginia Medical School, Norfolk, Virginia, USA

Marie Matte, BA, ART, MEd, PhD, Associate Dean, Compliance, Assessment, and Evaluation, Central Michigan University College of Medicine, Mount Pleasant Michigan, USA

Peter McCrorie, BSc, PhD, Professor of Medical Education, St George's, University of London, UK

Patrick McHugh, MB, ChB, FRNZCGP, FRCUC, FDRHM, Programme Leader, Tairawhiti Interprofessional Education Programme, University of Otago, New Zealand

Judy McKimm, BA, MA(Ed), MBA, Dean and Professor of Medical Education, Swansea University, UK

Eileen McKinlay, RN, MA(App), Senior Lecturer, Department of Primary Health Care and General Practice, University of Otago, Wellington, New Zealand

Michelle McLean, BSc(Hons), MSc, PhD MEd, Professor and Associate Dean, Faculty of Health Sciences and Medicine, Bond University, Gold Coast, Australia

Regina Helena Petroni Mennin, BS, CHES, MHS, DrPH, Professor of Human Sciences in Health, Department of Preventive Medicine, Federal University of São Paulo, School of Medicine, São Paulo, Brazil

Stewart Mennin, BS, MS, PhD, Principal, Mennin Consulting and Associates; Professor Emeritus, Department of Cell Biology and Physiology; Assistant Dean Emeritus, Educational Development and Research, University of New Mexico School of Medicine, Albuquerque, New Mexico, USA

Simeon Mining, DVM, MSc, PhD, DMed (h.c), Moi University, Department of Immunology, Kenya, Nairobi

Gary Mires, Dean of Medical Education, Professor of Obstetrics, School of Medicine, University of Dundee, Dundee, UK

Contributors

Veronica Mitchell, BSc(Physio) MPhil(HES), Facilitator, Faculty of Health Sciences, University of Cape Town, PhD Candidate, University of the Western Cape, Cape Town, South Africa

Alexandra Muller, Dr Med, Postdoctoral Research Fellow, Health and Human Rights Programme, School of Public Health and Family Medicine, University of Cape Town, South Africa

Richard Murray, MBBS MPH&TM DipRANZCOG FACRRM FRACGP, Dean and Head of College, College of Medicine and Dentistry, James Cook University, Townsville, Australia

Mark Muyingo, Lecturer Directorate of Obstetrics and Gynaecology, Makerere University College of Health Sciences, Kampala, Uganda

Elza Mylona, PhD, Professor of Medicine, Vice Dean of Faculty Affairs and Professional Development, Eastern Virginia Medical School, USA

Naghma Naeem, BSc, MBBS, MMed, PhD, Associate Professor and Head of Department of Medical Education, Batterjee Medical College, Jeddah, Saudi Arabia

Mathieu Nendaz, MD, MHPE, Associate Professor of Internal Medicine and Medical Education, University of Geneva Faculty of Medicine, Geneva, Switzerland

Jonas Nordquist, PhD, Director Medical Case Centre, Karolinska Institutet and Associate Director Residency Programs, Karolinska University Hospital, Sweden

Yosam Nsubuga, Lecturer, Directorate of Obstetrics and Gynaecology, Makerere University College of Health Sciences, Kampala, Uganda

S. Scott Obenshain, MD, Executive Dean, Ross University School of Medicine, Albuquerque, New Mexico, USA

Maree O'Keefe, PhD, MBBS, DCCH, FRACP, Professor and Associate Dean Learning and Teaching, Faculty of Health Sciences, University of Adelaide, Adelaide, Australia

Louricha A. Opina-Tan, MD, Diplomate, Philippine Academy of Family Physicians (DPAFP), Department of Family and Community Medicine, University of the Philippines-Philippine General Hospital, Manila, Philippines

Steve B. Pandey, MBBS, FRCS, Consultant Colorectal Surgeon, Worcestershire Royal Hospital, Worcester, UK

Jared Papa, MPAS, PA-C, Clinical Assistant Professor, Service Learning Coordinator, Idaho State University, Physician Assistant Program, Meridian, Idaho, USA

Elizabeth R. Paterno, MD, MPH, College of Medicine, University of the Philippines, Ermita, Manila, Philippines

Contributors

Fiona Patterson, BSc, MSc, PhD, CPsychol, AcSS, FRSA, FCMI, FRCGP(Hon), Professor, Principal Researcher, University of Cambridge, UK

Sheilla K. Pinjani, MBBS, MPHIL, MMedEd, Lecturer, Department for Educational Development, Faculty of Health Sciences, Medical College, Aga Khan University, Karachi, Pakistan

Anne Pitkäranta, Vice Dean (Education), Faculty of Medicine, University of Helsinki, Finland

Claire Pomeroy, MD, MBA, President, Albert and Mary Lasker Foundation, New York, New York, USA

Gominda Ponnamperuma, MBBS(Colombo), Dip. Psychology(Colombo), MMEd(Dundee), PhD(Dundee), Senior Lecturer in Medical Education, Faculty of Medicine, University of Colombo, Sri Lanka

Robyn Preston, MHSc(HealthProm) PGCertDisasRefugHlth BA(DevS)(Hons), Lecturer and PhD Candidate, General Practice and Rural Medicine, College of Medicine and Dentistry, James Cook University, Townsville, Australia

Sue Pullon, MBChB, FRNZCGP, MPHC, Associate Professor and Head of Department, Primary Health Care and General Practice, University of Otago, Wellington, New Zealand

Nancy Margarita Rehatta, MD, PhD, Professor in Anesthesiology; Head, Medical Education, Research and Staff Development Unit, Faculty of Medicine, Airlangga University, Indonesia

Stephen Reid, BSc, MBChB, MFamMed, PhD, Professor and Chair of Primary Health Care, Primary Health Care Directorate, Faculty of Health Sciences, University of Cape Town, South Africa

Harold I. Reiter, MD, MEd, FRCPC, DABR, Professor, Department of Oncology, Assistant Dean and Director, Program for Educational Research and Development, McMaster University, Hamilton, Canada

Arnoldo Riquelme, MD, MMed, Department of Gastroenterology, Centre for Medical Education, Faculty of Medicine, Pontificia Universidad Católica de Chile, Santiago, Chile

Trudie Roberts, BSc, MBChB, PhD, FRCP, FHEA, NTF, Hon FAcadMEd, Director, Leeds Institute of Medical Education University of Leeds, UK

Simone Ross, BPsych and MDR, Lecturer, General Practice and Rural Medicine, College of Medicine and Dentistry, James Cook University, Townsville, Australia

Jonathan Round, Dr, Reader in Clinical Education, Consultant in Paediatric Intensive Care, Institute of BioMedical Education, St George's, University of London, UK

Emma Rowett, BSc, MSc, Consultant Psychologist at the Work Psychology Group, UK

T. James Royle, MBChB, FRCS, MMedEd, National Laparoscopic Colorectal Fellow, Newcastle upon Tyne Hospitals, NHS Foundation Trust, Newcastle upon Tyne, UK

Contributors

Shazia Sadaf, BDS, MMEdEd, Visiting Faculty, Department for Educational Development, Faculty of Health Sciences, Medical College, Aga Khan University, Karachi, Pakistan

Farid Saleh, Department of Anatomy, College of Medicine, Al-Imam Mohammad Ibn Saud Islamic University, Riyadh, Saudi Arabia

John Sandars, MD, MSc, MRCP, MRCGP, FAcadMEd, CertEd, Professor of Medical Education, Director of Research, Medical Education, Medical School, University of Sheffield, UK

Antonio Sansevero, MD, MHPE, Pediatric Surgeon, Assistant Professor, Federal University of Roraima, Brazil

Michael Schmidts, MD, MME, Assistant Professor, Department of Medical Education, Medical University of Vienna, Austria

Lambert Schuwirth, MD, PhD, Professor of Medical Education, Flinders University, Adelaide, Australia, Professor for Innovative Assessment, Maastricht University, Maastricht, Netherlands

Mark Servis, MD, Senior Associate Dean for Medical Education, Roy Brophy Chair and Professor of Clinical Psychiatry, University of California, Davis, School of Medicine, USA

Ishtiyaq A. Shaafie, MBBS, MD, GradDipHPE, Professor and Head, Department of Biochemistry, College of Medicine, Gulf Medical University, Ajman, United Arab Emirates

Mohamed H. Shehata, MRCGP, MD, JMHPE, Associate Professor of Family Medicine, Suez Canal University, Medical Education Consultant at the Egyptian Fellowship – Ministry of Health, Ismailia, Egypt

Nicole Shilkofski, MD, MEd, FAAP, Assistant Professor of Pediatrics, Anesthesiology and Critical Care Medicine, Johns Hopkins University School of Medicine, Baltimore, Maryland, USA. Former Vice Dean for Education at Perdana University Graduate School of Medicine, Kuala Lumpur, Malaysia

Deborah Simpson, PhD, Director Medical Education Programs, Aurora Health Care and Professor, Family and Community Medicine (Clinical Adjunct), Medical College of Wisconsin and University of Wisconsin School of Medicine and Public Health, Milwaukee, Wisconsin, USA

Margot Skinner, PhD, MPhEd, DipPhty, FNZCP, Senior Lecturer, School of Physiotherapy, University of Otago, Dunedin, New Zealand

David Snadden, MBChB, MClSc, MD, FRCGP, FRCP(Edin), CCFP, Professor of Family Practice, Executive Associate Dean Education, University of British Columbia, Canada

Jennifer Soep, MD, Associate Professor and Pediatric Clerkship Director, Department of Pediatrics, University of Colorado School of Medicine, Aurora, Colorado, USA

Contributors

Rita Sood, MD, MMEd, FAMS, FRCP, Professor, Department of Medicine, All India Institute of Medical Sciences, New Delhi, India

Ruy Souza, Assistant Professor of Neurology and Medical Education, Federal University of Roraima, Boa Vista, Brazil

Carole Steketee, PhD, BEd(Hons), BA(Ed), Professor and Associate Dean of Teaching and Learning, School of Medicine, University of Notre Dame, Australia

Roger Strasser, MBBS, BMedSc, MClSc, FRACGP, FACRRM, FRCGP(Hon), Professor and Dean, Northern Ontario School of Medicine, Lakehead and Laurentian Universities, Thunder Bay and Sudbury, Canada

Abu Bakar Suleiman, MDBS, FRACP, MMed, President, International Medical University, Kuala Lumpur, Malaysia

Poh Sun Goh, MBBS(Melb), FRCR, FAMS, MHPE(Maastricht), Associate Professor and Senior Consultant Department of Diagnostic Radiology, Yong Loo Lin School of Medicine, National University of Singapore, Singapore

Adrianta Surjadhana, MD, Senior Lecturer Physiology, Department Physiology, School of Medicine, Airlangga University, Surabaya, Indonesia

David Talford, MPAS, PA-C, Clinical Assistant Professor, Department of Physician Assistant Studies, Idaho State University, Meridian, Idaho, USA

Kok Leong Tan, MBBCh, BAO, MPH, MPH Family Health, Senior Lecturer in Community Medicine, International Medical University, Kuala Lumpur, Malaysia

Mirella Youssef Tawfik, MD, PHPSMed, Assistant Professor of Public Health, Community Medicine, Former Director of Clinical Skills Lab, Faculty of Medicine, Suez Canal University, Ismailia, Egypt

Fred Tromp, PhD, Researcher, Department of Primary Care and Community Care, Radboud University Nijmegen Medical Centre, Netherlands

Betsy VanLeit, PhD, OTR/L, Associate Professor and Director, Occupational Therapy Program, Department of Pediatrics, Health Sciences Center, University of New Mexico, Albuquerque, New Mexico, USA

Jacqueline van Wyk, BSc(Ed), UWC, BEd, MEd(UN), PhD(UKZN), FAIMER, Consultant Clinical and Professional Education, Nelson R. Mandela School of Medicine, College of Health Sciences, University of KwaZulu-Natal, Durban, South Africa

Manda Venkatramana, MBBS, MS, FRCSEd, GradDipHPE, Clinical Professor of Surgery and Dean, College of Medicine, Consultant Surgeon, GMC Hospital and Research Center, Gulf Medical University, Ajman, United Arab Emirates

Contributors

Margit I. Vermeulen, MD, MSc, PhD, General Practitioner, Julius Centre for Health Sciences and Primary Care, University Medical Centre Utrecht, Netherlands

Aaron I. Vinik, MD, PhD, FCP, MACP, FACE, Murray Waitzer Endowed Chair for Diabetes Research, Professor of Medicine/Pathology/Neurobiology, Director of Research and Neuroendocrine Unit, Eastern Virginia Medical School, Norfolk, Virginia, USA

Nu Viet Vu, PhD, Professor of Medical Education and Director of the Unit of Development and Research in Medical Education, University of Geneva Faculty of Medicine, Geneva, Switzerland

Donna Waechter, PhD, LCME Assistant Secretary, Senior Director, LCME Surveys and Team Training, Association of American Medical Colleges, Washington, DC, USA

Michaela Wagner-Menghin, Priv.-Doz. Mag. Dr., Assistant Professor, Department for Medical Education, Medical University Vienna, Austria

David Wilkinson, MBChB, FRCP, PhD, DSc, Deputy Vice Chancellor (Corporate Engagement and Advancement), Macquarie University, Sydney, Australia

Ian Wilson, MBBS, FRACGP, MAssess&Eval, PhD, Dean of Medicine, University of Wollongong, NSW, Australia

Marianne Xhignesse, MD, MSc, Professor, Department of Family and Emergency Medicine, Centre de Pédagogie des Sciences de la Santé (CPSS), Faculty of Medicine and Health Sciences, Université de Sherbrooke, Sherbrooke, Quebec, Canada

Hematram Yadav, MBBS, MPH, MBA, FAMM, Professor in Community Medicine, International Medical University, Kuala Lumpur, Malaysia

Shajahan Yasin, MBBS, FRACGP, MAFP, Professor and Director of Curriculum, Jeffrey Cheah School of Medicine and Health Sciences, Monash University Malaysia

Mei Ling Young, BA, MA, PhD, Provost, International Medical University, Kuala Lumpur, Malaysia

Naveed Yousuf, MBBS, MBA, Adv Dip HPE, PhD, Assistant Professor, Department for Educational Development, Faculty of Health Sciences, Medical College, Aga Khan University, Karachi, Pakistan

Marko Zdravkovic, MD, Resident of Anaesthesiology and Intensive Care, University Medical Centre Maribor; Teaching Assistant in Physiology and formerly Head of Centre for Medical Education, Faculty of Medicine, University of Maribor, Slovenia

Rukhsana W. Zuberi, MD, FCPS-Med MHPE, The Noor Mohammad E Mewawalla Professor of Family Medicine and Associate Dean Education, Chair of Department for Educational Development, Faculty of Health Sciences, Aga Khan University, Pakistan

PREFACE

This is a time of unprecedented change in medical education around the world. Medical schools, postgraduate bodies and other organisations are responding to rapid advances in medicine, changes in healthcare delivery and public and governmental expectations, new education approaches, and technology and globalisation with greater doctor mobility. Differences in geography, culture, history and resources lead to diversity among education systems in the responses to these pressures. There is a need to exchange information about educational approaches from different situations, to learn from the experiences of others and how they have overcome the challenges they have faced. There is a growing interest in sharing best practices through the expanding literature on medical education and the increasing participation in international conferences such as the Association for Medical Education in Europe (AMEE) annual conference, which attracts more than 3,500 participants from over 100 countries. This book offers a unique perspective on how we can respond to the contemporary challenges that are common to educators internationally and also unique to different regions with variable resource limitations.

The *Routledge International Handbook of Medical Education* recognises and addresses the tensions between approaches to solutions relating to broad and general international practice and local adaptive approaches and solutions that meet the needs of different regions with different resources, cultures, healthcare delivery systems and politics. It recognises the need to maintain established successful practices when appropriate and to respond adaptively to the challenges facing healthcare and medical education with the possibility of disruptive innovation. The *Handbook* also recognises tension between being prescriptive with precise guidelines and specifications about what needs to be done and elicitation and distillation of the principles that enable a school to develop their own 'fit for function' solutions to their challenges. The *Routledge International Handbook of Medical Education* offers a unique international perspective based on 97 case studies that recognise and value cultural differences and their contributions and impact on medical education.

The book is a unique resource illustrative of best practices in medical education addressing regional and global challenges around the world. The book speaks directly to teachers, administrators and managers, researchers and policy makers in diverse scenarios working to improve medical education and to improve the health of societies. It aims to stimulate educators of present and future healthcare professionals to benchmark their own programmes. Leading authorities from different regions focus on present and future directions for medical education, and on a research agenda for health education practices and policy development. The chapter authors and case study contributors bring a rich and robust international perspective to the work and assure the relevance of the book to contemporary challenges among a wide range of stakeholders. The editors of the book have collaborated with chapter authors to synthesise and highlight best practices and to build on the case studies to frame current and future directions that promote sustainability and the adaptability of medical education.

The book is organised into seven parts: (1) the mission of the medical school; (2) the student; (3) the curriculum; (4) teaching and learning; (5) assessment; (6) the medical school; and (7) the future of medical education.

The chapters in each part outline key themes and issues relating to the topic while introducing different regional approaches and strategies that constitute best practice for a given set of problems through integrated case studies illustrating the diversity of practices in the face of regional and global changes. There are contributions from 199 authors from 26 countries across all regions of the globe.

Part 1: The mission of the medical school opens with a chapter by Trevor Gibbs exploring how the mission of medical schools has changed over the last century to include a growing emphasis on social accountability and responsibility, with illustrative case studies from Tunisia, Australia, Canada and the Philippines. The theme of change continues in Chapter 2 by Stefan Lindgren and David Gordon, who consider the evolving role of the doctor and the future competencies that will be required. Issues such as professionalism, the needs of society, lifelong learning and the global role of the doctor are discussed, with a case study from India. Ronald M. Harden takes up the theme and discusses the recent move to outcome- or competency-based education, with case studies from Switzerland, Indonesia, Australia, Canada, the USA and Saudi Arabia. This section concludes with a chapter by Victor Lim and colleagues exploring issues arising in relation to determining the number of medical students who should be admitted to study in different countries, with case studies from Malaysia, the Netherlands, South Africa and Saudi Arabia.

Part 2: The student begins with a chapter by Trudie Roberts and Tadahiko Kozu, who consider the comparative advantages of different entry points for medical students, with case studies from Australia, Argentina, Japan, Saudi Arabia, the UK and South Korea. Jon Dowell explores approaches and considerations for student selection given differing workforce needs and requirements across the globe, with case studies from Pakistan, the UK, Canada and the Netherlands. Khalid A. Bin Abdulrahman and Catherine Kennedy examine the growing emphasis being placed in many medical schools on student engagement within the institutions, curriculum, academic and local communities, with case studies from Finland, Slovenia, United Arab Emirates and Ireland. Athol Kent and Chivaugn Gordon consider the benefits and challenges of the increasing internationalisation of medical education and student mobility, drawing on the experience of contrasting approaches in South Africa.

Curriculum is the focus for *Part 3: The curriculum* of the book, with an opening chapter by Ronald M. Harden on planning curriculum in the 21st century. Key themes explored include authenticity, collaboration and the changing role of students and teachers, with case studies from the UK, Mozambique and Peru. The issue of authenticity is picked up by Hossam Hamdy, who compares different approaches to learning with case studies from Egypt, Bahrain, Malaysia, Peru and the United Arab Emirates. Ruy Souza and Antonio Sansevero examine contrasting approaches to the early integration of clinical experience with case studies from Australia, the United Arab Emirates, the UK, Egypt and the USA.

Integration continues as the key theme of *Part 3*, with chapters by Regina Helena Petroni Mennin on community-based medical education, with case studies from Australia, Indonesia, South Africa and Brazil; Stewart Mennin on the integration of the sciences basic to medicine within the whole curriculum, with contributions from Malaysia, Argentina and Saudi Arabia; and Dawn Forman and Betsy VanLeit on interprofessional education highlighted by examples from Australia, the Philippines, Kenya, New Zealand and Egypt.

Part 4: Teaching and learning addresses teaching and learning and contains chapters by Stewart Mennin, who considers how learning can be made more effective by combining theory and practice, with case studies from the USA and Singapore; and John Sandars, who explores ways in which new technologies can contribute to successful education programmes with cases from the UK, South Africa, USA, Uganda and Singapore.

Part 5: Assessment contains three chapters on assessment, beginning with a chapter by Lambert Schuwirth, who investigates the implementation of meaningful assessment with illustrative case studies from Saudi Arabia, Austria and the UK. Reg Dennick explores the range of computer-based objective written tests and Vanessa C. Burch examines the assessment of clinical competence with case studies from the UK, Argentina, Chile and Saudi Arabia.

Part 6: The medical school considers the future role of medical schools in the context of the enormous changes that have occurred in recent decades. John Hamilton and Shajahan Yasin examine the implications of the increasing internationalisation of medical education and the practical, contextual and cultural considerations with case studies from Malaysia and a US/Australian joint medical degree. David Wilkinson considers the issues of sustainability for medical schools, picking up the discussion of the importance of social accountability from Chapter 1. Khalid A. Bin Abdulrahman and Trevor Gibbs highlight the importance of leadership. The role of faculty development and question of recognition of teaching excellence are explored by Deborah Simpson, Maryellen E. Gusic and M. Brownell Anderson, supported by case studies from the USA, Pakistan and Singapore. Dan Hunt and colleagues conclude this part with an examination of accreditation and programme evaluation in that context, with case studies from the USA, Canada, Taiwan, South Korea and Indonesia.

The *Routledge International Handbook of Medical Education* concludes with a final chapter by Stewart Mennin, looking to the future of medical education and some of the key questions and challenges to be faced.

The *Routledge International Handbook of Medical Education* has been designed to be read in a number of different ways to suit the needs and demands of the readers. Each chapter is standalone and can be read and understood by itself. Relevant cross-reference is made to other chapters in the book when an issue arises that may be dealt with in further detail elsewhere. A subject index is available at the end of the book so that readers are able to dip in and out of chapters to suit their needs. The case studies provided in the book have been placed within chapters to demonstrate how a major theme is illustrated. However, most case studies, in medical education, as in life, can be related to more than one theme or issue and it is recommended that the reader takes the time to explore the range of practices demonstrated in the case studies to gain a truly global picture. Each chapter ends with a number of 'take-home messages' that summarise the key themes and issues that arise in the chapter.

ACKNOWLEDGEMENTS

We would like to acknowledge with thanks and appreciation the contributions of all the chapter and case study authors. Our thanks are also due to Cary Dick for helping to process the manuscripts and the publishers for their support. Compiling a book with such a diverse range of experiences and practices has been a challenging feat, made possible by the time and commitment of these dedicated teams and individuals.

ABBREVIATIONS

Chapters

AAMC	Association of American Medical Colleges	13, 24
ABMEK	Accreditation Board for Medical Education in Korea	24
AC	Academic Council	20
ACGME	Accrediting Committee on Graduate Medical Education (USA)	3
ACME-Tri	*Assessing Change in Medical Education – The Road to Implementation*	13
ADZU-SOM	Ateneo de Zamboanga University-School of Medicine (Philippines)	1
AFTA	Asia Free Trade Area	24
AIDS	Acquired immunodeficiency syndrome	4, 7, 12 22
AKU	Aga Khan University (Pakistan)	6, 22, 23
AMC	Australian Medical Council	20, 24
AMEE	Association for Medical Education in Europe	Preface, 21
AM•EI	Academic Medicine Education Institute (Singapore)	23
ANZAHPE	Australian and New Zealand Association for Health Professional Educators	14
ARC-PA	Accreditation Review Commission on the Certification of Physician Assistants	16
ASA	American Society of Anesthesiologists	19
ASEAN	Association of South East Asian Nations	12, 24
ASGE	American Society of Gastrointestinal Endoscopy	19
AUSSE	Australian Survey of Student Engagement	7
BC	British Columbia	21
BMAT	Biomedical Admissions Test (UK)	6
BRICS	Brazil, Russia, India, China and South Africa	19

List of abbreviations

CAAM-HP	Caribbean Accreditation Authority for Education in Medicine and other Health Professions	24
CAIPE	Centre for the Advancement of Interprofessional Education (UK)	14
CanMEDS	Canadian Physician Competency Framework	3, 6
CAS	Complex adaptive system	15
CAT	Computer-assisted training	11
CBE	Competency-based education	3
CBE	Community-based education	3, 14
CBL	Case-based learning	7, 10
CBME	Community-based medical education	12
CbD	Case-based discussion	19
CBT	Computer-based testing	18
CC	Curriculum Committee	22
CCC	Comprehensive Community Clerkship	1
CCC	Critical clinical competencies	21
CCP	Core clinical problem	9
CEC	Clinical encounter cards	19
CHDP	Community Health and Development Program (Philippines)	14
CHEER	Collaboration for Health Equity through Education and Research (South Africa)	1
CIDMEF	Conférence Internationale des Doyens des Facultés de Médicine d'Expression Française (International Conference of Deans of French-speaking Medical Schools)	1
CIHC	Canadian Interprofessional Health Collaborative	14
CIPP	Context, input, process and product (Stufflebeam 2003) evaluation model	3, 9
COBES	Community-based education and services	14
COM	College of Medicine	5
COME	Community-oriented medical education	12
COPC	Community-oriented primary care	12
CPU	Conceptualisation–production–usability model	1
CsR	Chart-stimulated recall	19
CWS	Clinical work sampling	19
DCEL	Distributed community-engaged learning	1
DED	Department for Educational Development (Pakistan)	22, 23
DOPS	Direct observation of procedural skills	19
DST	Digital story telling	16
Duke-NUS	Duke-National University of Singapore	15
E&P	Examinations and promotions	22
EBM	Evidence-based medicine	17
ECE	Early clinical exposure/experience	11

List of abbreviations

ECFMG	Educational Commission for Foreign Medical Graduates	24
EHEA	European Higher Education Area	7
EIT	Eastern Institute of Technology (New Zealand)	14
EMI	Extended matching item	18
EPA	Entrustable professional activity	3, 13, 25
EPC	Early patient contact	11
EVMS	Eastern Virginia Medical School (USA)	23
FAIMER	Foundation for Advancement of International Medical Education and Research	24
FMT	Faculty of Medicine, Tunis (Tunisia)	1
FMUA	Faculty of Medicine, University of Airlangga (Indonesia)	3, 12
FOAMed	Free open-access medical education	16
FOM-SCU	Faculty of Medicine, Suez Canal University (Egypt)	10
GAMSAT	Graduate Medical Schools Admissions Test (Australia)	6
GBP	Growing to be a Physician	7
GCC	Gulf Cooperation Council	4
GCSA/ GCSAMS	Global Consensus for Social Accountability of Medical Schools	1 21
GDH&D	Global Determinants of Health and Development	7
GDP	Gross domestic product	4
GEM	Graduate-entry medicine	11
GEP	Graduate-entry programmes	5
GMC	General Medical Council (UK)	9, 11, 13, 17, 20, 24
GMU	Gulf Medical University (United Arab Emirates)	11
GP	General practice	6
GP	General practitioner	4, 12, 17, 22
GPA	Grade point average	20
G-PAL	General peer-assisted learning	7
GPEP	General Professional Education of the Physician	13
GRAT	Group Readiness Assurance Test	10
HEFCE	Higher Education Funding Council for England (UK)	5
HIV	Human immunodeficiency virus	4, 9, 12, 22
HLTF	High Level Task Force	4
HPAT	Health Professions Admissions Test (Eire)	6
HPE	Health professional education	10, 22, 23
HPEQ	Health Profession Education Quality	24
ICBME	International Competency-Based Medical Educators	3
ICSAD	Imperial College Surgical Assessment Device	19
IIME	Institute for International Medical Education	9
IMC	International Medical College (Malaysia)	20
IMU	International Medical University (Malaysia)	20

List of abbreviations

IPC	Interprofessional collaboration	14
IPE	Interprofessional education	3, 14
IRAT	Individual Readiness Assurance Test	10
ISU	Idaho State University (USA)	16
JCSMHS	Jeffrey Cheah School of Medicine and Health Sciences (Malaysia)	20
JCU-SOM	James Cook University School of Medicine (Australia)	1
JHUSOM	Johns Hopkins University School of Medicine (USA)	13
JORT	*Journal Officiel de la République Tunisienne*	1
KHA	Korean Hospital Association	24
KIMEE	Korean Institute of Medical Education and Evaluation	24
KMA	Korean Medical Association	24
KSAU-HS	King Saud bin Abdul-Aziz University for Health Sciences (Saudi Arabia)	5
KSU	King Saud University (Saudi Arabia)	17
LAM-PTKes	Lembaga Akreditasi Mandiri Perguruan Tinggi Kesehatan (Independent Accreditation Body for Health Professional Education) (Indonesia)	24
LCME	Liaison Committee on Medical Education (USA and Canada)	24
LGBT	Lesbian, gay, bisexual and transgender	8
LI	Learning issue	5
LO	Learning outcome	5
LOCS	Learning Opportunities in the Clinical Setting	11
LPUK	Lembaga Pengembangan Uji Kompetensi (Indonesia)	24
MCAT	Medical College Admissions Test (USA)	6, 20, 24
MCQ	Multiple-choice question	10, 17, 18
MD	Medical doctor	24
MDG	Millennium Development Goals	4
MEDINE2	Thematic Network Medical Education in Europe	7
MEP	Mixed parallel-entry programmes	5
MEQ	Modified essay question	17
MHPE	Master's in Health Professions Education	22
Mini-CEX	Mini-clinical evaluation exercise	9, 17, 19
Mini-PAT	Mini-peer assessment tool	19
MIT	Massachusetts Institute of Technology	4
MLP	Mobile learning programme	16
MMC	Modernising Medical Careers	19
MMC	Malaysian Medical Council	20
MMI	Multiple Mini-Interview	6
MOVE	Medical Overseas Voluntary Electives charity	7
MSC-AA	Medical School Council Assessment Alliance	18

List of abbreviations

MSF	Multi-source feedback	19
MUM	Monash University Malaysia	20
NBE	National Board of Examiners (India)	18
NHS	National Health Service (UK)	4, 19, 22
NIVEL	Netherlands Institute for Health Services Research	4
NOSM	Northern Ontario School of Medicine (Canada)	1, 24
NSSE	National Survey of Student Engagement (USA)	7
NTCS	Northern Territory Clinical School (Australia)	5
NUMed	Newcastle University Medicine Malaysia	20
NZ	New Zealand	14
OBE	Outcome-based education	3
OHS	Ochsner Health System (USA)	20
OMR	Optical mark reader	18
OSCE	Objective Structured Clinical Examination	3, 5, 6, 7, 9, 11, 13, 16, 17, 19, 20, 24
OSPE	Objective Structured Practical Examination	10, 13
PA	Physician assistant	16
PAL	Peer-assisted learning	7
PBDI	Patterned Behaviour Descriptive Interview	6
PBL	Problem-based learning	1, 3, 5, 7, 9, 10, 11, 13, 14, 21
PBT	Paper-based testing	18
PCC	Primary Care Curriculum	15
PHEEM	Postgraduate Hospital Educational Environment Measure	19
PiP	Preparation in Practice	9
PMS	Partner medical school	20
PRCC	Parallel Rural Community Curriculum (Flinders, Australia)	5, 12
PRP	Postgraduate residency programme	19
PT	Peer tutor	7
PUCMS	Pontificia Universidad Católica de Chile Medical School	19
PUGSOM	Perdana University Graduate School of Medicine (Kuala Lumpur, Malaysia)	13
QAA	Quality Assurance Agency for Higher Education (UK)	7
RCPSC	Royal College of Physicians and Surgeons of Canada	3, 24
RHIP	Rural Health Interdisciplinary Program	14
RIME	Reporter, interpreter, manager, educator	3
SA	South Africa	8
SAQ	Short-answer question	10

List of abbreviations

SBA	Single best answer	17
SEARO	South East Asia Regional Office	12
SEP	School-leaver entry programmes/ Standard entry programmes	5
SIM	Mini-simulations	6
SingHealth	Singapore Health Services	23
SiP	Systems in Practice	9
SIUSOM	Southern Illinois University School of Medicine (USA)	21
SJT	Situational judgement test	6
SLE	Saudi Licensing Examination	5
SMART	Specific, measurable, achievable, realistic and timely	23
SOS	Subcommittee on Standards	24
SP	Standardised/simulated patient	13, 21
SPARQS	Student Participation in Quality Scotland (UK)	7
SRC	Student-run clinic	11
SSC	Student-selected components	3, 9
TB DOTS	Tuberculosis directly observed therapy	1
TBL	Team-based learning	9, 10, 15
TEPDAD	Association for Evaluation and Accreditation of Medical Education Programs (Turkey)	24
THEnet	Training for Health Equality Network	1
TkBL	Task-based learning	10
TMAC	Taiwan Medical Accreditation Council	24
TS	Tutorial system	7
UAT	University Admissions Test (Pakistan)	6
UBC	University of British Columbia (Canada)	21
UCAS	Universities and Colleges Admission Service	5
UCD	University of California, Davis (USA)	24
UCSF	University of California, San Francisco	11, 16
UGIE	Upper gastrointestinal endoscopy	19
UGIETP	Upper gastrointestinal endoscopy basic training programme	19
UGME	Undergraduate medical education	22
UKCAT	United Kingdom Clinical Aptitude Test	6
UKFP	UK Foundation Programme	19
UNIMAS	Universiti Malaysia Sarawak (Malaysia)	10
UNMHSC	University of New Mexico Health Sciences Center (USA)	14
UP	University of the Philippines	14
UPC-MS	Peruvian University of Applied Sciences Medical School	9, 10
UQSM	University of Queensland School of Medicine (Australia)	20
USMLE	United States Medical Licensing Examination	15, 20
UW	University of Washington (USA)	16

List of abbreviations

VDU	Visual display unit	18
VLE	Virtual learning environment	16
VPP	Virtual patient pool	7
WFME	World Federation for Medical Education	5, 11, 24
WHO	World Health Organization	1, 4, 9, 12, 14, 22
WPBA	Workplace-based assessment	17, 19
WWAMI	Washington, Wyoming, Alaska, Montana, Idaho	16

PART 1

The mission of the medical school

1
RETHINKING THE MISSION OF THE MEDICAL SCHOOL

Trevor Gibbs

Increasing attention is being focused on the social responsibility and accountability of a medical school internationally and in relation to the community for which they serve.

Michel Montaigne, a well-respected educationalist of his time, reflected that for many years we have worried over the state of education of our students and battled with the dichotomy that exists between didactic teaching and efficient learning.

> Since I would rather make of him an able man than a learned man, I would also urge that care be taken to choose a guide with a well-made rather than a well-filled head.
> *(Michel Montaigne (1533–1592), French Renaissance philosopher)*

Almost 400 years later, the Flexner Report (Flexner 1910) criticised the lack of scientific teaching in North American and Canadian medical schools, as well as questioning the didactic approach to medical education. As a result, we hope that our approach to student learning has changed for the better.

Although the Flexner Report (Flexner 1910) is more remembered for its success in creating a single and hopefully more efficient model of medical education, we should also note that it resulted in the closure of approximately half of the medical schools in America – perhaps a success for medical education in general but a travesty for many individual schools. As a result of the report, medical education became much more expensive, and by closing those schools that admitted African-Americans, women and students of limited financial means, it placed many appropriate students out of reach of graduating in medicine; schools became better but more elitist. That itself raised an important question: what is the relationship between a medical school and the community its graduates serve?

There is little doubt that the dynamic of the last century of medical education has seen a change of emphasis from process (how to educate) to product (the graduate) and, more latterly, to create a careful balance between the two to produce a 'fit for practice' graduate. More than a century after the seminal Flexner Report, the main challenge for health professions' educators is now to create medical and healthcare educational institutions that are responsible for graduating future healthcare professionals, who will be the change agents of the future (Global Consensus for Social Accountability of Medical Schools (GCSA) 2010).

Over the last three decades a variety of innovative educational interventions are deemed to have created 'better' doctors, with the implication that these doctors mean better healthcare. According to the American Board of Internal Medicine Foundation (2002), these doctors should be graduates who not only excel as excellent care providers, but also support patients' autonomy and are advocates of social justice; they are socially and community-aware.

Hence, as we move into an era where we pay as much attention to the product as we do the process, we find that we are paying increasing attention to what is described as the social accountability of a medical school – the obligation of schools to direct their education, research and service activities towards addressing the priority health concerns of the community, region and nation they have the mandate to serve (Boelen and Heck 1995). But what does social accountability mean, how should it be interpreted and acted upon by medical schools and, most importantly, how can its effectiveness be assessed?

By describing the concept of social accountability in greater detail and illustrating it with five case studies, each drawn from various parts of the globe, and schools at different stages of social accountability development, this chapter will attempt to answer those important questions.

Why social accountability?

Perhaps before addressing the question of what is social accountability, we should address an equally important question: why social accountability? In 2010, Frenk and colleagues, in referring to *The Independent Global Commission on Education of Health Professionals for the 21st Century*, suggested that the education of medical students should match the changing health system needs (Frenk et al. 2010). They suggested that medical school graduates' qualities must match the competencies and attitudes required to ensure they are able to solve priority health needs (Sen Gupta et al. 2009; Sales and Schlaff 2010), as well as developing the leadership skills that enable them to be 'enlightened change agents' of the future (Frenk et al. 2010). This thought or proposal is clearly seen in the case studies from Tunisia, Australia and Canada, which prompted change to 'reorienting their curriculum to the priority healthcare needs of their country'.

At the same time other authors were asking that we address the global shortage, medical migration and uneven distribution of healthcare workers and create curricula that better prepare graduates who are fit for purpose for the community (or communities) they are going to serve (Strasser and Neusy 2010; World Health Organization 2010; Gibbs and McLean 2011). This is clearly illustrated in the case study from the Ateneo de Zamboanga University-School of Medicine, Philippines, in which there was a large part of the country's population not served by any medical school or efficient healthcare provision.

Case study 1.1 The new mission of the Faculty of Medicine of Tunis, Tunisia, Africa

Ahmed Maherzi

The Faculty of Medicine of Tunis (FMT) had always been committed to train doctors with the triple mission of education, research and care, but had not verified the impact of its actions on Tunisian society (Boelen 2012). An internal assessment in 2002 and an external assessment by the Review Board of the International Conference of Deans of French-speaking Medical Schools in 2005 (CIDMEF 2006) pointed out deficiencies of the educational system: the choice of general practice as a career was made by default, usually resulting from students failing to be admitted for other specialty training; the clerkship training was mainly hospital-based teaching, with an emphasis on the specialties; research was not given its proper recognition; there was limited interaction with the poorest areas of the country; and there was a clear lack of independent assessment and performance procedures.

Subsequently, the FMT made it a priority to enhance family medicine by reorienting the curriculum towards the priority health needs of the country: to improve bedside training, to enhance clinical research, to set up an assessment department and develop a partnership strategy with regional hospitals.

A first step was to reform medical education at national level, promoting family medicine (JORT 2011) in the four Tunisian medical schools, and providing students with common core training in primary care which reflected the major health problems of the population.

To improve quality and equity for people living in most disadvantaged areas, the FMT initiated a partnership with several regional hospitals in north-western parts of the country. This project had several objectives: to coordinate and improve first, second and third levels of healthcare delivery; to support continuing medical education of local health professionals; and to organise formal collaborative ventures between the FMT with local medical and paramedical teams in order to improve professional competences. The medium-term goal was to establish, through a collaborative approach, centres for mother and child health, emergencies and medical specialties such as psychiatry and oncology. A working group including national and international experts is currently being formed to evaluate the initiative through specific indicators (Boelen 2012).

This new vision of social accountability has changed the training strategy of the school, and using the GCSAMS (2010) document has also initiated a national interest for improving quality through accreditation procedures. This endeavour has also been conducted in consultation with an international group of experts to ensure that the performance of Tunisian medical schools meets the best standards in education, research and service delivery for the well-being of its citizens.

Case study 1.2 James Cook University School of Medicine, Australia

Sarah Larkins, Richard Murray, Tarun Sen Gupta, Simone Ross and Robyn Preston

The James Cook University School of Medicine (JCU-SOM) (now the College of Medicine and Dentistry) was established in 2000 as the first new Australian medical school in over 20 years and the only school in the northern half of Australia. Northern Australia's population is dispersed over a huge geographical area, with no settlement larger than 200,000 people, and suffers from a maldistribution of health professionals. For example, in 2012, the ratio of doctors to population varied from one medical practitioner for every 246 people in major cities, to 1:425 in outer regional and remote areas (Australian Institute of Health and Welfare 2014b). Health status is in inverse proportion to this (Australian Institute of Health and Welfare 2014a).

The JCU-SOM originated with a clear mission to train doctors to respond to the health needs of rural, remote, Aboriginal, Torres Strait Islander and tropical populations, and with articulated values of social justice, excellence and innovation.

The JCU-SOM's social mission is to address the priority health needs of underserved populations using an approach aligning the selection of medical students, curriculum and clinical placements to

(continued)

(continued)

the health and healthcare needs of northern Australia. This role should extend beyond graduation, in particular through partnering with the health sector to create appropriate postgraduate training pathways to meet the needs of the region. The selection process favours students from rural origins and Aboriginal and Torres Strait Islander people. The students are exposed to early and substantial rural clinical placements studying a curriculum with a strong focus on primary care and rural, remote and tropical health issues in these geographical areas. The staffing profile, research activity, professional interests and advocacy of the school reflect these priorities. The school partners with the health sector to develop rural hospitals and practices as teaching health systems, and has been instrumental in developing postgraduate training pathways in rural generalist medicine. Likewise, research activities focus on health service strengthening, health workforce training and optimising the accessibility of health services for Aboriginal and Torres Strait Islander, rural and remote and other medically underserved populations (Figure 1.1).

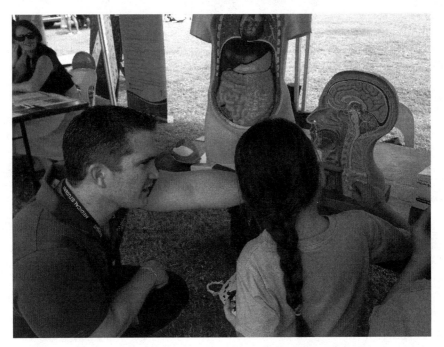

Figure 1.1 Year 5 medical students from James Cook University undertaking community-based health promotion. (Courtesy of A/Prof. Sophia Couzos. Reprinted here with the permission of the subject.)

The school also partners through the Training for Health Equity Network (THEnet) (www.thenetcommunity.org), with participating schools throughout the world. THEnet partners have developed, piloted and published an evaluation framework to measure progress towards socially accountable health professional education in real-world health professional school settings across contexts (Larkins et al. 2013). With its THEnet partners the school has implemented an international Graduate Outcome Study, following students at all 11 schools from entry to medical school, to graduation and for 10 years thereafter in terms of their origin, their practice intentions, actual practice destination (geographical and specialty) and attitudes to serving underserved groups.

The JCU model of medical education has been a success, with 65 per cent of graduates spending their first postgraduate year in non-metropolitan locations and this pattern continues in later postgraduate years (Sen Gupta et al. 2014). Around half of the graduates are undertaking generalist specialty training (general practice or rural medicine), considerably more than from most Australian universities, and they are already making a clear contribution to the northern medical workforce.

Case study 1.3 Northern Ontario School of Medicine, Canada

Roger Strasser

Northern Ontario is geographically vast, with a volatile resource-based economy, and 40 per cent of the population living in rural/remote areas and diverse cultural groups, most notably Aboriginal and francophone peoples. The health status in Northern Ontario is worse than in Canada as a whole and there is a chronic shortage of health professionals (Rural and Northern Health Care Panel 2010; Glazier et al. 2011). In 2001, the Ontario Government established the Northern Ontario School of Medicine (NOSM) with a social accountability mandate to contribute to improving people's health. NOSM is a joint initiative of Laurentian University, Sudbury (population 160,000) and Lakehead University, Thunder Bay (population 110,000). The university campuses are over 1,000 km apart and provide teaching, research and administrative bases for NOSM, which is a rural-distributed community-engaged school (Tesson et al. 2009).

Uniquely developed through a community consultative process, the holistic, cohesive MD programme curriculum is grounded in the Northern Ontario health context. The curriculum is organised around five themes: 'northern and rural health', 'personal and professional aspects of medical practice', 'social and population health', 'foundations of medicine' and 'clinical skills in healthcare' (Strasser et al. 2009) and it relies heavily on electronic communications and community partnerships to support distributed community-engaged learning (DCEL). In classrooms and in clinical settings, students explore cases from the perspectives of physicians practising in Northern Ontario. There is a strong emphasis on interprofessional education and integrated clinical learning, which takes place in over 90 communities and multiple health service settings, so that the students gain personal experience of the diversity of the region's communities and cultures (Strasser et al. 2009; Strasser 2010; Strasser and Neusy 2010).

NOSM was the first medical school in the world in which all students undertake a longitudinal integrated clerkship, the Comprehensive Community Clerkship (CCC) (Couper et al. 2011; Strasser and Hirsh 2011). During the year, students achieve learning objectives which cover the same six core clinical disciplines as in the traditional clerkships and live in one of 15 communities.

NOSM graduates have achieved above-average scores in national examinations, including top-ranking scores in the clinical decision-making and patient interaction sections. Most students chose family practice (predominantly rural). Almost all other MD graduates (94 per cent) are training in family medicine and other general specialties, with only 6 per cent training in subspecialties. A growing number of NOSM graduates are practising family physicians in Northern Ontario and have become NOSM faculty members. The socio-economic impact of NOSM includes: new economic activity, more than double the school's budget; enhanced retention and recruitment for universities and hospitals/health services; and a sense of empowerment among community participants, attributable in large part to NOSM (Strasser et al. 2013).

(continued)

(continued)

Implementing DCEL is challenging. The first challenge is to counter the conventional wisdom that universities are ivory towers separated from 'real-world' communities. Persuading community members that the medical school is serious about meaningful partnerships requires considerable discussion. Successful DCEL depends on empowering communities to be genuine contributors to all aspects of the school. This includes local health professionals who are full clinical faculty members. The partnerships are facilitated by formal collaboration agreements which set out the roles and functions of the partners, including the local steering committee, which provides the mechanism by which the school is a part of the community and the community is a part of the school.

Case study 1.4 The Ateneo de Zamboanga University-School of Medicine (ADZU-SOM), Philippines

Fortunato L. Cristobal

Zamboanga Sulu Archipelago is one of the most marginalised and medically underserved regions in the Philippines. Almost four million people live in its mountainous rural and island municipalities, with their lives punctuated by sporadic political unrest. Only 300 doctors served this region in the early 1990s and the nearest medical school is 600 km away. Frustrated by poor community health status and ongoing doctor shortages, a group of local doctors developed a non-profit medical school foundation to address the region's priority health needs; the Zamboanga Medical School Foundation was established to pioneer and implement an innovative health development and social equity-focused medical curriculum with the expressed purpose of providing solutions to the health problems of the communities in the region.

By 1993 professional development seminars had started to develop new teaching pedagogies and innovative curricular ideas about social and community models for illness and health development. The first students entered in 1994 and a spirit of institutional and individual volunteerism has existed since; faculty are paid a very modest honorarium dependent upon their responsibilities. A local private university initially contributed free teaching space and civic leaders raised local and international scholarships to keep student fees affordable. Students were purposely recruited from the region.

The five-year MD curriculum has the Philippines' most pressing national and regional health priorities at its core. All basic sciences, clinical content and social/community models for health are integrated within a longitudinal problem-based learning (PBL) approach; health development, social determinants of health and the social justice underpinnings for addressing health inequalities are highlighted. A community-based practicum begins in the first year and ends with students living and practising in small communities for the entire fourth year. Three-quarters of all clinical attachments are in remote rural communities, with only a quarter being hospital-based.

As a result of this social approach, the students' projects have included building community pit latrines; improving potable water access; developing solid-waste management policies; increasing immunisation rates in children; determining risk factors for tuberculosis directly observed therapy (TB DOTS)-defaulting patients; developing cottage industry-based income generation schemes; and creating home vegetable gardens to augment local food resources. Mobilisation of effective community health volunteers has improved the early detection of asymptomatic hypertension, adult diabetic patients and malnourished children.

Understandably, the changes were met with initial scepticism, with doubts cast about the quality of its graduating doctors. However, the results from the school speak loudly for themselves: to date, 220 students have graduated with an MD, more than 50 per cent with a combined MD/MPH degree; 200 have passed the Philippine National Medical Board examination, with a pass rate of 95.23 per cent, which is higher than the majority of Filipino schools with traditional curriculum and teaching methods. Over 97 per cent of the graduates are presently still practising in the Philippines. Seventy-five per cent of the graduates still practise within the region of the medical school, with 50 per cent based in rural and remote areas.

Developing an innovative medical school in pursuit of a social goal was a challenging and daunting project for all. However, social justice demands that the pressing, unfulfilled health needs of our marginalised communities receive our energetic collaboration, with all sectors contributing to this end; the volunteers at Zamboanga have shown a way forward for even the poorest of regions to assert that historic disadvantage does not have to be an ongoing destiny.

Case study 1.5   Lessons from eight medical schools in South Africa – the CHEER collaboration

Stephen Reid

The Collaboration for Health Equity through Education and Research (CHEER) was formed in 2003 to examine strategies that would increase the proportion of health professional graduates who choose to practise in rural and underserved areas in South Africa. Consisting of eight individuals – one from each of the universities in South Africa with a medical school plus one member from a health science faculty without a medical school – they undertook a literature review (Grobler et al. 2009), a qualitative study (Couper et al. 2007) and a case-control quantitative study (Reid et al. 2011) to address the original research question: how to increase the number of health professionals in rural Africa? Three series of peer reviews at each university addressing key issues of collective concern formed an integral process in the collaboration (Table 1.1).

The first round of peer reviews (Reid and Cakwe 2011), assessed each faculty in terms of 11 themes which would contribute to the preparation of graduates for service in rural and underserved areas (Table 1.2). The gap between the stated intention of the faculties and their graduate outcomes was clearly demonstrated, except in the area of technical clinical skills. There were noteworthy exceptions, however: at one faculty, for example, community members contribute not only to the recruitment and selection of medical students, but also to curriculum development and student assessment at community sites.

The second round of peer reviews tackled the issue of the relationships between universities and their health service partners. A scale was devised from formal 'transactional' relationships on the one

Table 1.1 CHEER peer reviews – research questions

Phase	Years	Question
Phase 1	2005–2008	How do health sciences faculties prepare their graduates for working in rural and underserved areas in South Africa?
Phase 2	2008–2012	What is the nature of the relationship between health science faculties and their health service partners?
Phase 3	2012–	What are the nature and extent of social accountability of health sciences faculties in South Africa?

(continued)

(continued)

Table 1.2 Themes used for peer review assessments of the preparation of graduates for practice in rural and underserved areas

1	Faculty mission statements
2	Resource allocation
3	Student selection
4	First exposure of students to rural and underserved areas
5	Length of exposure
6	Practical experience
7	Theoretical input
8	Involvement in the communit
9	Relationship with the health service
10	Assessment of students
11	Research and programme evaluation

hand, often circumscribed by legal memoranda of understanding, to less formal 'communal' relationships on the other hand. Central and tertiary hospitals tended towards the former, whereas the relationships at community health centres and other community-based sites were more informal. A consistent challenge that many programmes faced was balancing the need to provide health services to large numbers of patients in under-resourced situations with the simultaneous need to provide quality medical education and supervision of clinical placements for students.

Finally, a third round of peer reviews aimed to measure the social accountability of medical schools, using an adaptation of THEnet Social Accountability Framework (Training for Health Equity Network 2011) based on the 'CPU model' (Boelen et al. 2012; see below for further explanation).

There is a major disjuncture between health sciences education and health service needs in South Africa, both in terms of the numbers and the career choices of graduates, as well as the curative and specialist orientation of their skills. A fundamental realignment to South African context is needed, and the CHEER peer review and research project collaborations have been able to highlight and quantify the important gaps.

As a group of peers inclusive of every medical school in the country, a common purpose developed in supporting one another to find better ways of making our medical graduates more 'fit for purpose' in terms of the health needs of the country. Overall, the collaboration stimulated a number of successful collaborative research projects which contributed to national policy development as well as accreditation practices. In addition, the peer review approach was highly successful in sharing common challenges, spreading innovative practices and stimulating new ideas. In our experience with CHEER, 'what works' is comprehensive collaboration and peer support, in trying to find the best ways to tackle very complex issues in under-resourced circumstances in South Africa.

According to Boelen and Woollard:

> more than ever are we facing the challenge of providing evidence that what we [the medical schools] respond to are the priority health needs and challenges of the ones we intend to serve: patients, citizens, families, communities and the nation at large.
>
> *(Boelen and Woollard 2011: 614)*

But how do medical schools organise themselves to address these challenges, specifically through their education, research and service delivery functions? In part these questions are answered by the South African case study, in which a group of medical schools organised themselves into an effective group with the same mission; making their graduates 'fit for purpose' for the whole country.

What is social accountability?

The World Health Organization (WHO) defines social accountability in medical schools as:

> The obligation to direct their education, research and service activities towards addressing the priority health concerns of the community, region or nation that they are mandated to serve. The priority health concerns are to be identified jointly by governments, health care organisations, health professionals and the public.
> *(Boelen and Heck 1995: 3)*

Over the years social accountability has come to represent the ultimate in a spectrum of educational responses to social need. However, two other intrinsically related aspects of the spectrum, social responsibility and social responsiveness, have become apparent and need further explanation.

The term *social responsibility* simply implies an awareness of a school's duties towards learning from the community and society. An example of this would be for a school to run a course in public health or primary care, but have little or no purposeful engagement with or within the community. A *socially responsive* school takes this further and engages its students in community-based learning activities throughout the curriculum, creates educational outcomes related to the community and society, assesses these and hopefully encourages graduate students to practise within that community. In a *socially accountable* school, the school creates an even closer affiliation with its community; discusses health priority needs with its community to shape the curriculum; creates curricular programmes to respond to these needs; verifies whether anticipated outcomes and results have been attained in satisfying social needs; and bases their commitment to research and service delivery functions upon these needs.

This spectrum of socially oriented education can be further explained by referring to the Social Obligation Scale described by Boelen et al. (2012) (Table 1.3). As discussed by Boelen, the three concepts are not specifically distinct and flow from one to another through an incremental process, eventually focusing on a desired level of achievement or outcome. The social needs serve as references, whether implicitly in the case of responsibility, or explicitly in the case of responsiveness, or anticipatively, through collaboration, investigation and research, in the case of accountability. Social accountability asks that a medical school acts proactively to foresee its place in the development of medical graduates who will eventually fulfil a declared and dynamic social obligation. This important principle is seen in all five case studies, with each school recognising a need to shape its graduates to be able to fulfil the future needs of their region or country.

Once medical schools have agreed that they wish to move on from the levels of social responsibility and social responsiveness and accept the principles of social accountability, they need to change definitional descriptors into activities – translate the concept into actions. Using the WHO definition of social accountability (Boelen and Heck 1995), the activities required of the institution can be divided into four distinct groups: organisational management, educational policy, research and collaboration with community agencies and service providers.

Table 1.3 The Social Obligation Scale (modified from Boelen et al. 2012)

	Social Obligation Scale		
	Responsibility →	Responsiveness →	Accountability
Social needs identified	Explicitly	Anticipatively	Anticipatively
Institutional objectives	Defined by faculty	Inspired from data	Defined with society
Educational programmes	Community-oriented	Community-based	Contextualised
Quality of graduates	'Good' practitioners	Meeting criteria of professionalism	Health system change agents
Focus of evaluation	Process	Outcome	Impact
Assessors	Internal	External	Health partners

At this point readers may wish to re-read the five case studies within this chapter, so that they can match the actions/activities described below with how the schools in the studies implemented the concept of social accountability.

Organisational management

Social accountability should be a prime directive in a medical school's purpose and mandate and integrated in its day-to-day management. This would imply that:

- the subject of social accountability becomes a priority in the medical school's mission statement and strategic plans;
- through discussion with its local, region and national contacts, the school uses the information gained to shape its vision and mission in all the areas of education, research and service delivery;
- the school's contacts for active engagement and consultations are drawn from all levels of its community and health system organisation.

In the JCU-SOM case study, the school started with a clear mission to train the doctors to be responsive to the health needs of its community. This was clear from its mission statement, which also articulated with the school's values of social justice, excellence and innovation; social accountability permeated throughout the school, so that their staffing profiles, research activities, professional interests and advocacy matched and reflected this mission. In the FMT case study, the school specifically worked with its community and patient associations, while the NOSM case study made formal collaborative agreements with the community, the school becoming part of the community, and the community part of the school.

Educational policy

Admissions

Where possible a medical school's graduates should reflect the demographics of the population served, which means that a school should attempt to recruit, select and support medical students who reflect the social, cultural, economic and geographic diversity of the community served, which in turn may mean recruiting from disadvantaged and under-represented areas. The hope is that those students are more likely to commit to future work within the school's immediate community and region. The JCU-SOM specifically targeted potential students from rural and Aboriginal backgrounds and cultures, while ADZU-SOM successfully created scholarships to help local students from poor backgrounds.

Education programmes

To match the concept of social accountability, a school's educational curriculum must create opportunity for students to learn from, participate in and work with the communities within which the school resides, whether at a local, regional or national level. Thus medical students are offered early and longitudinal exposure to community-based and community-oriented learning experiences to understand and act on health determinants and gain appropriate community clinical skills; the concept of professionalism, ethics, teamwork, cultural competence and leadership features highly in the curriculum, together with interprofessional learning and communication skills. In all of the five case studies, it is clear that a major part of their curriculum lies within the community, not simply placing students within that community, but encouraging learning activities that put as much back into the community as they take out.

In a medical school's curriculum, the concept of social accountability should feature through core structured activities and voluntary elective periods, link programmes and cultural exchanges. Specific attention must be given to key health problems found in the community, and the students should have opportunities to learn within underserved and disadvantaged communities and populations, either through structured teaching and learning opportunities or by student-led projects designed to improve the health and healthcare of local, underserved and disadvantaged communities. The students in the ADZU-SOM case study created multiple developmental opportunities for their community.

Faculty development, continuing medical education and professional development

The aim of a medical school should be to promote lifelong learning in its faculty, which should be shaped and driven by the needs of the community and underpinned by an awareness of social accountability. Hence, faculty development programmes should focus on developing teachers who are socially aware and shape their teaching around social accountability; the same rules apply to continuing medical and professional development. Inherent within all of the case studies, but clearly demonstrated in the JCU-SOM, ADZU-SOM and NOSM, is the effect that a socially accountable curriculum has on the faculty. In each case, there has been an ability to retain faculty within the area of most need, and to retain a high grade of practitioners ready to facilitate student learning within the community.

Research

Research activities

In order that a medical school can be considered as socially accountable, it is important that the community, regional and national needs from research inspire and formulate the medical school's research, including knowledge translation. Hence, dominant and prevalent patterns of disease and eradication of local or regional illnesses should take priority in research programmes.

To do this a medical school should actively engage with and partner the community in developing their research agenda. Research from the school should be measured by its impact upon the community which the school serves.

However, a careful balance needs to exist that allows the school to benefit from available research monies from providers divorced from the community; much research is not related directly to community need since important community issues are not always seen as innovative areas for research. However, all five of our case studies have implied that their research is directed to the community needs; their community will benefit from their research activities. In these early days of social accountability, research results are not yet forthcoming, but building into the remit of the school the need to tailor research towards the needs of the local community suggests that it will not be long before this very specific activity bears fruit.

Collaboration with community agencies and service providers

A medical school's graduates and its health service partnerships should have a positive impact on the healthcare and the health of its community. Inevitably this means that the school should form effective collaborative partnerships with other community stakeholders, including other health professional and governing bodies, to optimise its performance in meeting the requirement for the quality and quantity of trained graduates. A school's postgraduate training programmes should be targeted towards producing a variety of generalists and specialists, appropriate both in quality and quantity to serve the medical school's community, and towards the creation of 'change leaders', active in population health and health-related reforms, with an emphasis on coordinated person-centred care, health promotion, risk and disease prevention and rehabilitation for patients and communities. A medical school should work in partnership with potential employers of graduates to enable them to provide care in under-resourced specialties and to underserved and disadvantaged communities. In all of the case studies, active, effective partnerships were formed with their community. In the FMT case study, the healthcare providers were the local hospitals, specifically in socially deprived areas. JCU-SOM and ADZU-SOM chose to partner more rural hospitals and community teaching centres, while at NOSM a more rural and socially deprived community became an active partner of the medical school. In South Africa the CHEER partnership has been one of collaborative medical schools working together to improve the healthcare of their country.

Assessing the effectiveness of a socially accountable medical school

If medical schools are responsible for producing graduates with competencies and attitudes to address health inequities and respond to priority health needs, there needs to be a way of demonstrating that they have achieved their goal. At the present time there is one set of principles that can be applied to the assessment of a socially accountable medical school and one validated framework of assessment based upon those principles. In 2009, Boelen and Woollard described a set of three expressions of social accountability; they introduced what is now known as the CPU model. This has subsequently been placed into a framework and validated by a number of international medical schools that have critically evaluated the progress of their schools towards social accountability using the THEnet Evaluation Framework (Palsdottir and Neusy 2010; Larkins et al. 2013; Ross et al. 2014). Recently the CPU has been described, in greater detail and with more descriptors, by Boelen et al. (2012), in order to aid accreditation of medical schools that wish to express their ability to be a socially accountable school.

The CPU framework focuses on three 'expressions of social accountability':

1. C – conceptualisation; what sort of graduate the school needs to produce;
2. P – production; the type of teaching, learning and assessment methods used;
3. U – usability; the methods that are used to investigate the effectiveness of the graduates in providing the required service.

Extensive examples of each of the three expressions are beyond the scope of this short chapter. However, readers who are interested in a more detailed approach to the CPU model are recommended to read the paper by Boelen and colleagues (2012).

The full effect of a socially accountable curriculum has yet to be demonstrated, but early results suggest that the concept at least is meaning that more students are staying in the area of their medical school to practise (see JCU-SOM, ADZU-SOM and NOSM case studies).

Conclusion

If effective healthcare is related to the standard of training of doctors, then it appears logical that the training should also be related to the specific needs of the community, region or nation those doctors will eventually serve, rather than towards a more generic graduate whose skills may not be used to maximum effect. The concept of social accountability focuses on these specific needs and forms a framework for the medical school to work within to produce that graduate. It also extends the principles further into the areas of postgraduate education, continuing professional development, research and service delivery. When the CPU model is applied to social accountability it can assist in designing indicators that can help medical schools build their own benchmarks to assess progress towards accreditation in the area of social accountability and within the context of their particular environment.

Take-home messages

- Medical education has changed its emphasis from the process (how to educate) to the product (the graduate) and, more latterly, to a careful balance created between the two in order to create a 'fit for practice' graduate.
- Today's medical schools and their educational programmes need to address priority health problems, anticipating the health and human resource needs of their community and ensuring that graduates are employed where they are most needed.
- Medical schools need to be socially accountable, to recognise their obligation to direct their education, research and service activities towards addressing the priority health concerns of the community, region and nation they have the mandate to serve.
- To match the concept of social accountability, the school's educational curriculum must create opportunity for students to learn from, participate in and work with the communities within which the school resides, whether at a local, regional or national level.
- The medical school's graduates and its health service partnerships should have a positive impact on the healthcare and the health of its community.
- If medical schools are responsible for producing graduates with competencies and attitudes to address health inequities and respond to priority health needs, there needs to be an effective way of demonstrating that they have achieved their goal.

Bibliography

American Board of Internal Medicine Foundation, American College of Physicians Foundation, European Federation of Internal Medicine (2002) 'Medical professionalism in the new millennium: A physician charter', *Annals of Internal Medicine*, 163(3): 243–6.

Australian Institute of Health and Welfare (2014a) *Australia's health 2014. Australia's health series no. 14*, Canberra: AIHW.

Australian Institute of Health and Welfare (2014b) *Medical workforce 2012. National health workforce series no. 8*, Canberra: AIHW.

Boelen, C. (2012) 'Making an academic institution more socially accountable: The case of a medical school', *Presse Médicale*, 41(12): 1165–7.

Boelen, C. and Heck, J. (1995) *Defining and measuring the social accountability of medical schools*, Geneva: World Health Organization.

Boelen, C. and Woollard, R. (2009) 'The CPU model: Conceptualisation–production–usability', *Medical Education*, 43(9): 887–94.

Boelen, C. and Woollard, R. (2011) 'Social accountability: The extra leap to excellence for educational institutions', *Medical Teacher*, 33(8): 614–19.

Boelen, C., Dharamsi, S. and Gibbs, T. (2012) 'The social accountability of medical schools and its indicators', *Education for Health*, 25(3): 180–94.

CIDMEF (Conférence Internationale des Doyens des Facultés de Médecine d'Expression Française) (2006) *Politique et méthodologie d'évaluation des facultés de médecine et des programmes d'études médicales*. Online. Available HTTP: http://www.cidmef.u-bordeaux2.fr/sites/cidmef/files/st_ev03_v2.pdf (accessed June 2013).

Couper, I.D., Hugo, J.F.M., Conradie, H. and Mfenyana, K., Members of the Collaboration for Health Equity through Education and Research (CHEER) (2007) 'Influences on the choice of health professionals to practise in rural areas', *South African Medical Journal*, 97(11): 1082–6.

Couper, I., Worley, P. and Strasser, R. (2011) 'Rural longitudinal integrated clerkships: Lessons from two programs on different continents'. *Rural and Remote Health*, 11: 1665. Online. Available HTTP: www.rrh.org.au (accessed June 2013).

Flexner, A. (1910) *Medical education in the United States and Canada: A report to the Carnegie Foundation for the Advancement of Teaching, bulletin no. 4*, New York City: The Carnegie Foundation for the Advancement of Teaching.

Frenk, J., Chen, L., Bhutta, Z., Cohen, J., Crisp, N., Evans, T., Fineberg, H., Garcia, P., Ke, Y., Kelley, P., Kistnasamy, B., Meleis, A., Naylor, D., Pablos-Mendez, A., Reddy, S., Scrimshaw, S., Sepulveda, J., Serwadda, D. and Zurayk, H. (2010) 'Health professionals for a new century: Transforming education to strengthen health systems in an interdependent world', *Lancet*, 376(9756): 1923–58.

Gibbs, T. and McLean, M. (2011) 'Creating equal opportunities: The social accountability of medical education', *Medical Teacher*, 33(8): 620–5.

Glazier, R.H., Gozdyra, P. and Yeritsyan, N. (2011) *Geographic access to primary care and hospital services for rural and northern communities: Report to the Ontario Ministry of Health and Long-Term Care*, Toronto: Institute for Clinical Evaluative Sciences (ICES).

Global Consensus for Social Accountability of Medical Schools (2010) *Consensus document*. Online. Available HTTP: http://healthsocialaccountability.sites.olt.ubc.ca/files/2011/06/11-06-07-GCSA-English-pdf-style.pdf (accessed June 2013).

Grobler, L., Marais, B.J., Mabunda, S., Marindi, P., Reuter, H. and Volmink, J. (2009) 'Interventions for increasing the proportion of health professionals practising in rural and other underserved areas', *Cochrane Database of Systematic Reviews*, Issue 1.

JORT (*Journal Officiel de la République Tunisienne*) (2011) *Décret N°90 du 25 novembre 2011 fixant le cadre général des études médicales, habilitant à l'exercice de la médecine de famille et à la spécialisation en medicine*. Online. Available HTTP: http://www.ordre-medecins.org.tn/pdf/bulletin-2013-def.pdf (accessed 23 March 2015).

Larkins, S.L., Preston, R., Matte, M.C., Lindemann, I.C., Samson, R., Tandinco, F.D., Buso, D., Ross, S.J., Palsdottir, B. and Neusy, A.J. (2013) 'Measuring social accountability in health professional education: Development and international pilot testing of an evaluation framework', *Medical Teacher*, 35(1): 32–45.

Palsdottir, B. and Neusy, A.J. (2010) *Transforming medical education: Lessons learned from THEnet*. Commission Paper June 2010.

Reid, S.J. and Cakwe, M. on behalf of the Collaboration for Health Equity through Education and Research (CHEER) (2011) 'The contribution of South African curricula to prepare health professionals for working in rural or under-served areas in South Africa: A peer review evaluation', *South African Medical Journal*, 101(1): 34–8.

Reid, S.J., Volmink J. and Couper, I.D. (2011) 'Educational factors that influence the distribution of health professionals in South African public service: A case control study', *South African Medical Journal*, 101(1): 29–33.

Ross, S., Preston, R., Lindemann, I., Matte, M., Samson, R., Tandinco, F., Larkins, S., Palsdottir, B. and Neusy, A-J. (2014) 'The training for health equity network evaluation framework: A pilot study at five health professional schools', *Education for Health*, 27(2): 116–26.

Rural and Northern Health Care Panel (2010) *Rural and northern health care framework/plan, stage 1 report. Final report*. Toronto: Ministry of Health and Long-Term Care. Online. Available HTTP: http://www.health.gov.on.ca/en/public/programs/ruralnorthern/docs/report_rural_northern_EN.pdf (accessed June 2013).

Sales, C.S. and Schlaff, A.L. (2010) 'Reforming medical education: A review and synthesis of five critiques of medical practice', *Social Science and Medicine*, 70(11): 1665–8.

Sen Gupta, T.K., Murray, R.B., Beaton, N.S., Farlow, D.J., Jukka, C.B. and Coventry, N.L. (2009) 'A tale of three hospitals: Solving learning and workforce needs together', *Medical Journal of Australia*, 191(2): 105–9.

Sen Gupta, T., Woolley, T., Murray, R., Hay, R. and McCloskey, T. (2014) 'Positive impacts on rural and regional workforce from the first seven cohorts of James Cook University medical graduates', *Rural and Remote Health*, 14(1): 2657.

Strasser, R. (2010) 'Community engagement: A key to successful rural clinical education', *Rural and Remote Health*, 10(3): 1543.

Strasser, R. and Hirsh, D. (2011) 'Longitudinal integrated clerkships: Transforming medical education worldwide?', *Medical Education*, 45(5): 436–7.

Strasser, R. and Neusy, A.J. (2010) 'Context counts: Training health workers in and for rural areas', *Bulletin of the World Health Organization*, 88(10): 777–82.

Strasser, R.P., Lanphear, J.H., McCready, W.A., Topps, M.H., Hunt, D.D. and Matte, M.C. (2009) 'Canada's new medical school: The Northern Ontario School of Medicine – social accountability through distributed community engaged learning', *Academic Medicine*, 84(10): 1459–64.

Strasser, R., Hogenbirk, J.C., Minore, B., Marsh, D.C., Berry, S., McCready, W.A. and Graves, L. (2013) 'Transforming health professional education through social accountability: Canada's Northern Ontario School of Medicine', *Medical Teacher*, 35(6): 490–6.

Tesson, G., Hudson, G., Strasser, R. and Hunt, D. (eds) (2009) *Making of the Northern Ontario School of Medicine: A case study in the history of medical education*, Kingston, Ontario: McGill-Queen's University Press.

Training for Health Equity Network (2011) *THEnet's social accountability evaluation framework version 1. Monograph I (1 ed.)*, Belgium: The Training for Health Equity Network. Online. Available HTTP: http://thenetcommunity.org/wp-content/uploads/2013/05/The-Monograph.pdf (accessed June 2014).

Training for Health Equity Network, THEnet (2013). Online. Available HTTP: http://thenetcommunity.org/ (accessed June 2013).

Wilson, N., Couper, I., de Vries, E., Reid, S., Fish, T. and Marais, B. (2009) 'A critical review of interventions to redress the inequitable distribution of healthcare professionals to rural and remote areas', *Rural and Remote Health*, 9(2): 1060.

World Health Organization (2010) *Increasing access to health workers in remote and rural areas through improved retention: Global policy recommendations*, Geneva: World Health Organization.

2

THE ROLE OF THE DOCTOR AND THE COMPETENCIES EXPECTED FROM THE DOCTOR OF THE FUTURE

Stefan Lindgren and David Gordon

The role of the doctor is changing in response to advances in medicine, developments in healthcare delivery and changes in patients' expectations.

Medical education must prepare students for the needs of the world of tomorrow

Medical education is a lifelong process. It begins when the student enters medical school and ends on the last day of professional life. Medical students of today, both undergraduate and postgraduate, will see unimaginable changes in medical practice and the delivery of healthcare during their future career. These changes will follow developments in science and clinical practice; but they will also relate to new health priorities and threats to public health, to rising expectations from patients and the public and changing attitudes in society.

Traditional roles of the doctor will change, and new roles will emerge. Healthcare is changing from the unique doctor–patient relationship to the interaction of the patient with the entire healthcare team. Within this team, the doctor must have the competence and responsibility for definitive decisions in uncertain and complex situations, based on his or her scientific and clinical knowledge and experience.

The various stages of this lifelong learning have different responsibilities and offer different windows of opportunity (Table 2.1). Undergraduate medical education leading to a licence to practise should be planned and executed with the expected needs of the future in mind rather than based on history or the organisation of medicine in yesterday's society. Undergraduate education must prepare students for the next steps in their professional education, and demonstrate and document the competence they have achieved, ready for employment as professional and trustworthy physicians.

Medical schools, and their partners in postgraduate medical education, share the responsibility of all universities to foster members of society who will contribute to democratic and global development, both social and economic. Students must understand the needs of healthcare in different societies and the need for growth, development and improvement of regional healthcare systems.

Table 2.1 The various stages of lifelong learning for a doctor

Stage of education	Undergraduate	Specialist education	Continuing professional development	
What is the doctor doing?	Studying with supervised clinical responsibilities	Training as a specialist by today's specification: clinical practice with increasing personal responsibility and decreasing supervision	Early independent professional practice, and educating and training the next generation	Established independent professional practice Continuing to educate and train the next generation Leading in clinical practice and in teaching
What is the doctor learning?	Professional attitudes Scientific attitudes Scientific principles, and principles of disease and of clinical practice Psychological and social attitudes and principles 'Learning how to learn'	Enhanced professional attitudes Additional scientific and clinical principles and knowledge Continuing to 'learn how to learn' as a specialist and a practitioner	A future that we cannot predict . . . Understanding and absorbing new knowledge and practices Learning how to teach, how to lead and how to disseminate knowledge and good practice for the general benefit of society	

This relates to the education of a doctor as a medical professional, the needs of society worldwide and lifelong learning – all relevant to the future global role of the doctor.

What do we mean by professionalism in medicine?

A profession is, by definition, a vocation (not just a trade) in which the practitioner acknowledges that he or she has knowledge and skill that must be applied for *good*, not just for *gain*. A good analogy is the priesthood: a priest must use wisdom, knowledge and skill for the good of all; similarly, a doctor has a moral obligation to use his or her understanding and expertise for the good of society and (in particular) of the individual patient.

Professionalism is the basis of the contract of medicine with society. It demands placement of the interests of patients above those of the physician, the setting and maintenance of standards of competence and integrity, and provision of expert advice both to society and to the individual patient on matters of health. The principles and responsibilities of medical professionalism must be clearly understood by both the profession and society. Essential to this contract is public trust in physicians, which depends on the integrity of both individual physicians and the entire profession. In the face of changes in society and of globalisation, reaffirmation of the fundamental and universal principles and values of professionalism becomes all the more important for all doctors.

Development of professional attitudes in tomorrow's doctors is an important responsibility of the medical school. In addition to professionalism, fostering understanding of the need for continuing professional development; a critical and scientific approach; the ability to function in multiprofessional teams and systems as a leader and as a member; and a culture of creativity, innovation, continuous improvement and global social accountability are central to the educational responsibilities of universities. Because there is an increased focus on team-based delivery of healthcare, the definition of the professional role of the doctor cannot be done in isolation from other professions. To achieve all this, medical schools must work in close partnership with other important stakeholders in health and related areas, to improve the performance of the healthcare system. The competencies that doctors must acquire include those relating to ethics, teamwork, cultural competence, leadership and communication. The case study from India reviews the experience of introducing an orientation programme for new graduates about to embark on their internships, which included many of these vital competencies.

Case study 2.1 Easing the transition to clinical work – the role of an internship orientation programme in India

Rita Sood

The All India Institute of Medical Sciences is a premier tertiary-care institute in India offering undergraduate, postgraduate and postdoctoral courses in medicine and its various branches. The undergraduate curriculum is largely traditional and discipline-based with integrated organ- and system-based modules offered from the third semester onwards. The course content is heavy on biomedical sciences, with only limited teaching on professionalism, ethics, communication and psycho-social issues. Four-and-a-half years of training are followed by a year of compulsory internship rotation during which students rotate through various departments to learn practical skills and the art of doctoring. In this phase of training new graduates are expected to acquire and extend their skills under supervision, to become capable of functioning independently without direct supervision.

Quite often, new graduates go through this period without a clear aim as they are also preparing for the postgraduate entrance examinations, which are largely knowledge-based.

An orientation programme was conducted before these new graduates started their 1-year internship to familiarise them with their clinical tasks and their roles in society and the community. Interns were invited to participate in a 2-day programme conducted by a team of faculty members and administrators. The key objectives of the programme were to enable the interns to:

- focus on the need for developing effective communication skills essential for healthy doctor–patient interactions;
- assess the psycho-social needs of patients while providing care;
- identify the ethical and medicolegal issues involved in patient care;
- enhance their written communication skills;
- review the principles of rational drug therapy;
- familiarise themselves with universal precautions and biomedical waste management;
- develop and refine the skills and understanding necessary for the appropriate use of laboratory services;
- identify their role in multidisciplinary healthcare teams;
- develop a sense of belonging, responsibility and accountability.

The programme included interactive lectures, structured panel discussions, small-group discussions and role plays. Multiple case studies involving ethical principles applied to dilemmas and professional conduct and various scenarios for practising communication skills, including breaking bad news and communication across different cultures, were used for role play by the interns and facilitated by faculty. All the interns were highly engaged using an interactive process in a friendly, non-threatening environment. Most of the faculty participated in the sessions allocated to them while the author, as the programme coordinator, was available to students throughout the full programme. Participation in this programme was voluntary. Forty-one out of 44 eligible interns joined the programme on day one and 28 interns participated on day two. A formal evaluation of the programme was done at the end of day two, to which 19 interns contributed. Evaluation was done using a feedback questionnaire, and an interactive session, during which most faculty were present. The pre- and post-test comprised of 20 multiple-choice questions that tested theoretical knowledge and clinical problem-solving skills. The final analysis was done on the pre- and post-test responses of 19 interns.

The responses from the interactive session and the feedback questionnaire suggested that the workshop was successful in achieving its objectives and was useful for the interns' professional activities. Almost all the participants suggested such a programme should be mandatory for all.

It is important for new medical graduates to get opportunities for hands-on training and experiential learning in a safe environment where they can practise and internalise skills required to become an effective doctor. This programme is now being carried out regularly and many medical schools are conducting such orientation programmes for interns and new postgraduates. The Medical Council of India (2011) in its new curriculum reform initiative (*Vision 2015*), has introduced a mandatory foundation course spread throughout undergraduate training and the internship, incorporating most of the above elements of training.

Note: This case study was first published in *The National Medical Journal of India* (NMJI) 2010; 23: 160–2.

The needs of society from the doctor of the future

Medical knowledge continues to increase dramatically, but inequities in health persist both within and between countries. New challenges mean that healthcare systems worldwide have to struggle to keep up, as they become more complex and costly. Medical education has not kept pace with these challenges, and the mismatch between competencies achieved and the needs of patients and population grows (Global Consensus for Social Accountability of Medical Schools 2010). There remains too much focus on episodic encounters and acute events compared to continuous care and the management of chronic conditions. Education remains oriented to the hospital at the expense of primary care. The Lancet Commission (Frenk et al. 2010) put forward the vision that all health professionals in all countries should be educated to mobilise knowledge and to engage in critical reasoning and ethical conduct, so that they are competent to participate in patient- and population-centred health systems as members of locally responsive and globally connected teams. Although the evidence base of the Lancet Commission report is incomplete (Gordon and Karle 2012), the aim to assure universal coverage by those high-quality comprehensive services that are essential to advance opportunities for health equity within and between countries cannot be disputed.

Much of the challenge for the future is based around the gap between the richest and poorest in society. Since long-term trends are for spending on health to increase faster than the growth in national income, doctors will be asked to play a central role in 'doing more with less' and addressing preventive issues.

Promotion of health

The future role of the doctor will include an enhanced focus on health promotion and on the prevention of illness. The future doctor must understand and contribute to the improvement of those conditions in society that affect the health of individuals and of different population groups, from both a national and global perspective. The doctor must be responsive to society in meeting the needs of people and populations in the area in which he or she works, and at the same time must expand this social accountability to a global perspective. It is not enough for medical schools, today, to educate the doctors of tomorrow solely to meet the needs in their own society. Doctors of the future must be prepared to take on a more global role, and be ready to practise in other, and particularly poorer, parts of the world.

The global view

In less developed parts of the world, medical care is often deficient, and in richer countries the costs and complexities of healthcare are rising unsustainably. Both rich and poor societies need to understand what can only be done by doctors, and what should be done by other members of the healthcare team, in order to plan their health workforce efficiently. In this rapidly changing environment, an implicit understanding of what doctors do without a proper analysis of their function is no longer acceptable. In defining this role of the doctor, it is essential to avoid being culture- or region-specific and not to define the role of the doctor in isolation from other professions.

This definition must not solely comprise cognitive and technical competences, but also must include more complex attitudes and skills, for example the competence to change, to learn, to improve and develop personally. Once this complex role is defined, the content and process of medical education and of lifelong learning, to produce a person equipped to fulfil that role, can be decided. Above all, medical education at all levels must respond to health challenges in the society of today and of the future, and this definition of the role of the doctor must not be bound to one particular culture or region.

Subjects of particular importance for the global roles and values of future doctors are summarised in Table 2.2. The role of the doctor as a communicator to patients, to other doctors and to healthcare professionals is obvious, but this role in relation to society is generally not often considered. The duty to teach is self-evident in the daily life of doctors, but often considered more of an added-on skill in special situations than part of their everyday role, and this duty to teach is not just to students and other health professionals: it is widely in society. Several commissions and publications have in recent years addressed the role and competence of future doctors and the implications for medical education. They come to generally shared conclusions, summarised in Table 2.3.

Freedom to move is an indisputable human right, but migration makes it necessary to address the global imbalance of healthcare resources. Migration of health professionals from less-developed regions to wealthy parts of the world has contributed to a global health workforce crisis. This illustrates the essential need to expand the global medical health workforce, and the need to build healthcare teams appropriate for the circumstances of the particular country or region, for

Table 2.2 Subjects of particular importance for the roles and values of future doctors

- Professionalism: its meaning and significance today, and its relevance for personal development
- The doctor as communicator, educator and researcher
- Demographic changes, migration and the future of medicine
- The doctor as a manager of healthcare within society, and as a community health leader
- The social accountability of medicine and the doctor
- Leadership and membership within the healthcare team

Source: Originally published in Lindgren and Gordon (2011).

Table 2.3 Generally agreed priorities for the future doctor and medical education

- Matching of competencies to patient and population needs
- Teamwork
- First-line healthcare
- Leadership
- Leadership to improve health-system performance
- Partnership approach with patients for long-term health gain
- Social accountability
- Difficult decisions in situations of complexity and uncertainty
- Communication
- Professionalism
- Physician-scientist
- Generalist
- Capacity to change
- Profound ethical understanding
- Lifelong learner
- Habits of inquiry and improvement
- Striving for excellence

Source: Originally published in Lindgren and Gordon (2011), where references to other sources are shown.

the delivery of health and medical services. Doctors also need continual educational, professional, administrative and personal support so as not to feel isolated or disillusioned. This is also a problem in richer countries, where many graduates, motivated by social factors, are lost to other occupations.

Lifelong learning

Medical students of today will see huge and continuing changes in medical practice and the delivery of medical care during their careers. Furthermore, the healthcare needs of different populations and societies will change. Thus, each student must be educated for a lifelong career and not simply trained for a job. This includes the need to strive for excellence continuously, both on a personal level and in the systems and teams in which the doctor will work throughout his or her professional life. Only when doctors are competent in the skills that underpin lifelong learning will they be well placed to adapt to changes in knowledge, update their practice in line with the changing evidence base and continue to contribute effectively as societal needs change.

Perhaps the most important challenge for medical education is to address this understanding of what it means to be a medical doctor, and at the same time adopt the socially responsible position of meeting society's long-term needs in relation to healthcare.

Medical education for the future global role of the doctor

Medical schools must anticipate these future needs of society, educating competent doctors with professional attitudes, able to act as agents for change in society, understanding health promotion, with a global view, and prepared for lifelong learning. They will be able to work in teams, with the skills always to be a member, and only sometimes to be the leader, of the team. The interaction of the patient with the healthcare team will often be such that the patient is also a member of that team: the doctor must understand and welcome this. It is a challenge to preserve the doctor–patient relationship in this setting, with respect for the patient's integrity, needs, knowledge and experience.

Education for leadership is not just for leadership of the healthcare team. Flexible leadership and management by the doctor offer ways to develop healthcare systems in different parts of the world in context, based on available resources and competencies, and medical schools should not produce doctors with only local, special or restricted characteristics.

The duty of doctors to examine their responsiveness and accountability to society as a whole is important, because without such self-analysis the profession may blindly continue to do what it believes has always been done. This analysis particularly includes the cost of medical actions and interventions, in relation to overall indirect societal costs for loss of health and to the total resources available for healthcare.

The structure of undergraduate medical education will include longer continuous periods of integrated clinical training than are the norm today. This will give priority to education in, and assessment of, professional competencies as well as developing the ability of students to work together with other professional groups in health and medical services. The clinical settings for student education may affect the choice of their future vocational direction and specialised service. More sustained periods of learning in first-line healthcare with high-quality role models from those services is one way of stimulating the students to choose that – a prerequisite for the worldwide need to develop high-quality first-line healthcare.

Medical education with an appropriate content of first-line healthcare is one way to ensure that there is not an excess of doctors with only narrow specialism. The future doctor, whether generalist or specialist, must take more responsibility for the overall management of resources and be an advocate of the health needs of the particular population he or she serves. By sometimes leading in a management role, doctors may fulfil an important function in population needs-based healthcare, promoting effective achievement of health outcomes, efficiency and equity, with emphasis on prevention and on patient and public satisfaction. The doctor has multiple roles in society, particularly in community health leadership and the management of healthcare.

In many parts of the world there is an obvious mismatch between medical school graduates, the distribution of specialists and the needs of the healthcare system. Medical education has not kept pace with this need and has a regrettable history of producing doctors fit for the past, and perhaps for the present, but not for the future. This need to change, to meet the needs of patients, society, learners and teachers, must involve postgraduate medical education and continuing professional development as well as medical schools. Educational development and reform, related to healthcare systems and their improvement, to enhance the global roles and values of the doctor, are needed.

Undergraduate medical education must always be devoted to the needs of the future and not to the pressures of today. Education of the doctor for an ever-changing and developing career, which may extend for 40 or more years, is required, and simple training for the here and now of medical practice today is not enough. In considering how medicine will develop we need to know what is meant by medical professionalism; to understand the needs of society and how medicine should respond to them, particularly the needs for disease prevention and health promotion; to think of all the future roles of the doctor; and to think globally rather than parochially.

This gives us the vision of lifelong learning and development. Not only will this help medical care continuously to improve, but it can also inspire the medical students and young doctors of today that their professional lives will not be fixed and stagnant, but always be going forward, to the benefit of society, and of the individual patient.

Take-home messages

- The traditional role of the doctor is changing. We must prepare our students to be lifelong learners, adaptable to the changing health needs and practices of the future.
- Ensuring that professionalism remains the key contract of medicine with society is vital; that doctors retain a moral obligation to use their skills for the good of society and not just for personal gain.
- The globalisation of society and the medical workforce requires the role of the doctor to be global, not regional or culture-specific. In addition, greater attention needs to be given to opportunities for health equity within and between countries.
- Population growth and the increasing cost of healthcare require a refocusing of attention to health promotion and disease prevention; of working within teams and across professions for the benefit of all.

Bibliography

Frenk, J., Chen, L., Bhutta, Z., Cohen, J., Crisp, N., Evans, T., Fineberg, H., Garcia, P., Ke, Y., Kelley, P., Kistnasamy, B., Meleis, A., Naylor, D., Pablos-Mendez, A., Reddy, S., Scrimshaw, S., Sepulveda, J., Serwadda, D. and Zurayk, H. (2010) 'Health professionals for a new century: Transforming education to strengthen health systems in an interdependent world', *Lancet*, 376 (9756): 1923–58.

Global Consensus for Social Accountability of Medical Schools (2010) *Consensus document*. Online. Available HTTP: http://healthsocialaccountability.org (accessed 23 August 2013).

Gordon, D. and Karle, H. (2012) 'The state of medical and healthcare education: A review and commentary on the Lancet commission report', *World Medical & Health Policy*, 4(1): 1–18.

Lindgren, S. and Gordon, D. (2011) 'The doctors we are educating for a future global role in healthcare', *Medical Teacher*, 33(7): 551–4.

Medical Council of India (2011) *Vision 2015 New Delhi: Medical Council of India*. Online. Available HTTP: www.mciindia.org/tools/announcement/MCI_booklet.pdf (accessed 8 April 2014).

3

WHY OUTCOME-BASED EDUCATION (OBE) IS AN IMPORTANT DEVELOPMENT IN MEDICAL EDUCATION

Ronald M. Harden

A key development in medical education in the past decade has been the move to outcome-based or competency-based education.

The importance of outcome-based education

It has been argued, and for good reasons, that outcome-based education (OBE) represents the most important development in education in the past two decades. A clear specification of the end product of training and the associated learning outcomes is essential for effective curriculum planning. We would not commission an architect to build a new house until we had approved the plans. The seeds we plant in our garden and how we cultivate them, including the growing conditions we create and the fertilisers we use, will depend on the plants we expect to grow. In the same way, in OBE recognition is given to the importance of the end product of the training programme and the competencies expected of the doctor trained. Who could disagree with that? In this OBE backward or reverse-planning model, the course content and the teaching, learning and assessment methods are derived from the expected learning outcomes.

Curriculum development in medical education traditionally is associated with a forward-planning approach, with course content and teaching methods determined first. This approach, however, has failed to meet the needs of the population and systems of healthcare (Frenk et al. 2010) and there is compelling evidence and an overall global consensus that it is no longer appropriate for the training of a 21st-century doctor.

As described in Chapter 9, OBE is an important element in the move away from the perception of the curriculum as a syllabus comprising a body of knowledge and skills to be transmitted to the student. Set out in OBE are the expected learning outcomes and the competences or abilities required in healthcare professionals if they are to move on to the next stage of their training programme or be accredited to practice independently as healthcare professionals. The rapid development of an outcome-based approach to education was recognised in the March 2002 issue of *Medical Teacher,* which had OBE as a theme with international developments in the field highlighted. A subsequent issue of the journal in 2010 featured a series of papers on competency-based education (CBE) authored by the International Competency-Based Medical

Educators (ICBME) collaborative. In this chapter we will not distinguish between the concepts of OBE and CBE and for practical purposes will treat them as the same.

Despite critics, OBE has become part of mainstream education through initiatives such as the Tuning Project and has been recognised by regulating bodies in medicine such as the General Medical Council in the UK, the Accrediting Committee on Graduate Medical Education (ACGME) in the USA, the Royal College of Physicians and Surgeons of Canada (RCPSC: the CanMEDS initiative) and other bodies internationally. The Geneva case study illustrates how a curriculum was constructed around the CanMEDS competency framework.

Case study 3.1 An integrated and community-oriented curriculum at the University of Geneva Faculty of Medicine, Switzerland

Anne Baroffio, Nu Viet Vu and Mathieu Nendaz

The 6-year Geneva curriculum was constructed to prepare students for medical roles, as defined in the CanMEDS competency framework:

- *Medical expert* – To develop clinical competence, students acquire basic knowledge in the first year, then integrate basic, clinical and psychosocial knowledge to explain the mechanisms underlying clinical cases (problem-based learning (PBL)), together with an early practice of clinical skills among students and with simulated patients in the second and third years, and finally progressively shift to clinical reasoning by solving clinical cases during the fourth year, and practising in an integrated clinical environment until the end of the sixth year.
- *Communicator* – To develop their doctor–patient communication skills, students are trained in communication skills while practising history taking and clinical examination with simulated patients in the second and third years, then with real patients in the fourth, fifth and sixth years.
- *Collaborator* – To develop students' ability to work with other healthcare professionals, we are currently developing interprofessional training in the fourth and fifth years. Some students collaborate with nutritionists and physiotherapists during practicum in the community (third year). In addition, small-group working, inherent to the PBL practice, trains students to work with peers during the second and third years. This is also true on the wards, where they regularly collaborate with nurses, midwives and other allied health professions during the fourth, fifth and sixth years.
- *Health advocate* – The central choice of our medical school is to train students for primary care. They are introduced to the links existing between patients, society and illness during the first year, then to public health issues such as the Swiss healthcare system, and preventive and social medicine during the second and third years. They practise with patients in private primary care settings and public institutions during the second and third years.
- *Scholar* – To develop an autonomous and lifelong learning, students get self-readings complementary to the lectures during the first year and regularly practise self-directed learning with PBL from the second to the fourth years. Moreover, they are initiated to scientific research through a master's thesis during the fourth and fifth years and an optional research programme for medical students during the second and third years.

- *Professional* – The importance of developing professional values is present throughout the curriculum and students are assessed in a summative way by validated criteria. The Medical Humanities programme includes biomedical ethics and medicolegal teaching during the first 3 years.
- *Manager* – Although this dimension is little developed in our pregraduate curriculum, students are introduced to organisation and challenges of healthcare systems during the first 3 years.

Our present curriculum, implemented in 1995 and refined over the years, responds to many dimensions of the 21st-century physician. It has been accredited twice (2006, 2012) and is supported by alumni.

Our future challenges consist of continuing our efforts to promote primary care medicine, reinforcing interprofessional training and valuing test-enhanced learning, based on the best available evidence. This approach must remain an important preventive remedy against the danger of 'curriculum sclerosis'.

OBE and new approaches to medical education

This has been a time of change in medical education, with the introduction of curriculum strategies such as PBL, vertical and horizontal integration and interprofessional learning; new teaching methods, including e-learning and simulation; and new approaches to assessment, including a greater emphasis on performance and work-based assessment. Many of these approaches are described in this book. Embedded in these developments is the need for the recognition of clearly defined learning outcomes and competences to be achieved by the end of the training programme. Table 3.1 lists examples of changes in education in the health professions and highlights the relevance of OBE to each trend.

Learning outcomes describe what is expected of the student and provide a vocabulary to support the use of the different curriculum approaches. OBE empowers students to take more responsibility for their own learning and supports the move to greater student engagement with the curriculum and to student-centred approaches. The teacher works with the student in planning a course of study to meet his or her personal needs – a move in the direction of an adaptive curriculum which is likely to be a feature of education in the future.

Benefits of OBE

OBE offers important benefits to all of the stakeholders – teachers, curriculum developers, students, healthcare professionals and the public. Some of the benefits are described below.

Quality control of the curriculum

The learning outcomes define the end product of training and are a statement as to the relevance of the curriculum and how the doctor entering practice meets the needs of the community which he or she is to serve. The learning outcomes are at the heart of quality assurance and accreditation of a school or an education programme. They can be used to support curriculum renewal and to support the revision of professional accreditation standards.

Table 3.1 Examples of trends in medical education and the relevance of learning outcomes

1	Interprofessional education (IPE)	IPE works best when the expected learning outcomes are appreciated. These include an understanding of the roles and values of other members of the healthcare team and generic competences relating to communication skills, teamwork and professionalism
2	Community-based education (CBE)	In the education programme, some learning outcomes are best achieved in the community setting and others in the hospital setting. For example, in relation to the management of abdominal pain, the investigation and treatment can be addressed in the hospital setting while decisions about the early management and when a patient needs to be referred for further investigation are best achieved in the community setting
3	Electives and student-selected components (SSCs)	Electives and SSCs allow students not only to study a subject in more depth than is possible in the core curriculum, but importantly also contribute to the core learning outcomes, including self-regulated learning
4	Personalised adaptive learning	A detailed explicit statement of the exit learning outcomes allows a learning programme to be planned and tailored to meet the needs of individual students
5	The flipped classroom	Clearly defined learning outcomes inform the students' personal study before the whole-class session and guide the teacher's preparation of problem-solving activities to be undertaken in class
6	The use of simulators	A consideration of learning outcomes can extend the use of simulators beyond the acquisition of clinical skills, to include, for example, the application of the basic sciences to clinical practice
7	Progress tests for student assessment	Progress tests assess how students progress to achieve the expected standards in each of the outcome domains. Milestones relating to each learning outcome can be identified against which the student's progress can be judged
8	Portfolio assessment	Portfolios are being used increasingly as an assessment tool. Through the portfolio, students can demonstrate their mastery of each of the learning outcomes
9	Provision of feedback to students	The provision of effective feedback to students is on the agenda today. Feedback is most valuable if it is related to the student's progress in relation to the mastery of each of the learning outcome domains

Case study 3.2 Implementing an outcome- or competency-based approach in practice in Indonesia

Nancy Margarita Rehatta and Adrianta Surjadhana

In 2006, based upon a study of society and health needs in Indonesia, a task force on primary healthcare set out the minimum competencies to be achieved by graduates. Seven areas of competence were identified: professionalism; self-awareness and self-development; effective communication; information management; scientific foundation of medicine; clinical skills; and health problem management (Figure 3.1). This was the starting point for Indonesia to implement a National Standard for Medical Education and National Standard Competency in medicine. With a subsequent revision, the standards were approved in 2012 by the Indonesian Medical Council. The curriculum model was competency-based and implemented through a SPICES approach to curriculum planning. The SPICES model is based on six educational strategies that can be implemented within a curriculum along a spectrum from innovative to traditional (further discussion can be found in Chapter 9 of this Handbook).

All medical schools in Indonesia are required to base their education programme and curriculum on these standards. Twenty per cent of the curriculum is allocated to take into account local needs and areas of excellence. Faculty of Medicine, University of Airlangga (FMUA) decided to include in the curriculum tropical medicine, mass disaster training and research that related to these topics. Tropical diseases are still a problem for Indonesia and mass disaster training was chosen as Java is in the ring-of-fire pathway of natural disaster.

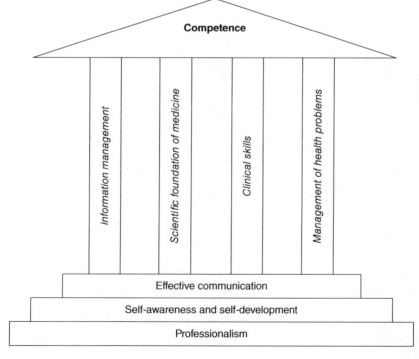

Figure 3.1 Standard competence of Indonesian doctor, 2012.

(continued)

> *(continued)*
>
> Changing from content-based to competency-based was not a smooth process as, although it was believed the outcome would be better as the competences identified related to health needs in the country, at that time the concept of competence-based curriculum was not clearly understood by most teachers. Many teachers were concerned that the word 'standard' would mean a limitation of the competence to be achieved and that the revised curriculum with fewer lectures would be associated with a decrease in the graduate quality compared to the graduates of the previous content-based curriculum. Over time the problems associated with the approach diminished, the educational climate became more supportive and more teachers became willing to become involved.
>
> An example of the difficulties faced can be seen in the implementation of an integrated module. In delivering an integrated lecture, teachers were confused about the goal of the lecture, lacked training in working as an interprofessional team and found it difficult to align the lecture with learning outcomes and identify appropriate achievement to test the specified outcomes.
>
> National Board examinations for medical students began in 2006 and since 2012 all the graduates of medical school in Indonesia have to pass the national exit examination based on the national standard of competence. The test consists of a computer-based test for knowledge and an Objective Structured Clinical Examination (OSCE) for skills.
>
> In 2012, FMUA conducted a study of customer's opinions regarding the achievement by graduates of the specified competences. This provided valuable feedback and indicated where further efforts are needed to improve the students' learning and the curriculum. There is no doubt regarding the advantages of the competence-based curriculum, but the transition needs time. For a traditional medical institution like FMUA, it is necessary to change the mindset of the stakeholders.

As shown in the case study from Indonesia, the determination of a set of learning outcomes can be the starting point for the specification of national standards for medical education. Clearly defined learning outcomes, as shown in the Australian case study, can lead to harmonisation of professional accreditation and quality assurance processes across a range of healthcare professions.

The case study from Canada relates learning outcomes and the curriculum to the school's mission to train physicians with the necessary competences, including a humanistic view and the ability to respond as necessary to change.

> ## Case study 3.3   Sharing learning outcomes across health disciplines in Australia
>
> *Maree O'Keefe and Amanda Henderson*
>
> Australian higher education operates within a quality and regulatory environment with legislated higher-education standards (Australian Government Tertiary Education Quality and Standards Agency 2012). In preparation for this new era of academic quality assurance, the Australian Learning and Teaching Council in 2010 undertook a national learning and teaching academic standards project. Health was included as a single discipline group and, as project leaders in health, the authors were tasked with developing four to six learning outcome statements. These learning outcome statements (or threshold learning outcomes) would then represent the capabilities and competencies to be expected of every Australian health graduate (O'Keefe et al. 2011).

Twenty-six individual disciplines were included in the work: inter alia medicine, dentistry, nursing, veterinary science, osteopathy and Western Chinese medicine. The professional accreditation standards/competencies for each of these individual health disciplines were then compared using qualitative thematic analysis techniques to identify common content domains. As a result, six threshold learning outcomes were developed and refined.

Discipline engagement was a critical factor in the acceptance of the emerging threshold learning outcomes as a true representation of disciplinary expectations for student learning. Considerable reliance was placed on deans and chairs of individual professional and accreditation councils (of which there were over 70) to disseminate information and provide feedback to the project leaders at various stages of the thematic analysis. Nationally, 37 meetings and workshops were conducted to explain the purpose and value of the project and to refine the emerging threshold learning outcome statements. A project email database of key academic contacts grew to over 1,000 in just months.

At national meetings and workshops, representatives from different institutions and healthcare disciplines came together to focus on commonalities in healthcare education. One of many positive outcomes of the workshops and meetings was the attendant fostering of interdisciplinary dialogue and sharing of good educational practice. At one meeting, for example, seven different institutions and health disciplines were represented at a round-table discussion of common student learning outcomes. Academics from veterinary science, medicine and exercise physiology affirmed the centrality of good communication skills, while colleagues from nursing, osteopathy and dentistry confirmed the importance of delivering safe, collaborative healthcare. For the project leaders this experience, repeated multiple times around the country, was one of the truly rewarding aspects of the project.

The utility of project outcomes has extended beyond the original intent of the project. A framework of common health graduate learning outcomes has contributed to government health workforce planning and harmonisation of professional accreditation and higher-education quality assurance processes. It has also been of use as an organising framework for revisions of professional accreditation standards and curriculum renewal, and has provided a robust platform to support interprofessional education initiatives.

Focus and simplicity in capturing key learning outcomes proved a critical factor in relation to ensuring relevance and resonance across disciplines. Anchoring the threshold learning outcomes to existing accreditation standards/competencies gave weight and credibility to the project outcomes. The project also underlined the complex and interrelated nature of health disciplines.

Case study 3.4 Towards a competency-based curriculum – the focus of undergraduate medical education curriculum renewal at the Université de Sherbrooke, Canada

Marianne Xhignesse, Denis Bédard, Ann Graillon, Sharon Hatcher, Frédéric Bernier, Sylvie Houde, Daniel Gladu, Paul Chiasson and Ève-Reine Gagné

The Faculty of Medicine and Health Sciences, Université de Sherbrooke greeted its first students in 1966 with an organ system-based curriculum. The 4-year undergraduate medical programme underwent an initial PBL reform in 1987, followed by a 'reform of the reform' in 1997, with tutors becoming more active and students receiving problem objectives. A clerkship reform was implemented in 2007

(continued)

(continued)

featuring an integrated competency-based framework. Ninety-eight key clinical situations and related tasks focusing on four types of competencies – diagnosis, investigation, treatment and education – were identified. Students were required to maintain a log book of the tasks with which they engaged across the different clerkships in a transdisciplinary fashion. Formative and summative assessments removed from specific disciplinary contexts, including OSCEs, were developed to evaluate clerks. They were designed to reflect various professional roles – clinical reasoning, communicator, collaborator, manager, health advocate and lifelong learner.

Due to organisational limitations the clerkship reform was carried out in relative isolation from the pre-clinical curriculum, where disciplinary teaching remained predominant and evaluation methods unchanged. The impetus for the present pre-clerkship renewal process in 2010 stemmed not only from current literature regarding medical education reform and evolving national standards, but also from a local situational portrait based on multiple consultations with different stakeholders. Through this process it became clear that there was a widening gap between the curriculum as planned by designers, the enacted curriculum by teachers and the curriculum experienced by students (Bédard and Béchard 2009).

Inspired by Stufflebeam's context, input, process and product (CIPP) evaluation model (2003), needs, opportunities and threats were defined, general orientations and actions selected and implementation scenarios drafted. Six broad orientations to shape the curriculum and student assessment were identified: (1) acting with competency; (2) generalism/global approach to health; (3) trans-disciplinary perspective; (4) interprofessional collaboration; (5) flexibility; and (6) comprehensive and coherent management. Significant modifications were proposed, including the integration of competency assessment into authentic clinical practice throughout the curriculum; provision of a roadmap for physician cognitive and professional development; and the establishment of milestones to situate better the gradual acquisition of professional competencies. Clerkship competencies will be used as the basis for this development. Regular communications with key stakeholders maximise buy-in as the process unfolds.

Pre-clinical curricular changes since 1987 have had a primarily methodological focus on the enacted curriculum. The current changes are focusing rather on the planned curriculum. The curriculum experienced by students will serve to inform the latter (rather than the former) such that fundamental principles of competency will not be lost and remain congruent with our mission (to train competent physicians with a humanistic view, dedicated to lifelong learning and committed to responding to evolving community needs) and values (professionalism, quality, dynamism, humanism, autonomy, collaboration).

Although previous curricular changes shared similar positive intentions, a drift occurred over time. In implementing any sort of change, we need to be mindful of the gap that can develop between what was initially planned and what is experienced by students in the end. Regular 'product' evaluations by those in charge of curricular planning are essential to ensure that things remain on track by monitoring outcomes (both intentional and unintentional).

Assessment of the competencies of students, trainees and doctors

The learning outcomes provide a framework for the assessment of the competence and abilities of the learner during and at the end of the medical school programme, of the trainee at the end of specialist training and of the doctor in practice. In a spiral curriculum (Harden and Stamper 1999: 141), students demonstrate that they have achieved the specified milestone and appropriate level of mastery at each phase of the curriculum. Related to this is the concept of the 'entrustable professional activity (EPA)', a task that an individual can be trusted to perform unsupervised in a given healthcare context, once sufficient competence has been acquired (ten Cate 2005).

The case study from Indonesia describes the development of a national examination for medical students based on agreed competencies. The USA case study describes how the assessment of paediatric residents at the University of Colorado School of Medicine was based on the ACGME competencies.

Case study 3.5   Assessment of paediatric residents based on ACGME competencies in the USA

J. Lindsey Lane, Jennifer Soep and M. Douglas Jones, Jr

A system of assessing residents in the Department of Pediatrics, University of Colorado School of Medicine Pediatric Residency programme has been introduced based on the ACGME Pediatric Milestones. The Milestones provide detailed descriptions of components of clinical work sequenced in a quasi-developmental progression from novice to master. They are nested under each of the six ACGME competencies – patient care; medical knowledge; interpersonal and communication skills; professionalism; systems-based practice; and practice-based learning and improvement.

Difficulties had been experienced in implementing a numerical rating scale based on the six ACGME competencies, with descriptive anchors of each element of the competencies aligned with a number rating scale. Faculty found it difficult to relate ratings to the capabilities of residents in the workplace, and found it challenging to analyse and deconstruct what they observed in order to match observations to one of the six ACGME competencies. In addition, it was impossible to develop a shared understanding of the context of work and expectations for performance among over 600 faculty evaluating almost 90 residents. Number ratings conveyed nothing meaningful about performance other than to identify who was at the top and who was at the bottom and provided little information that residents could use to set goals for learning.

A revised assessment system was introduced which focused on performance. We developed a framework for assessment based on the reporter, interpreter, manager, educator (RIME) model while continuing to incorporate language reflecting the six ACGME competencies and the new Pediatric Milestones introduced by ACGME.

Our new framework relies on tasks that faculty routinely observe and make sense in the clinical practice workplace. The new assessment form has no numbers and asks for descriptions of observed work and up to three feedback points. We use qualitative data analysis software to code and link each comment/description to the appropriate milestone or milestones. Teachers are able to go online and complete a descriptive comments form from any computer in our institution, and residents are able to send forms electronically to their teachers requesting descriptive comments. When a descriptive comments form has been completed, the resident is notified and can review the information immediately instead of waiting for a meeting in the indefinite future.

(continued)

> *(continued)*
>
> We undertook intensive faculty development about the new approach to assessment prior to launch. Faculty development is ongoing. Since implementation, the number of useful descriptions of resident performance has increased fourfold. Comments are electronically assembled for review by residency programme leadership and individual residents. Residents, in consultation with faculty, set individual learning goals based on the descriptive data.
>
> The assessment system introduced provides richer evidence of capability to facilitate judgements about progression to competence and independent practice. Residents appreciate receiving timely information about their performance that they can use to create learning goals and improve their practice.

There is a move to change from the current time-based system of training, where what is fixed is the time or duration of training with standards that are variable, to a standard-based approach where what is fixed is the standards or outcomes achieved and what varies is the time for training. This may apply to an element within a training programme such as the acquisition of skills using a simulator or to a shortening (or lengthening, where necessary) of the time required for mastery of the overall training programme.

Empowering the student and the teacher

A statement of the expected learning outcomes empowers both students and teacher –students to take more responsibility for their own learning and the teacher or trainer to innovate and select the most appropriate content and teaching methods from the rich menu of choices now available.

A curriculum blueprint helps to ensure that both the learning experiences provided and the student assessment instruments are matched to the learning outcomes. The curriculum map and the learning outcomes provide the learner with information about his or her progress and what further or remedial study is required. The case study from the University of Colorado School of Medicine illustrates how, based on a competency framework, paediatric residents were assessed and given feedback as to their performances. The residents working with faculty were able to set their individual learning goals.

Priorities and information overload

A major challenge facing educators is how to respond to curriculum demands associated with the 'information explosion' and the doubling of knowledge in the biomedical sciences every 2 years, along with the recognition of new topics such as patient safety and personalised medicine. A consideration of the expected learning outcomes assists the teacher and curriculum designer in assigning priorities as to what is to be included in the curriculum and to ensure that no important aspects are ignored or left out.

Support for collaboration

The value of collaboration in the development and delivery of education programmes in the healthcare professions has become increasingly appreciated and will feature increasingly in health professions education. Collaboration may be between the different disciplines within a medical school, between the different phases of education – undergraduate, postgraduate and continuing education – and between the different healthcare professions. Learning outcomes provide a vocabulary which facilitates discussion among the stakeholders.

Examination of the expected learning outcomes across the different healthcare professions may demonstrate, as illustrated in the case study from Australia, the commonalities in healthcare education and encourage interprofessional dialogue and the sharing of good educational practice. An agreement about common core outcomes also facilitates mobility of doctors and students, an increasingly important aspect due to the globalisation of the medical profession.

The challenges of OBE

OBE has featured prominently on the education agenda over the past two decades. Alongside a sometimes extravagant enthusiasm for the subject, one finds rants and raves against an OBE approach. Both extreme positions risk distorting the picture, as in a hall of mirrors in some circus show, confusing or hiding the real power of OBE. This conflict was highlighted by Harris et al. (1995) and by Bowden (1995).

Those occupying both sides of the argument – the strong protagonists or champions for the cause and the highly vocal critics or opponents – in general agree that there needs to be some sort of direction in an education programme with clarity about the nature of the end product. No one wants to return to the situation when what was covered in the education programme depended entirely on the whims of a teacher or trainer. So if there is a measure of agreement about OBE, where then does the problem or confusion lie? Why is it that what seems to be an attractive idea is not universally accepted? The answer lies in a misunderstanding or misinterpretation of the concept.

The big picture and fragmentation of learning

Problems have arisen where the specification of learning outcomes has been confused with behavioural instructional objectives (Harden 2002). Grant (1999) has argued that:

> behavioural objectives, or competencies, can never describe complex human behaviour. The sum of what professionals do is far greater than any of the parts that can be described in competence terms. They are making judgements, managing cases in the absence of definitive information.
>
> *(Grant 1999: 273)*

OBE, however, if correctly implemented, is about the larger picture. Indeed, one of the strong arguments for an OBE approach is that the broad frameworks of competencies specified identify and represent what is expected today of the doctor, including metacompetencies such as decision making, attitudes and professionalism (Harden et al. 1999).

The expected learning outcomes provide a holistic perspective on the curriculum. Each discipline is challenged to consider not only what is expected of the student in relation to the discipline, whether it is a clinical subject such as obstetrics or a basic medical science subject such as physiology, but also how the discipline contributes to the generic competencies as set out in the school's exit learning outcomes.

Teacher autonomy

Concern has been expressed that OBE leads to teachers being told what they must teach with no freedom for them to use their personal experience and intuition. At an extreme of this view, the teacher is turned into some sort of automaton, programmed to follow automatically and mechanically a predetermined course. One reason that the move to OBE more generally attracted fierce opposition was that it was believed that education should be open ended, not constrained by outcomes. While this liberal notion of education may be appropriate in the arts and humanities, the difficulty in the healthcare professions is that we do not have the luxury of being vague about the product of the training.

An agreement as to the expected learning outcomes, rather than disempowering the teacher, gives the teacher the freedom to determine and implement a programme that will result in students achieving the required level of mastery. Teachers have the freedom to devise and create appropriate learning opportunities and experiences and to introduce their own individuality and perspective to this. The case study from Indonesia shows how local needs can be accommodated within a national statement of learning outcomes with 20 per cent of the curriculum specified locally.

A challenge, however, is to provide the necessary staff development, as for many teachers OBE will be a new concept and assistance will be required as to how learning outcomes can best be embedded in the curriculum. The case study from Indonesia shows how over time a competency-based approach is accepted by teachers.

Level of competence

A criticism of OBE is that minimum levels of competence are promoted. This need not be so. Learning outcomes can be specified at different levels, as demonstrated at Brown University (Smith and Dollase 1999). Competence was defined in nine domains at three levels – beginner level, intermediate level and advanced level. Students were required to attain a beginner- and intermediate-level competence in all nine abilities. An advanced level of competence in problem solving and three other abilities of the student's choice were also required. The model of progression described by Harden (2007) is easily translated into the specification of learning outcomes at different levels of competence. The idea of progression in terms of learning outcomes can be seen in the Australian case study, where the 'threshold learning outcomes' indicate a baseline of competence.

Implementation of OBE

How OBE is best implemented will depend on the local context. Almost certainly, however, steps in the process will include those described below, although the order or attention to detail will vary in different situations. All of the stakeholders should be involved in the process, as described in the Australian case study. The introduction of an outcome-based approach is most easily achieved as part of a curriculum review, as illustrated in the Canadian case study. There are major benefits, as demonstrated in the Indonesian and other case studies, relating the learning outcomes to national accreditation standards and in so doing give credibility to the outcomes specified.

Decide on an overall framework

Key to the success of OBE is a user-friendly, intuitive framework which covers the key domains to be addressed. One option is to choose an existing framework such as the Scottish Doctor,

CanMEDS or ACGME frameworks. This approach has been adopted successfully in many institutions. Amendments can be made and each domain expanded to meet local needs. An alternative is to start *ab ignitio* and develop a framework designed to meet local needs. The Saudi Arabia case study describes how the national framework of Saudi Arabia was used along with recommendations from the UK General Medical Council as a basis for the identified learning outcomes.

Case study 3.6   Basic science integration into the whole curriculum at the Faculty of Medicine, King Abdulaziz University, Saudi Arabia

Abdulmonem Al-Hayani

The new curriculum in the Faculty of Medicine, King Abdulaziz University started in the academic year 2006–2007. The curriculum follows an outcome-based approach to curriculum design and development, where significant outcomes or attributes of students at graduation were well defined at the start. The programme attributes take into account Saudi MED and the General Medical Council's *Tomorrow's Doctors* (2009). The programme clearly defines the graduate attributes, which include: practice and maintenance of good standards of clinical care and professional communication; establishment of good relationships with patients, colleagues and senior and junior staff; acquisition of teaching and training skills; lifelong learning attitude; and humbleness, punctuality and honesty. Graduates' attributes are compatible with community needs and employability skills required for the medical field practice as well as the National Qualifications Framework set by the National Commission for Academic Accreditation and Assessment.

The specific learning outcomes informed the phase 1 curriculum, which appeared over 2 years – a system-based course including the basic medical sciences and the clinical clerkships and electives in phase 2. A feature of the curriculum has been the introduction of problem-based learning (PBL) through constructed cases, which become the focus for 2 weeks of study. The cases were designed in such a way that students must draw on knowledge, ideas and concepts from across the discipline, integrating basic and clinical sciences in order to generate and pursue learning goals. PBL, in particular, emphasises elaboration of learning goals and their discussion in small groups, calling on all relevant knowledge across the disciplines.

Populate the framework with the agreed learning outcomes

The desired outcomes should be established for each of the framework domains. For example, in relation to practical procedures, a decision has to be taken as to which procedures should be included and, in relation to communication skills, which aspects of communication and the level of mastery required at the completion of the education programme.

Prepare a grid or preferably a curriculum map relating the learning outcomes to the phases and courses in the curriculum

It is important to recognise that OBE does not stop with the specification of the learning outcomes. The content of the curriculum and the aspects addressed in each stage of the curriculum must be determined by the expected learning outcomes (Figure 3.2). How each course contributes

Why OBE is an important development

to the exit learning outcomes should be specified and the milestones or what is expected of a student at each phase of the curriculum should be determined.

Prepare a grid or curriculum map identifying for each learning experience the expected learning outcomes

Learning outcomes should be specified for all learning experiences, including lectures, tutorials, PBL sessions, practical classes, clinical experiences and work in a simulation laboratory. The work may be completed over a period of time, with responsibility given to the individual in charge of the session.

Relate the assessment to the learning outcomes

Prepare a grid or curriculum map identifying how each learning outcome is assessed at the different stages in the curriculum, e.g. through a written assessment, an OSCE or as part of a portfolio assessment. As discussed in Chapters 17–19, important advances have been made in the assessment of outcomes such as professionalism, attitudes and team working. The case study from the University of Colorado illustrates how the assessment of trainees was built round the ACGME competencies for paediatrics residents and the milestones in the move from novice to master.

Arrange a faculty development programme

It is essential to engage the faculty in the specification of learning outcomes and in the implementation of an OBE approach. The concept of OBE will be new to many faculty and faculty must be involved and made familiar with the approach, with the learning outcome framework and how the course for which they are responsible contributes to this.

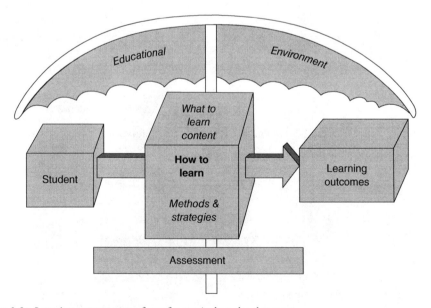

Figure 3.2 Learning outcomes as a focus for curriculum development.

Take-home messages

- The principal focus for medical education should be on the product and the desired learning outcomes rather than on the programme structure and education process. Quite simply, outcome-based and competency-based education mean clearly focusing and organising the educational programme around what are deemed to be the essential competencies and abilities for the learner at the end of the educational programme.
- OBE is a powerful education strategy that should be used as a focus for curriculum planning, as a means of making informed discussions about the approaches to teaching and learning be adopted, and as a basis for the assessment of students/trainees and of the education programme itself. This means starting with a clear picture of what it is important for the healthcare professional to be able to do and then organising the curriculum, learning opportunities and assessment to make sure that this learning happens.
- OBE is at the cutting edge of curriculum development and an understanding of the expected learning outcomes can contribute to our appreciation and success of newer approaches to medical education, such as team-based learning and interprofessional education.
- OBE is not a magic bullet that on its own can address the problems facing medical education. As with all developments or tools and as illustrated in the case studies, how it is implemented and how staff are engaged with the process matter.
- OBE requires a regular revision of the curriculum to ensure that competencies outlined continue to meet the needs of the student, profession and wider community.

Bibliography

ACGME Paediatric Milestones. Online. Available HTTP: http://www.acgme.org/acgmeweb/Portals/0/PDFs/Milestones/320_PedsMilestonesProject.pdf (accessed 10 April 2014).

Australian Government Tertiary Education Quality and Standards Agency (2012) Online. Available HTTP: http://www.teqsa.gov.au/ (accessed 28 March 2013).

Bédard, D. and Béchard, J.P. (2009) 'Quelques conditions pour un curriculum en développement au supérieur'. In D. Bédard and J.P. Béchard (eds) *Innover dans l'enseignement supérieur*, Paris: Presses Universitaires de France.

Bowden, J.A. (1995) *Competency-based education: Neither a panacea nor a pariah*. Paper presented to TEND 97, Abu Dhabi, 6–8 April. Online. Available HTTP: http://crm.hct.ac.ae/events/archive/tend/018bowden.html (accessed 10 April 2014).

Faculty of Medicine, University of Airlangga (2012) *Summary of tracer study*. Unpublished.

Frenk, J., Chen, L., Bhutta, Z.A., Cohen, J., Crisp, N., Evans, T., Fineberg, H., Garcia, P., Ke, Y., Kelley, P., Kistnasamy, B., Meleis, A., Naylor, D., Pablos-Mendez, A., Reddy, S., Scrimshaw, S., Sepulveda, J., Serwadda, D. and Zurayk, H. (2010) 'Health professionals for a new century: Transforming education to strengthen health systems in an interdependent world', *Lancet*, 376(9756): 1923–58.

General Medical Council (2009) *Tomorrow's doctors: Outcomes and standards for undergraduate medical education*, London: GMC. Online. Available HTTP: http://www.gmc-uk.org/education/undergraduate/tomorrows_doctors_2009_foreword.asp (accessed 29 April 2014).

Grant, J. (1999) 'The incapacitating effects of competence: a critique', *Advances in Health Sciences Education: Theory and Practice*, 4(3): 271–7.

Harden, R.M. (2002) 'Learning outcomes and instructional objectives: Is there a difference?', *Medical Teacher*, 24(2): 151–5.

Harden, R.M. (2007) 'Learning outcomes as a tool to assess progression', *Medical Teacher*, 29(7): 678–82.

Harden, R.M. and Stamper, N. (1999) 'What is a spiral curriculum?', *Medical Teacher*, 21(2), 141–3.

Harden, R.M., Crosby, J.R. and Davis, M.H. (1999) 'From competency to meta-competency: A model for the specification of learning outcomes', *Medical Teacher*, 21(6): 546–52.

Harris, R., Guthrie, H., Hobart, B. and Lundberg, D. (1995) *Competency-based education and training: Between a rock and a whirlpool*, Melbourne, Australia: Macmillan Education.

Indonesian Medical Council (2006) *The National Standards competencies of Indonesian medical doctors*, Jakarta: Indonesian Medical Council.

Indonesian Medical Council (2012) *Standard for Indonesian medical education*, Jakarta: Indonesian Medical Council.

O'Keefe, M., Henderson, A. and Pitt, R. (2011) *Learning and teaching academic standards: Statement for health medicine and veterinary science*, Australian Learning and Teaching Council. Online. Available HTTP: http://www.olt.gov.au/resources (accessed 28 March 2013).

Smith, S.R. and Dollase, R. (1999) 'Planning, implementing and evaluating a competency-based curriculum. AMEE education guide no. 14 part 2', *Medical Teacher*, 21(1): 15–22.

Stufflebeam, D.L. (2003) 'The CIPP model for evaluation'. In T. Kellaghan and D.L. Stufflebeam (eds) *International handbook of educational evaluation*, Boston, MA: Kluwer.

ten Cate, O. (2005) 'Entrustability of professional activities and competency-based training', *Medical Education*, 39(12): 1176–7.

Zaini, R.G., Bin Abdulrahman, K.A., Al-Khotani, A.A., Al-Hayani, A.M.A., Al-Alwan, I.A. and Jastaniah, S.D. (2011) 'Saudi meds: A competence specification for Saudi medical graduates', *Medical Teacher*, 33(7): 582–4.

4

HOW MANY MEDICAL STUDENTS?

Matching the number and types of students to a country's needs

Victor Lim, Abu Bakar Suleiman and Mei Ling Young

> *The number of students admitted to study medicine in a different country has been a matter of speculation and controversy.*

Anticipating physician supply for future health needs is crucial for policy planners, the public and for medicine itself. However it is a complex and complicated issue for which there have been no clear answers. There is no universal norm or standard for a minimum density or coverage of human resources for health recommended by the World Health Organization (WHO). However, the 2006 *World Health Report* estimated that countries with a density of fewer than 2.28 doctors, nurses and midwives per 1,000 people generally fail to achieve a targeted 80 per cent coverage for skilled birth attendance and child immunisation (WHO 2006). In 2009, the High Level Task-Force (HLTF) on Innovative International Financing for Health Systems offered two estimates of the number of health workers required to achieve the health-related Millennium Development Goals (MDGs) (Taskforce on Innovative International Financing for Health Systems 2009). One, developed by the WHO, found that 3.5 million more health workers (including additional managers and administrators) across 49 low-income countries were required to accelerate progress towards – and in many cases to achieve – the health-related MDGs, while also expanding coverage for other diseases and contributing to the hunger target in the first MDG (WHO 2013). The other set of calculations, by the World Bank and other institutions, found that these 49 countries required 2.6–2.9 million additional health workers, including managers, whose critical role is too often overlooked (World Bank et al. 2009). Dreesch et al. (2005) have proposed a methodology in human resource planning aimed at achieving the WHO's MDGs.

The number of physicians in any country is often driven by government to create more healthcare activity or to control public expenditure. Moreover, whether more doctors improve patients' health outcomes is still unclear. What is more certain is that more doctors will increase healthcare expenditure.

Who determines the number of medical students in a country is often not clear. In many countries medical schools come under the purview of the ministry responsible for higher education, while planning for health manpower is the responsibility of the ministry responsible for health. Ideally the planning of medical schools and medical school numbers should be undertaken collaboratively between the two ministries so that the provider organisation can give input into decisions on student intakes, but this may not always be the case.

Number of doctors required

The number of doctors needed to be trained by the country depends on many factors, including demographic patterns; disease pattern; level of medical technology and worker productivity; changing roles of support staff; affordability; distribution of doctors; gender issues; and migration of doctors.

Demographic patterns

The number of doctors required is driven to a great extent by the population in the country, although it is difficult to ascertain what an ideal doctor-to-population ratio should be. According to WHO (2013), the world mean for the period 2005–2012 is 14.2 physicians per 10,000 population or approximately one physician to 704 persons. There is considerable variation from country to country. Afghanistan has only 1.9 physicians per 10,000 population, while the Russian Federation has 43.1 physicians per 10,000 population (WHO 2013).

Although, as a tool, a worker-to-population ratio is easy to understand and to apply, it has important limitations. It provides no insight into personnel utilisation and does not allow any explorations into interactions between numbers, mix, distribution, productivity and outcomes. Moreover, any base-year maldistribution will likely continue into the target year.

The number of doctors required will also depend on the age profile of the population. Countries with a higher proportion of the elderly would require more medical services. In the USA more than three-quarters of persons over the age of 65 have at least one chronic disease that would require regular medication and care. In 2011 the first of the 78 million baby-boomer generation reached the age of 65 and concern has been raised that the health system in the USA may not be adequate to meet the demands of increasing numbers of the elderly (Institute of Medicine 2008).

Disease pattern

The pattern of disease seen in a country has an impact on the demand on health services. This is particularly so in the case of chronic diseases, which become more prevalent as the population ages. Worldwide there is an increasing prevalence of chronic diseases like hypertension, diabetes and coronary heart disease. In the USA the percentage of healthcare spending that is associated with people with chronic conditions has increased from 78 per cent to 84 per cent in the 7 years between 2002 and 2009 (Robert Wood Johnson Foundation 2010).

Level of medical technology and worker productivity

Advances in medical technology, including genetics, nanotechnology and information technology, will radically alter the practice of medicine. It is difficult to predict what number of doctors or which skills are required for optimal functionality in the new age of medicine. Technological advances may lead to greater productivity. Productivity can have a profound effect on numbers. A study by Birch et al. (2007) on predicting the number of nurses to be trained illustrates the effect of productivity in determining the optimum number of nurses to be trained in Canada. In their simulation study, they calculated that they would need to increase the number by 2,975 places per year to avoid future shortages. However, if a productivity improvement of 0.5 per cent per year was achieved, the required intake increase would drop to 825 places.

Changing roles of support staff

Health workforce planning is not merely a numbers game. The future functionalities of supporting staff will also play a role in determining the number of doctors required. The rise of the allied health professions would mean that tasks previously considered the exclusive purview of physicians can now be performed as effectively, safely and, importantly, more cheaply by allied health professionals.

Affordability

A country must be able to afford to employ all the doctors it produces. According to the Action for Global Health (2011), in El Salvador in 2008 as much as 53 per cent of the population had no access to healthcare, not because there was a lack of trained and prepared professionals – hundreds of doctors qualify every year but are unable to find a position in the public health system.

Distribution of doctors

In many countries, both developed and developing, the primary challenge may not be the number of doctors but the maldistribution of doctors. There is a tendency for doctors to gravitate to the more affluent urban centres. A study from Ghana revealed that, although most Ghanaian medical students are motivated to study medicine by the desire to help others, this does not translate into willingness to work in rural areas. Students from families with higher parental education and professional status are significantly less willing to serve in rural areas (Agyei-Baffour et al. 2011).

Gender issues

A report from the Royal College of Physicians published in 2009 predicted that within 8 years most doctors in the UK will be women (Elston 2009). Forty per cent of doctors in the UK were already women. In general practitioner (GP) clinics, 42 per cent were female. The General Medical Council reported that in 2013 women made up 44 per cent of all licensed doctors in the UK. Women accounted for 49 per cent of GPs and 32 per cent of specialists. Between 2010 and 2013, there had been a significant increase in the number of women on the Specialist Register and this increase was twice the increase in numbers of male doctors. In surgery, the number of women increased by 42 per cent compared with 12 per cent for men, although 90 per cent of surgeons were still male in 2013. In Emergency Medicine the number of female doctors grew by 44 per cent, compared with 28 per cent for males, and women accounted for a third of doctors in emergency medicine in 2013 (General Medical Council 2013).

These changes raise some major planning issues for the National Health Service (NHS) as, among female GPs, almost half (49 per cent) work part-time. Nearly a third (30 per cent) of female hospital consultants also work part-time. This could mean that more doctors will need to be trained and employed to ensure adequate care for patients.

The shift of the medical profession from a male-dominated profession to a female one is a pattern not only in the UK but also in many other countries, including Malaysia.

The gender issue reported in the UK is important and research is needed to assist in national planning of human capital development in the health sector. This issue may reflect concerns beyond the health sector, as Easton points out in her commentary on 'America's wayward sons' (2013), citing research by Autor and Wasserman (2013) from the Massachusetts Institute of Technology (MIT) and work done by other social scientists. There are broader social issues for which much research needs to be done.

Migration of doctors

The migration of trained healthcare personnel from less-developed to more-developed countries is an issue faced by the poorer developing countries. In France, the Netherlands and Germany, increasing immigration of medical practitioners is seen as a means to maintain an adequate stock of physicians. German hospitals recruit abroad for doctors, particularly in Eastern Europe (Bourassa Forcier et al. 2004).

The UK has also been a country that used migration in a significant way to meet staffing needs. The Department of Health explicitly described international recruitment as a sound and legitimate strategy for the development of its workforce. In 2002 a third of the 71,000 doctors working in NHS hospitals had their primary medical qualification from outside the UK. In 2003, two-thirds of the 15,000 new registrants with the General Medical Council were from other countries (Buchan 2006).

In 2010, the sixty-third World Health Assembly adopted the *WHO Global Code of Practice on International Recruitment of Health Personnel* (WHO 2010). Ministers of health agreed to stop recruiting health workers from developing countries unless agreements are in place to protect the health workforce, and to provide technical and financial assistance to these countries as they strengthen their health systems. Whether this measure will alleviate the challenges faced by developing countries remains to be seen. Implementation of the WHO code by itself may not stop the 'brain drain' completely unless other factors are also addressed.

Tools for forecasting physician supply

A number of forecasting tools are available and have been used to predict the future supply of physicians needed, but the methods employed and the benefits and shortcomings of these tools have not been well appraised. There is currently no universal agreement or 'magic formula' for this purpose. Health workforce planning is particularly complex because of the long lead times associated with the training of health professionals – in particular, doctors. This has an important consequence, as what might be considered best evidence or best judgement at a given time might be dramatically wrong at some time in the future as a result of unforeseen changes in the financial, political or clinical environments.

In a review of forecasting tools by Roberfroid et al. (2009), four main approaches have been identified.

1. The *supply projection* model is based on doctor-to-population ratios and takes into account total health services currently delivered by the entire pool of doctors. The total number of physicians needed in the future is calculated on the premise that the current level of services will be met on a per capita basis. This model can be further refined to take into account other parameters like anticipated changes in demographic profiles, future health service targets, changes in worker productivity and skills mix.

2   In the *demand-based* approach the quantity of health services demanded by the population is determined. The number of required doctors is estimated based on the number and types of projected services.
3   The *needs-based* approach projects the number of health workers and the quantity of services needed to maintain an optimum level of healthcare in the country and to keep the population healthy. Information required for this approach would include the local prevalence of disease, demographic patterns and defined appropriate standards of care.
4   In the *benchmarking* approach a reference country or region is identified and planning for workforce resources is made after adjustments for factors like demography, health system and population health. In the past Malaysia had used Canada as a benchmark in health workforce resource planning.

In practice a combination of the four above approaches is often employed. However, forecasting the required number of doctors remains an inexact science. Many assumptions have to be made in the forecasting model. It is no surprise that many countries perform rather poorly in this. As O'Brien Pallas et al. (2001) have lamented, 'Health human resources planning in most countries has been poorly conceptualized, varying in quality, professions specific in nature, and without adequate vision or data upon which to base sound decisions' (2001: 2).

The following case studies illustrate the different approaches taken by four countries: Malaysia, the Netherlands, South Africa and Saudi Arabia.

Case study 4.1   Malaysia

Kok Leong Tan, Ankur Barua, Sami Abdo Radman Al-Dubai, Hematram Yadav and John Arokiasamy

Malaysia is an emerging economy in Southeast Asia, with a population of 28.8 million in 2011. The gross domestic product (GDP) for 2012 was slightly over USD 300 billion, with a per capita gross national income purchasing power parity of nearly USD 17,000. Healthcare in Malaysia is provided by both public and private sectors. The major provider is the Ministry of Health, with funding through general taxation. In 2011, the 132 government hospitals and six medical institutions provided a total of 33,812 acute beds and 4,582 chronic beds respectively. In addition, there are 985 health clinics and around 2,000 community clinics that provide adequate cover for both urban and rural populations. The private health sector complements the government health services. In 2011 there were 220 private hospitals with 13,568 beds. Private healthcare is funded primarily through out-of-pocket payments and third-party payers. Around 6,500 private GP clinics also provide a range of primary healthcare services.

Healthcare in Malaysia is generally adequate, as demonstrated by marked improvements in vital health statistics since becoming an independent nation in 1957. Notwithstanding the improvements in health indices over the last six decades, Malaysia faces new health challenges in its transition from a developing to a developed nation. With improvements in health and socio-economic indicators, the elderly population will increase with anticipated increases in healthcare spending. There is also an increase in the prevalence of chronic diseases.

(continued)

(continued)

> Malaysia has employed the doctor-to-population ratio in health resource planning. The target is to achieve a ratio of 1:600 by 2020. This figure has improved steadily over the last decade, from 1:1,490 in 2000 to 1:791 in 2011. As of December 2013, this ratio was 1:633 based on 46,916 doctors in the country (Ministry of Health Malaysia 2014). Consequent to the number of medical schools in the country increasing dramatically over the last 10 years, the 1:600 ratio is expected to be achieved earlier. To ensure the quality of medical education an accreditation system for medical programmes has been established jointly by the Malaysian Medical Council and the Malaysian Qualifications Agency (Lim 2008).

Using a benchmark target of doctor-to-population ratio on its own is a simple but rather crude tool for health resource planning. Other factors, like the changing demographic profile, future service targets and the varying functionalities of the different categories of future healthcare professionals, have not been taken into account. There has been a lack of coordination between the Ministry of Higher Education, which grants licences for the establishment of medical schools, and the Ministry of Health, which is responsible for health resource planning. The rapid increase in medical schools in Malaysia raises the possibility of Malaysia producing more doctors than it requires. This will also have implications for placement of interns and opportunities for employment and postgraduate training. Concern has also been raised on the quality of medical education. There is a shortage of qualified faculty as well as a heavy reliance on Ministry of Health facilities for clinical training places, which are becoming increasingly scarce. The main challenge in Malaysia is no longer that of producing an adequate number of doctors but the capacity to produce quality doctors who can best serve the health needs of Malaysia's transformed healthcare system.

Case study 4.2 The Netherlands

Kok Leong Tan, Ankur Barua, Sami Abdo Radman Al-Dubai, Hematram Yadav and John Arokiasamy

The Netherlands has a relatively long tradition of workforce planning in healthcare. Workforce planning is an important instrument in controlling shortages (or oversupply) within the Dutch healthcare labour market. The Dutch government is advised by the Capacity Body (*Capaciteitsorgaan*) regarding all issues related to the intake of medical students and the training capacity in all recognised medical specialties (including general practice). The Capacity Body, which was established in 1999, is the exclusive advisory body to the government on the inflow into all undergraduate medical and specialised postgraduate training programmes.

The Capacity Body employs a stock-and-flow model that was developed by NIVEL (Netherlands Institute for Health Services Research). The model is used in planning the required number of doctors to be trained to meet the projected demand for doctors in the Netherlands. This model is based on setting an equilibrium year. Statistics, as well as expert estimations about future developments on the demand and supply sides for doctors, are collected until the target year. To project the supply of doctors, surveys are undertaken among different cohorts of doctors, to measure their working capacity, primary activities and expected age of retirement. To estimate the demand for doctors, trends in the demand for healthcare services based on demographic and epidemiological factors are predicted. The difference between the required and available supply of doctors is then used to calculate the number of doctors that are required to be trained until the target year. This calculation takes into account the length of study and drop-out rates. Forecasting and planning data are also calculated, using scenarios with different demand growth parameters, as well as factors that include the shortening of working hours and task delegation.

This model was evaluated after 10 years of use and appears to have been successful in stabilising the labour market for physicians in the Netherlands (Van Greuningen et al. 2012). The model also appears suitable for use in the projection of training needs of other categories of healthcare workers. A weakness of this model is that it is unable to take into account substitutions between different categories of healthcare professionals from a skill-mix perspective.

The Netherlands appears to have succeeded in developing a model that meets most requirements for health workforce planning. The model takes into account many of the factors that determine the number of doctors required by a country. Application of this model would require some amount of expertise, as many parameters are based on expert estimations. Resources are also needed to conduct surveys. Equally important is access to good-quality data on demographics and inflow and outflow patterns of trained personnel. All these are crucial for the calculation of projections and estimates. Developing countries may not have the resources or the necessary data in order to utilise this model effectively.

Case study 4.3   South Africa

Kok Leong Tan, Ankur Barua, Sami Abdo Radman Al-Dubai, Hematram Yadav and John Arokiasamy

South Africa is an emerging economy, with a population of 51 million people. In 2010 it had a GDP of USD 363.7 billion and a per capita GDP of USD 7,254. The overall population growth was 1.87 per cent between 2010 and 2011 and more than 60 per cent of the population is under 30 years. South Africa faces a major challenge in human immunodeficiency virus (HIV) infection and acquired immunodeficiency syndrome (AIDS). The infant mortality rate is 35 deaths per 1,000 live births. The under-5 mortality rate is 47 deaths per 1,000 live births (40 per cent due to HIV infection). The maternal mortality rate is 310 deaths per 100,000 births (50 per cent due to HIV infection). In 2010 the prevalence of HIV was 17.9 per cent (5.575 million). Of these, an estimated 518,000 were children under 15 years and 2.95 million were adult females over 15 years. HIV prevalence measured among pregnant women attending public health antenatal clinics has increased from 0.7 per cent in 1990 to 30.2 per cent in 2010. It was reported that 73 per cent of tuberculosis patients were HIV-positive. Around 35 per cent of all deaths in South Africa result from non-communicable conditions and 31 per cent result from AIDS (National Department of Health 2013).

According to the WHO *World Health Statistics* report for 2013, there are only 7.6 doctors per 10,000 population. There is a maldistribution of physicians, with some provinces having as few as 2.6 doctors per 10,000 population, while in some other provinces there are as many as 14.7 doctors per 10,000. In October 2011, there was a shortfall of all healthcare professionals in the country of

(continued)

(continued)

over 80,000 (Human Resources for Health South Africa 2011). In 2006 a total of 33,220 medical practitioners were registered. This represented a 14 per cent increase since 1999 and an annual average growth of 1.76–1.9 per cent. However, among African countries, South Africa has the highest number of doctors abroad, with 12,136 working in the USA, Canada, the UK and other developed countries. This is equivalent to one-third of its total workforce at home (Breier 2007). Since 1996, 37 per cent of South African doctors and 7 per cent of nurses have migrated (Naicker et al. 2009). Conversely, South Africa is the most popular destination for migrating health workers within Africa and, in 2004, 16 per cent of registered medical practitioners were graduates from other African countries.

South Africa has eight medical schools which at any one time train close to 7,500 students. The medical schools in the country have been asked to increase their intake to overcome the shortage of doctors in the country. The University of Witwatersrand increased their intake of medical students by an additional 38 students in 2012.

Unlike Malaysia, South Africa faces the challenge of inadequate number of doctors. It has a low doctor-to-population ratio (around 1:1,500). This problem is aggravated by marked maldistribution of doctors, a high prevalence of HIV infection and significant outflows of trained personnel due to migration to developed countries. The solution would appear to be to increase the number of medical students through higher intakes in each school and the establishment of new schools. It would be equally important to put in place measures to retain trained personnel in the country.

Case study 4.4   Saudi Arabia

Mohammad Yahya Al-Shehri

Medical education in Saudi Arabia is relatively new. Prior to 1967 most physicians working in the Kingdom were expatriates. The few exceptions were Saudi citizens who were educated in other parts of the world, mainly in Egypt, the UK, Germany, France, the Indian subcontinent and the USA.

The first medical college was established at King Saud University, Riyadh in 1967. The college was affiliated with London University, and the affiliation agreement lasted until 1979. The first student intake was enrolled in 1969 and 23 students graduated 6 years later. The medical college in Riyadh later facilitated the establishment of two new colleges, which opened in 1975 at King Abdulaziz University: Jeddah on the west coast and at King Faisal University in Dammam on the east coast. A fourth medical college was established in Abha in the southern part of Saudi Arabia in 1980 and all of their founding deans were former faculty members of King Saud University. Fifteen years later a fifth medical college was established at Um AlQura University, Mecca.

In the mid-1990s, these five medical colleges produced about 450 medical graduates per year and only 15 per cent of this workforce was local doctors. With an annual growth rate of 3.6 per cent, it was estimated that the local medical colleges would need to produce at least 1,000 graduates per year to maintain the status quo and increase the number of doctors. The mass media highlighted the issue and medical educators were in the hot seat, which placed pressure to admit more students into the medical schools. Certainly there was no shortage of applicants among high-school graduates, but there were significant challenges. Local faculty members or educators were in short supply;

the importance of maintaining a reasonable staff-to-student ratio was recognised; and there were a limited number of teaching hospitals and clinical facilities available.

Recognising this, the medical colleges took several steps. The Medical Colleges Deans' Committee of the Gulf Cooperation Council (GCC) countries and the Saudi Medical Colleges Deans' Committee were formed and later in 2002 the Saudi Society for Medical Education was established; several national and GCC-wide meetings, seminars and workshops were held; and forums and committees were formed. It was suggested that the country needed up to 12 new medical colleges and the consensus was to establish more medical colleges in different parts of the country to meet the shortage of medical doctors.

By 2005, 21 per cent of physicians in the country were local. A new strategic plan organised by the Ministry of Higher Education suggested that the targeted physician-to-population ratio should be 1:500 population, with 60 per cent Saudization by the year 2030. The adopted physician-to-population ratio was midway between 1:334 (of high-income countries) and 1:685 (of intermediate-income countries). The WHO recommends a ratio of 1:600. To meet the target, the Kingdom needs to graduate 2,500–3,000 doctors per year. The estimations were based on the Kingdom's population of 22 million and an annual growth rate of 2.5 per cent in 2005, and an estimated population of 40 million in 2030.

By 2011, the government had established 29 medical colleges in the Kingdom, including for the first time six private colleges that are run by either for-profit or non-profit private bodies. Private medical colleges are expected to play an important role in the future development of medical education in the Kingdom.

The number of medical colleges that were established in such a short period will most likely have a very positive effect on the number of Saudi physicians in Saudi Arabia in the future. But it brought with it some new challenges. Staffing, infrastructure issues and clinical facilities are some of the challenges facing these colleges. Private medical education is a new experience in the country. Accreditation, certification and licensing are some of the issues that are currently being worked out.

Thus, it seems that the problems related to the shortage of Saudi doctors are on the way to being solved, but maintaining quality with this number of medical colleges established in such a short period and the introduction of private medical education are new challenges.

Like South Africa, Saudi Arabia faces the challenge of an inadequate number of doctors. In addition to this, the majority of doctors in the country had been, and are still, non-Saudis. The country has therefore embarked on an ambitious plan to increase the number of locals to be trained as doctors. From a single school in 1967 there are now 29 medical schools in the country. The plan appears to be working but, as in Malaysia, the rapid increase in medical schools over a relatively short period of time has led to new challenges, such as having an adequate number of qualified trainers as well as training facilities. Equal emphasis should be placed on ensuring the quality of the medical graduates.

An additional complexity is the globalisation of medical education and healthcare services. Besides the international migration of doctors and nurses, there has been an increase in various types of health-related flows, including international accreditation, financing, patient movements and trade in health services. Chapter 8 discusses some of the problems and opportunities that arise from medical student mobility.

Patients have always travelled to developed countries for high-quality medical treatment, and now patients are travelling for quality low-cost treatment (Frenk et al. 2010). In a recent and interesting development, innovative hospitals in India are moving to the developed countries, such as the Cayman Islands, to deliver world-class care affordably (Govindarajan and Ramamurti 2013).

Some proposals for an approach to determining future number of medical students

From the case studies above, it would seem that any solution, if there is one, is probably unique for each country. The first step would be to estimate the number of doctors the country needs. This planning will have to take into account the health philosophy of the country; the emphasis given to 'curative vs preventive' as well as the health financing model and its sustainability. Other factors would include the pattern of population growth and the demographic profile, the pattern of disease and case-mix. The functionality of the doctors would have to be clearly defined based on the need for primary care doctors as opposed to specialists and subspecialists. The planning should also take into cognisance the country's policy on upgrading and enhancing the roles of nurses and other healthcare professionals.

The number of medical students to be trained is based on the number of doctors required (calculated as full-time equivalents instead of a head count), but taking into account:

- attrition rates in medical schools;
- gender bias in medical students;
- capacity of the country to produce intended number of doctors without compromising on quality;
- capacity to provide internship training for all the medical graduates and subsequently to provide employment for them;
- capacity to provide specialist and subspecialist training.

Planning for the number of medical students to be admitted requires the engagement of all key stakeholders: education and health sectors, industrial and professional organisations and consumers. The interests of the various stakeholders may not all coincide, but the approach must be transparent in terms of potential policy choices and their consequences, and the assumptions that have to be made in the workforce forecasting model.

There is no universally accepted approach to planning for physician demand and therefore the number of medical students to be trained. All approaches are based on many assumptions and therefore have limitations and inaccuracies. Each country needs to be explicit in its health vision and philosophy of access and equity, taking into account the social, political and financial realities. Forecasting models have to be responsive to the rapid changes taking place. It is clear that no one hat will fit all, and each nation has to adopt an approach that is pragmatic and best meets its needs.

Take-home messages

- Estimating the future number of physicians required by a country is a complex issue and requires the consideration of demographic patterns, disease patterns, the level of medical technology and worker productivity, the changing roles of support staff, affordability, the distribution of the workforce, the gender composition of the workforce and the migration of doctors.
- Various forecasting approaches are available, including the supply projection model, the demand-based approach, the needs-based approach and benchmarking.

- The solution to future physician needs is likely to be unique to each country. Planning would take into consideration the health philosophy of the country, whether the emphasis is on preventive or curative medicine, the health financing model and its sustainability.
- Planning requires the involvement of all key stakeholders: education, health, industrial and professional organisations and healthcare users.

Bibliography

Action for Global Health (2011) *Addressing the global health workforce crisis: Challenges for France, Germany, Italy, Spain and the UK*. Online. Available HTTP: http://www.actionforglobalhealth.eu/fileadmin/AfGH_Intranet/AFGH/Publications/HRH_REPORT_-_SCOPE_WEB_LORES_.pdf (accessed 13 May 2013).

Agyei-Baffour, P., Kotha, S.R., Johnson, J.C., Gyakobo, M., Asabir, K., Kwansah, J., Nakua, E., Dzodzomenyo, M., Snow, R.C. and Kruk, M.E. (2011) 'Willingness to work in rural areas and the role of intrinsic versus extrinsic professional motivations: A survey of medical students in Ghana', *BMC Medical Education*, 11: 56. Online. Available HTTP: http://www.biomedcentral.com/1472-6920/11/56 (accessed 13 May 2013).

Autor, D. and Wasserman, M. (2013) *Wayward sons: The emerging gender gap in labour markets and education*. Thirdway. Online. Available HTTP: http://content.thirdway.org/publications/662/Third_Way_Report_-_NEXT_Wayward_Sons-The_Emerging_Gender_Gap_in_Labor_Markets_and_Education.pdf (accessed 23 March 2015).

Birch, S., Kephart, G., Tomblin-Murphy, G., O'Brien-Pallas, L., Alder, R. and MacKenzie, A. (2007) 'Health human resources planning and the production of health: A needs based analytical framework', *Canadian Public Policy*, 33(Supp): S1–S16.

Bourassa Forcier, M., Simoens, S. and Giuffrida, A. (2004) 'Impact, regulation and health policy implications of physician migration in OECD countries', *Human Resources for Health*, 2(12): 1–11.

Breier, M. (2007) *The shortage of medical doctors in South Africa. Case study report forming part of the HSRC study: A multiple source identification and verification of scarce and critical skills in the South African labour market*. Online. Available HTTP: http://www.labour.gov.za/DOL/downloads/documents/research-documents/Medical%20Doctors_DoL_Report.pdf (accessed 23 March 2015).

Buchan, J. (2006) 'Migration of health workers in Europe: Policy problem or policy solution?' In C. Dubois, M. McKee and E. Nolte (eds) *Human resources for health in Europe*, Maidenhead: Open University Press.

Dreesch, N., Dolea, C., Dal Poz, M.R., Goubarev, A., Adams, O., Aregawi, M., Bergstrom, K., Fogstad, H., Sheratt, D., Linkins, J., Scherpbier, R. and Youssef-Fox, M. (2005) 'An approach to estimating human resource requirements to achieve the Millennium Development Goals', *Health Policy and Planning*, 20(5): 267–76.

Easton, N. (2013) 'America's wayward sons: Why they can't carry on', *Fortune, Asia Pacific Edition*, 11 April 2013. Online. Available HTTP: http://fortune.com/2013/04/11/americas-wayward-sons-why-they-cant-carry-on/ (accessed 15 June 2015).

Elston, M.A. (2009) *Women and medicine: The future. A report prepared on behalf of the Royal College of Physicians*, London: Royal College of Physicians.

Frenk, J., Chen, L., Bhutta, Z.A., Cohen, J., Crisp, N., Evans, T., Fineberg, H., García, P.J., Ke, Y., Kelley, P., Kistnasamy, B., Meleis, A., Naylor, D., Pablos-Mendez, A., Reddy, S., Scrimshaw, S., Sepulveda, J., Serwadda, D. and Zurayk, H. (2010) 'Health professionals for a new century: Transforming education to strengthen health systems in an interdependent world', *The Lancet*, 376(9756): 1923–58. Online. Available HTTP: http://www.thelancet.com/journals/lancet/article/PIIS0140-6736(10)61854-5/fulltext?_eventId=login (accessed 15 May 2013).

General Medical Council (2013) *The state of medical education and practice in the UK 2014*. Online. Available HTTP: http://www.gmc-uk.org/publications/25452.asp (accessed 24 March 2015).

Govindarajan, V. and Ramamurti, R. (2013) 'Delivering world class health care, affordably', *Harvard Business Review*, November. Online. Available HTTP: https://hbr.org/2013/11/delivering-world-class-health-care-affordably (accessed 15 June 2015).

Human Resources for Health South Africa (2011) *HRH strategy for the health sector 2012/13–2016/17*. Online. Available HTTP: http://www.gov.za/sites/www.gov.za/files/hrh_strategy_0.pdf (accessed 23 March 2015).

Institute of Medicine (2008) *Retooling for an aging America: Building the health care workforce*, Washington, DC: National Academies Press.

Lim, V.K.E. (2008) 'Medical education in Malaysia', *Medical Teacher*, 30(2): 119–23.

Ministry of Health Malaysia (2014) *Health facts*, Planning Division, Health Informatics Centre. Online. Available HTTP: http://www.moh.gov.my/images/gallery/publications/HEALTH%20FACTS%202014.pdf (accessed 6 April 2015).

Naicker, S., Plange-Rhule, J., Tutt, R.C. and Eastwood, J.B. (2009) 'Shortage of healthcare workers in developing countries – Africa', *Ethnicity and Disease*, 19(1 Supp 1): S1–60–4.

National Department of Health; South Africa (2013) *Annual performance plan 2012/13–2014/15*. Online. Available HTTP: http://advocacyaid.com/images/stories/rrdownloads/Health_annual_performance_plan_2012-2014.pdf (accessed 10 June 2014).

O'Brien-Pallas, L., Birch, S., Baumann, A. and Murphy, G.T. (2001) *Integrating workforce planning, human resources, and service planning*, Geneva: World Health Organization. Online. Available HTTP: http://www.who.int/hrh/documents/en/Integrating_workforce.pdf (accessed 13 May 2013).

Roberfroid, D., Leonard, C. and Stordeur, S. (2009) 'Physician supply forecast: Better than peering in a crystal ball?' *Human Resources for Health*, 7:10. Online. Available HTTP: http://www.human-resources-health.com/content/7/1/10 (accessed 13 May 2013).

Robert Wood Johnson Foundation (2010) *Chronic care: Making the case for ongoing care*, Princeton, NJ: Robert Wood Johnson Foundation. Online. Available HTTP: http://www.rwjf.org/content/dam/farm/reports/reports/2010/rwjf54583 (accessed 11 June 2014).

Taskforce on Innovative International Financing for Health Systems (2009) *More money for health and more health for the money*. Online. Available HTTP: http://www.internationalhealthpartnership.net/fileadmin/uploads/ihp/Documents/Results___Evidence/HAE__results___lessons/Taskforce_report_EN.2009.pdf (accessed 13 May 2013).

Van Greuningen, M., Batenburg, R.S. and Van der Velden, L.F.J. (2012) 'Ten years of health workforce planning in the Netherlands: A tentative evaluation of GP planning as an example', *Human Resources for Health*, 10:21. Online. Available HTTP: http://www.human-resources-health.com/content/10/1/21 (accessed 13 May 2013).

World Bank/UNICEF/UNFPA/Partnership for Maternal, Newborn and Child Health (2009) *Background document for the Taskforce on Innovative International Financing for Health Systems. Working group 1: Constraints to scaling up and costs*. Online. Available HTTP: http://www.internationalhealthpartnership.net/fileadmin/uploads/ihp/Documents/Results___Evidence/HAE__results___lessons/Working%20Group%201%20Technical%20Background%20Report%20%28World%20Bank%20UNICEF%20UNFPA%20PMNCH%29.pdf (accessed 11 June 2014).

World Health Organization (2006) *Working together for health: The world health report 2006*, Geneva: World Health Organization. Online. Available HTTP: http://www.who.int/whr/2006/whr06_en.pdf (accessed 13 May 2013).

World Health Organization (2010) *WHO global code of practice on international recruitment of health personnel*. Online. Available HTTP: www.who.int/hrh/migration/code/WHO_global_code_of_practice_EN.pdf?ua=1 (accessed 10 June 2014).

World Health Organization (2013) *World health statistics 2013*, Geneva: World Health Organization. Online. Available HTTP: http://apps.who.int/iris/bitstream/10665/81965/1/9789241564588_eng.pdf (accessed 23 October 2013).

PART 2

The student

5

SHOULD STUDENTS BE ADMITTED TO MEDICAL SCHOOL DIRECTLY FROM HIGH SCHOOL OR AS UNIVERSITY GRADUATES?

Trudie Roberts and Tadahiko Kozu

The decision as to whether students should be admitted to medical school directly from high school or as a university graduate will depend on a number of factors.

Across the world outside North America, where it is the norm, there has been a noteworthy shift from traditional high-school entrance to medical school towards graduate entry to study medicine. The philosophy behind this move is varied; some schools feel that the life experience that graduates bring will help them understand the issues that patients face better than school-leavers, who have little experience of life's challenges or coping with them. Others feel that graduates, having already succeeded in their studies, will have developed good adult learning methods and be more resilient to the stress of study and working in emotionally charged situations. For some schools, the opportunity to bring into medicine excellent scientists who might take forward future research is an important consideration, and finally for some, the possibility of completing medical training in a reduced timeframe has influenced the introduction of graduate-entry programmes. One of the core purposes of undergraduate medical education is preparation for postgraduate training and continuing lifelong, self-directed learning in order to deliver good medical practice. In this chapter, we examine the question of graduate versus school-leaver entry to medicine and how this might affect that purpose.

Definitions

Cullen et al. (2007) found that there was confusion around the understanding of graduate entry. In this chapter three kinds of medical education programmes as means of entry to study medicine are distinguished: school-leaver entry programmes (SEP), graduate entry programmes (GEP) and mixed parallel-entry programmes (MEP).

In SEP, the basic requirement for entrants is the satisfactory completion of secondary education in high schools or equivalent. The length of the medical programme is usually 5 or 6 years.

This type of medical education is the norm in many countries of the world. The case studies from Australia and Argentina present examples of SEP. Not infrequently, graduates may also be admitted to SEP from the beginning and study together with school-leaver entrants. These students are better understood as graduate entrants in SEP and will not be considered further here.

Case study 5.1 Catering for the school-leaver, Bond University, Gold Coast, Australia

Michelle McLean

Bond University, a private, not-for-profit organisation, offers one of only four undergraduate medical programmes in Australia. The MBBS course is 'accelerated' in that students enter in May and graduate 4.8 years later. Year 1 comprises two 12-week semesters, followed by 2 years of three 12-week trimesters before clinical rotations begin in January of Years 4 and 5. School-leavers make up about one-quarter of the annual intake, with at least one-third of the cohort having no prior experience in biology. Graduate entrants are often from other health professions, such as nursing, physiotherapy and pharmacy.

A revised curriculum began in May 2013. We describe our Year 1 (2 × 12-week semesters, May and September) as a guided, hybrid problem-based learning (PBL) approach, allowing us to accommodate the lowest common denominator (i.e. a school-leaver with no biology). Each week, cases have been specifically designed to address the basic sciences required for the more traditional PBL approach in Year 2, an organ systems course. The 'guided' aspect relates first to the generic/transferable skills to which students are exposed during a 'middle' PBL session, scheduled between the traditional tutorial one (case opening) and tutorial two (case closing). To the best of our ability, the activities students undertake in this 'middle' PBL (often in small groups with their facilitator in a large venue) are related in some way to the content covered in the week's case in one or more of the programme themes (i.e., doctor as scientist, practitioner or professional and health advocate). The transferable skills include information literacy, critical thinking, group work, communication skills, technical and numeracy skills and self-management.

To give an example of how this worked for the first iteration:

- In Week 1, the 'middle' PBL is group work. It involved students in their newly formed groups, under the guidance of their trained facilitator, getting to know each other, drawing up their ground rules, exploring the various roles that they will be carrying out each week (e.g. chair, scribe, recorder, reflector, learning issue (LI) tracker) and clarifying any issues they may not have understood from the PBL guidebook they had been asked to read prior to the session and the training they had received during orientation.
- In Week 5 (Information Literacy 2), two colleagues from the university's Teaching and Learning Office provided students with a critical reading for the week's case on Day 1 (case opening) and then discussed with them the strategies they had used to read and summarise the information. These were explored further during the session. Additional exercises allowed students in their PBL groups the opportunity to try different strategies, including graphic organisers.
- In Week 8 (Critical Thinking 2), groups reviewed some of their earlier LIs, as command terms (i.e. Bloom's taxonomy) were introduced as a means of better defining the breadth and depth expected. For the next cohort, this session has been scheduled earlier, as the feedback suggested that it helped learners to define better the expectations of self-directed learning required for the week.

A particularly useful additional role in PBL that has been introduced at Bond is the LI tracker. At the outset of the semester, via BlackBoard, students are provided with the learning outcomes (LOs) for the semester and the year. These form the blueprint for continuous assessment. Each week, under the guidance of the trained facilitator, the LI tracker maps the LIs generated by the group for the case, as well as those generated from other activities (e.g. clinical skills, placements), to the faculty LOs. At the end of each semester, these are checked by the group to ensure that all LOs have been addressed.

The second aspect of the 'guided' approach to PBL relates to the training and direction provided to facilitators, who are largely casual. Each week, they attend a briefing session, both for the new case and for the 'middle' PBL session. Each case has a facilitator guide, which follows the eight steps of PBL, for example:

- Step 1 – Identify unfamiliar terms.
- Step 2 – Identify the major phenomena.
- Step 3 – What are the major questions that arise from this trigger?
- And so on.

The notes provide guidance to the facilitators in terms of the expected depth and breadth, and identify links to past and future cases to assist learners with the concept of spiral learning.

The student feedback received for the first semester of the renewed curriculum was overwhelmingly positive. Although a few of the graduate students felt that they had already developed some of the generic skills addressed during the 'middle' PBL, most school-leavers appreciated the opportunity to apply new strategies to their learning, whether this be concept mapping or time management. Facilitators too felt that the guided approach was beneficial, particularly for students entering directly from school.

Having covered most of the first spiral in terms of generic skills, the 'middle' PBL in Semester 2 was more integrated into the case. Students needed to apply the skills that they began developing in Semester 1 to data released in the case, e.g. interpreting graphs, statistics. We believe that our guided, hybrid approach has provided a supportive learning environment in which students, particularly those entering directly from school, have been exposed to a range of transferable skills that will be developed further as they progress through their studies.

On the other hand, true GEPs are usually 4 or 5 years in length and students are required to have a tertiary or higher degree at the point of entry. GEPs were unanimously adopted in all medical schools in the USA after the Flexner Report (Flexner 1910). The case studies from Saudi Arabia and South Korea discuss the experience of GEPs.

The third model of medical student recruitment is where graduates are admitted as a different cohort from SEP entrants and learn at first in a shortened course before merger with SEP cohort at a later point in the course. These parallel programmes should be identified as mixed MEP in order to distinguish them from pure GEP. The case studies from St George's, London, UK and Japan provide examples of MEPs.

A move from SEP to GEP

Following the movement to a more student-centred approach to learning, and a change from didactic lectures to self-directed, discussion-based indepth learning in medical education that started at McMaster University, Canada, in 1969 (Barrows and Tamblyn 1980), an intense debate emerged chiefly in Australia and the UK in the 1990s as to whether school-leavers are mature enough to benefit fully from an updated medical education for the 21st century (Charton and Sihota 2011; Geffen 1991; Horton 1998; Searle 2004; Sefton 1995). Transitions are known to be stressful for many individuals, and the transition period from high school to medical school has been shown to be particularly stressful. Additionally the medical course itself, with its intensive study and knowledge acquisition, together with its high-stakes assessments, has been shown to produce stress in medical students (Radcliffe and Lester 2003). Clinical attachments, often involving challenging and emotionally charged issues relating to patient care, have also been shown to provoke anxiety in medical students. Indeed, issues relating to a lack of maturity, discipline, life skills and direction amongst school-leavers have led some universities to introduce pre-entry or access courses to allow students time to adapt to university life (see the Argentina case study).

Conversely, rationales for graduate entry often promote the advantages to be gained from additional maturity and experience of study, almost regardless of the subject area, alongside notions of having a 'second chance' at achieving a vocation. In this section we review the uptake of GEP in a sample of countries from around the world.

Case study 5.2 Supporting transition to university study, Austral University, Argentina

Angel Centeno

In Argentina the medical degree lasts for 6 years and students apply to medical school after finishing their high school, when they are 17 or 18 years old. Entry at this age brings with it some challenges to effective university studies, as students often come to medical school without the educational and learning skills required for a career like medicine, can be immature and unsure of what they want, and are usually vulnerable due to the new and tough requirements for studying medicine. Moreover, strong generational identities and differences are an additional obstacle to entrance into medical school.

Our institution is young, only 18 years old. During this time we have had to make many changes to the admissions process and to the first year of the degree in order to facilitate student adaptation to university life. Our approach involves a short entrance course of two parts: first, a biological section to refresh some basic aspects of chemistry and biology, and to introduce students coming from schools with a social or liberal arts orientation to these subjects; second, a course called 'Introduction to academic life' that provides a brief introduction to logic, text analysis, and some effective study methods essential to facilitate the adaptation to the new studying paradigm. This entire course lasts 1 month.

Despite completing this course, half of the students admitted had poor academic performance in their first year. This led us to incorporate a seminar on study methodology and a change in the curriculum, placing subjects requiring description and recognition skills into the first year, and those that demand greater capacity for abstraction into the second year.

Over time we have recognised that many students need more time to adapt in the transition to university. In response to this, we have now introduced a new year-long programme, which involves the same orientation, and adds learning materials from the first year of the medical course. This allows us to make first year not so demanding, and helps potential students learn in a slow, yet progressively complex, way with a longer period of time for adaptation. During this extended programme, we expect our students to mature, and to discover and develop those skills they will definitely need during their first year of medical studies.

To be admitted to medical studies the students need to complete these two courses, and have an admission interview that focuses on motivational aspects, interests and personal characteristics that may support or delay these students' entry into university life. Those students who are admitted after this schema, either long or short, are afterwards monitored closely to avoid drop-outs caused by difficulties adapting to medical school. Retention is still a concern due to career issues, as many potential students do not know what they want to do in their future professional life. However, by the end of the second year most students were able to improve their academic performance and the drop-out rates decreased.

Japan

Some medical schools with SEP implemented GEP in parallel as MEP. As is outlined in the case study from Japan, in 1975 Osaka University Faculty of Medicine, one of the leading traditional schools, introduced an MEP. Twenty graduates were accepted onto a 5-year course and joined the 6-year SEP for 80 school-leavers (Kiyohara et al. 2005; Nara et al. 2011). By 2011 MEP has been implemented in 36 of 80 Japanese medical schools. The total number of GEP students in Japan is 2.8 per cent of a total of around 9,000 medical students.

Case study 5.3 A 30-year history of graduate-entry medical education programmes in Japan

Tadahiko Kozu

There are 80 Japanese medical schools: 42 national, eight prefectural (founded by local government), 29 private and one national Defense Medical College. High-school-leavers are eligible to enter medical school, and study a 6-year curriculum followed by the National Licensing Examination for Physicians on graduation, and 2-year obligatory postgraduate training. There were places for 8,932 new enrollees in 2011, in a country with a total population of 127.5 million.

The GEP started at Osaka University Medical School, a traditional national university, in 1975 with the purpose of creating a better merger of medicine and the natural sciences, and nurturing leading medical scientists, physician educators and good, mature clinicians. The GEP was partially changed in 2000 to MD-PhD course where the eligibility was having Master's degree or higher, and consent to proceed to Osaka Graduate School of Medicine after graduation. There were places for 20 GEP entrants (reduced to 10 from the year 2000) and 80 places for the SEP. Applications for the GEP were more than ten times over the available places each year. Graduate entrants were incorporated into the third-year class, with some electives only for graduates. Their mean age was 26 years old, and economic and family problems were big stressors for the graduate entrants.

Between 1975 and 2004, academia became the workplace for 32.8 per cent of GEP and 39.5 per cent of SEP graduates, 9.3 per cent of GEP and 6.2 per cent of SEP in departments of basic medicine. Full professors were 5.6 per cent of GEP and 2.2 per cent of SEP. Associate professors were 3.6 per cent of GEP and 2.8 per cent of SEP. Hospital directors were 6.1 per cent of GEP and 2.9 per cent of SEP. Private clinical practitioners were 15.7 per cent of GEP, and 7.9 per cent of SEP (Kiyohara et al. 2005).

(continued)

(continued)

In 2011, 36 Japanese medical schools offered GEP, 45 per cent of all 80 medical schools (Nara et al. 2011). The total number of GEP places available was 2.8 per cent of 9,000 medical school places in 2012. The number of places available in individual schools was on average five: 1–5 in 24 schools, 6–10 in seven schools, 11–15 in one school and 16–20 in three schools. The graduate entrants are incorporated into Year 1 of SEP in two schools, Year 2 in 29 schools, and Year 3 in four schools, with various amounts of elective introductory programmes (data supplied by Associate Professor Tetsuya Urano of Tokai University).

The purpose of GEP is not necessarily uniform: the development of mature learners, physician scientists and shortened tracks for rural community medicine are just some of the many reasons. The selection process also varies: independent selection for GEM; recommendation by deans; admission office selection.

In Japan enthusiasm for GEM is lacking and, in the absence of persuasive evidence, an exploration of its value continues.

Australia

In 1996–97, three Australian medical schools, Flinders University, University of Queensland and University of Sydney, started to implement GEP (Prideaux et al. 2000). It is noteworthy that they formed a consortium, collaborated effectively and shared information on curriculum planning, staff development, admission processes and used staff from partner institutions in the process of converting SEP to GEP (Prideaux et al. 2000). Elements of this planning have also been exported as some medical schools utilised the work of this consortium in developing their own GEPs (see Saudi Arabia and UK case studies). Currently, there are 14 GEPs in Australia and most of them are MEPs (Powis et al. 2004).

Case study 5.4   The experience of graduate entry into a medical programme – the case of College of Medicine, King Saud Ben Abdul-Aziz University for Health Sciences, Riyadh, Saudi Arabia

Ali I. Al Haqwi and Ibrahim A. Al Alwan

The College of Medicine (COM), King Saud bin Abdul-Aziz University for Health Sciences (KSAU-HS), was established by Royal Decree in January 2004. Initially, studying at COM began by enrolling only graduate students who had obtained their bachelor degrees from colleges of sciences, applied medical sciences, pharmacy and veterinary. Four years later, the COM accepted high-school graduates as another stream of students.

The curriculum of the University of Sydney was initially adopted, as it was designed to be a graduate-entry level, problem-based and community-oriented curriculum. This curriculum was then modified to meet the needs of the college and our community. The COM at KSAU-HS is a leader in enrolling graduate students locally and regionally. The annual intake of graduate students ranges between 25 and 30 students.

The evaluation of the student experience of enrolling for graduate entry was satisfactory for both students and decision makers at the COM. Subjectively, for some graduate students their life's dream was to be a doctor, but for one reason or another it had not been possible at the time of their graduation from high school. The COM at KSAU-HS helped these students to achieve their dream. The COM found that most of these students showed a high level of interest, enthusiasm and maturity. Their previous degrees also enriched the discussion in the lectures, tutorials and in the clinical setting.

On an objective level, the COM successfully achieved international accreditation by the World Federation of Medical Education (WFME) in 2010. Moreover, at graduation from the COM, our students achieved the highest marks amongst graduates from all medical colleges in Saudi Arabia, in the national Saudi Licensing Examination (SLE), for 3 consecutive years. At present the intake of graduate students continues, and there are plans to expand it further. This may give another indication about the success of this approach.

The challenges associated with accepting graduate students are mainly due to the fact that some of them have already begun their professional life, taken the decision to change their career and resume the role of being a student. This decision can be associated with significant financial and social burdens on students, which can often subject them to significant stress. Graduate students should be supported and offered counselling services to help them to overcome these challenges.

At present the COM continues to accept high-school and graduate students. This approach is likely to continue, as it is in line with national trends in accepting high-school graduates and continues to offer a unique opportunity that is not available, nationally or regionally, for selected graduate students to continue their studies in medicine.

UK and Eire

In 2000, the move to GEP in Australia was followed by an MBBS graduate-entry programme at St George's Medical School in the UK, in collaboration with Flinders University (McCrorie 2001). This MBBS programme is a 4-year curriculum and is implemented in parallel with the pre-existing 5-year SEP (see UK case study). Other medical schools adopted GEP and currently there are 15 GEPs in the UK offering approximately 10 per cent of admissions in the UK (Garrud 2011; Medical Schools Council 2014). In Eire, the University of Limerick started the first GEP in 2007, admitting 61 entrants (Finucane et al. 2008).

Case study 5.5 Graduate entry – the St George's experience, London, UK

Peter McCrorie

In 2000, St George's started the first UK GEP, admitting students with degrees from any discipline. It was felt that medical schools were missing out on potentially good doctors, just because they didn't have the right A-levels, or because they wanted to make a career change. This course provided them with the opportunity they needed.

In 1999, a team was put together, consisting of a senior experienced course director, a skilled administrator and six young educationally sound, enthusiastic clinicians from a generalist background. The broad principles and outline of the curriculum were created at a series of away days. Funding was secured from St George's and Higher Education Funding Council for England (HEFCE)/General Medical Council approval for the course obtained. Appointments were made in areas where there was insufficient expertise or work overload in both academic and support staff. This was crucial for the acceptability of the programme.

(continued)

(continued)

The first 2 years of the programme involved PBL using the progressive-release format. To overcome the very short course design time before the first students arrived, PBL cases were purchased from Flinders University in Adelaide and adapted for UK use. Training on PBL facilitation and writing PBL cases was provided by Flinders staff. The course was divided into a series of modules and themes and teams were assembled to flesh out the course content and timetable. The PBL cases were allocated to specific modules and put in an appropriate order. All teaching was contextualised and time was created in the timetable for self-directed learning. There were no individual courses in any discipline, though there were curricula for each; the overall curriculum was therefore both horizontally and vertically integrated.

A key principle of the course was meaningful early patient experience, linked to the case of the week, mostly in general practice. The whole course was centrally controlled, each year having its own academic lead. The overall course was planned as a 4-year entity, although the detailed yearly course content was created on a step-by-step basis. Clinical attachments followed the module structure as far as possible, with students being given greater opportunity to plan their own learning. Assessments were theme-based, but run within modules, with formative assessments always preceding summative assessments. Assessments tested scientific and clinical reasoning, maturing into diagnostic reasoning, management and treatment in the later years, clinical and communications skills and professional behaviour, including medical ethics and evidence-based medicine.

Problems encountered mostly related to interaction with the 5-year school-leaver programme, which was running in parallel to the GEP. It proved burdensome to run two completely separate programmes, especially because of the confusion on clinical placements where two sets of students were present at the same time but for different periods and using different educational philosophies. The two courses were eventually combined into a single course with two entry points, one for school-leavers and one for graduates, with students coming together for the final 3 years. Inevitably some of the key educational innovations were lost during this exercise. A decision to move to graduate entry only would likely have been a better solution.

The first two years of the graduate entry programme have been sold to new medical schools in two other countries (Ireland and Portugal) and franchised to a third (Cyprus). All are running successfully. The success of the original GEP was shown by the students being required to sit the same final assessments, and being at least as successful as their school-leaver counterparts, winning prizes, merits and distinctions and publishing papers on a range of research topics undertaken while on the course. The drop-out rate was close to zero and, when this occurred, was related to personal issues and rarely to academic performance. Almost all graduates of the programme are in full employment and have gone on to achieve successful careers in a wide range of specialties.

Graduates, being more mature, are generally more self-directed and motivated than school-leavers. They find it easy to relate to patients and are academic high achievers. Students with non-science degrees perform at least as well in final examinations as those with science degrees. The mix of backgrounds makes for a much richer learning experience. Graduates of whatever discipline – art or science – make good medical students and successful doctors. But design a course specifically to match their skills, and avoid running a parallel course for school-leavers.

South Korea and Iran

In 2002, GEPs were introduced to ten of 41 medical schools in South Korea (see South Korea case study). It is interesting that, in South Korea, it was political pressure from the government that urged medical schools to implement GEP. At its height, 27 out of 41 medical schools converted

SEP to GEP or MEP. After a change of government, there was a reversal of this policy and only five medical schools in South Korea will be left as GEPs in 2015.

Case study 5.6   External influence in medical education, South Korea

Ducksun Ahn

There are 41 medical colleges in South Korea. Since 2006, 15 colleges have admitted only college graduates (GEP: 4 + 4), 14 have admitted only high-school-leavers (SEP: 2 + 4) and 12 have admitted an equal number of both college graduates and high-school-leavers (dual-entry system).

The GEP was first introduced by the Korean government to ten colleges in 2002, with the intention of producing better doctors. However, the Korean government never defined what they meant by the term 'better doctor'. In fact, the aim of introducing GEP was to ease the current university entrance examination fervour. The government's original plan was to force every college to implement the GEP. However, many medical colleges refused to change their admissions system/criteria, due to the fact that GEPs only serve to lengthen the time needed to earn the medical degree and there is no evidence that the graduates of GEP perform better than those of SEPs. For the medical colleges that refused to accept the government's request, the Ministry of Education threatened to cut their research funds. Consequently, 27 out of 41 medical schools converted into either a strict GEP or a lateral (dual)-entry system. However, there was also a very significant appeal from the Faculty of Natural Sciences and Engineering that they are losing their graduates to medical school. In addition, professional societies appealed that the process of change was not democratic. Finally, the former government (under the Lee Myung-Bak administration) decided to leave this decision to each medical school. Eventually, only five medical schools will be left as GEP medical schools in 2015. This is after the two public hearings in 2009 and 2010, held at the National Assembly of Korea.

Having GEPs has nothing to do with the quality of doctors. In Australia, where half of all medical schools have GEP, the aim of having GEP is to allow the late-decision-making students to be admitted to GEP schools. These students are definitely older and more mature, but age does not affect school performance. In Taiwan, the government forced five medical schools to convert to GEP in the 1980s. However, all five GEP schools closed down within 5 years except one, which continued as a dual-entry programme.

The experience of implementing GEP in Korea really was, and is, a costly war of attrition. It is not simple to change a standard entry programme (high-school-leaver system) to GEP. It is not a matter of just changing the name of the school. It is a very complex and complicated matter which needs very careful pre-planning, and requires ample time for changes to organisational culture as well.

The future of GEPs is not quite clear yet in Korea. So far, there has been no evidence that GEP schools are superior to SEP schools.

In 2008, 21 students were admitted in Tehran University of Medical Sciences in Iran. This move had three stated objectives: (1) strengthening the links between basic and clinical sciences; (2) selecting the students on the basis of a wider range of criteria instead of strictly academic ones; and, as graduate applicants are older and have previous academic experience, (3) providing a chance for applicants to make a more informed choice of medicine (Majdzadeh et al. 2009).

Comparing SEP and GEP: students and performance

As detailed in the case studies from Saudi Arabia and the UK, the increased maturity and improved learning skills of graduates are often seen as the benefits of GEP, while possible increased stressors of life stage and personal responsibilities can be a disadvantage. In addition the possibility for enabling access to a vocation to skilled and able people who have previously not had the opportunity, whether by timing or circumstance, is a powerful argument for GEP. In contrast, the additional costs incurred by students in terms of additional study, and by institutions in terms of adapting and running additional courses, are arguments against. Further, entry level has become a political issue in some countries, with GEP being introduced without the support of the medical schools (see Japan and South Korea case studies).

Ultimately, it may be argued that whichever entry level is adopted, solid research evidence of the benefits to be gained in terms of performance and outcomes is required. However, direct comparison of the success of different entry systems is complicated by a multitude of factors, including different curricula, teaching and assessment methods, and the context in which the research takes place. In their 2004 study Wilkinson et al. discovered that a change to graduate entry was often accompanied by a change in admission criteria and a change in curriculum, therefore it was not certain if the difference in student performance, if any, could be due to students having a prior degree, exclusion of less motivated students via admission process or to the changes in the curriculum. For meaningful direct comparisons of performance of the two groups it is important that the studies are undertaken of students on the same education programme.

Comparison of SEP and GEP performance should involve not only the academic aspects but also the perspectives of stakeholders; such as patients, student/family, society, academia, government and international world. Ideally, evidence would be available from controlled, large-scale longitudinal datasets, setting some staged endpoint such as pre-clinical, full-time clinical attachment, postgraduate board certification, workplace and lifelong performances as final outcomes, in a wider range of countries. However, such studies have still to be reported. This section will explore some of the key research findings that are available.

Demographic profiles of GEP candidates and entrants

Graduate entrants tend to be on average 7 or 8 years older than school-entry students (Harth et al. 1990; Rolfe et al. 2004). An analysis of the 2002–2003 data obtained from the Universities and Colleges Admission Service (UCAS) by the University of Nottingham Medical School in the UK found that applicants and successful entrants to their GEP were significantly more likely to be male and more socio-economically deprived and had a lower UCAS tariff point score when compared with applicants to the SEP (James et al. 2008). Additionally the researchers found that Caucasians were significantly fewer in number as entrants from this route. A second longitudinal study at Nottingham Medical School using 2003–2009 UCAS data of their GEP showed that applicants and entrants were older, marginally more likely to be female, and more likely to come from white and black UK communities rather than southern and Chinese Asian groups than their SEP counterparts. In this study again the secondary educational achievement of the GEP cohort was poorer in comparison with the SEP cohort (Garrud 2011).

In 2007 an analysis in Eire of 61 Irish/EU GEP students showed a slight male preponderance: over 90 per cent were still in their 20s, all had a first or upper second class honours degree, fewer than 20 per cent had a higher degree and 24 per cent were from a non-science background (Finucane et al. 2008).

Maturity and stress

Evidence relating the differences in levels of maturity and experience of stress between SEP and GEP students is ambivalent. A study by Hayes et al. (2004) found that graduate entrants on the course were significantly less anxious when compared to traditional undergraduates. However, in another report, mature-age entrants experienced greater stress throughout the medical course, but the stressors in the graduates appeared to be related to personal issues such as financial difficulties, loneliness and family problems (Harth et al. 1990). The academic advantage for GEPs was identified within the Saudi Arabia and UK case studies, with both suggesting that graduate entrants were more mature and self-directed and enriched the learning environment. Both also highlighted the challenges of studying later in life, with the UK case study highlighting that, while the drop-out rate for graduate entrants was close to zero, when it did occur it was for personal rather than academic reasons.

Motivation

Some evidence exists on the differing motivation of students entering SEP and GEP. Rolfe et al. (2004), in their study of 16 years of graduates at Newcastle University, Australia, found that, while the motivation for studying medicine was not substantially different between the two groups, the level of parental expectations was greater among school-leaver entrants, and the wish for professional independence and desire to prevent disease were found more frequently in graduate entrants. In Finland, a comparison of 25 students with prior degrees and 120 school-leaver classmates studying the same curriculum suggested that graduate students had stronger theoretical and practical commitment to their studies with a strong work-life orientation (Kronqvist et al. 2007). Wilkinson et al. (2004) showed that a prior degree predicted distinct goal orientation and cooperativeness, but postulated that entry to the course at an older age might be more important than having a prior degree in this regard. The case studies from Saudi Arabia and the UK both comment on the increased and more altruistic motivation of graduate students.

Overall student performance

In a controlled study at the University of Queensland (Harth et al. 1990), comparing 121 mature-age (7 years older) and 270 normal-age entrants of the same curriculum it was found that course grades were similar in both groups, but normal-age entrants tended to win more honours/prizes and postgraduate diplomas/degrees, including specialist qualifications. A cross-sectional mail-out survey to graduates from the first 16 graduating years (1983–98 inclusive) at Newcastle University, Australia revealed there were no differences in academic performance, awarding of research degrees, publication of scientific papers, holding career positions, choice of general practice or another specialty, practice location or employment sector between graduate and school leaver entrants (Rolfe et al. 2004). The authors concluded that there were no clear differences between the two groups based on the outcomes measured in this study.

Subject of previous degree

In some cases students entering medical studies, whether on SEP or GEP, do not have a scientific background, which may be considered to have some bearing on performance in medical school. Researchers at Newcastle University in the UK looked at the performance of graduate students who joined an SEP. They found that those students with a previous degree in arts and nursing were significantly more likely to receive a 'not satisfactory' assessment in the first year. The arts students made up the deficit by the end of the first year, but the reasons the nursing students struggled with the course were not clear and as a group they were more likely to get an unsatisfactory at the level of the final examination (De Clercq et al. 2001). Similarly, Craig et al. (2004) concluded that there was a small positive difference between the performance of science graduates and non-science graduates early in the programme, but that this tendency lessened with time. The case study from Argentina reports on the development of biology and chemistry teaching in their pre-entry programme as an introduction or refresher for students. The Australian case study discusses how a PBL approach is utilised to accommodate students with no biological background.

Type of programme

It is interesting to consider whether the type of programme, in addition to level of entry, may have an influence on student performance. In a more recent analysis at the University of Newcastle, UK, GEP students performed significantly better in the knowledge assessments than both 5-year programme students and graduate students on the 5-year programme (Price and Wright 2010). At the University of Birmingham, UK, where GEP entrants and SEP entrants are merged in the final 3 years (MEP), analysis of 19,263 student assessments revealed that MEP students showed better academic performance than mainstream students and obtained more 'honours' awards (Calvert et al. 2009).

Stage of education

It is also interesting to consider whether any differences identified between student performance on SEPs or GEPs are sustained over time. Leicester-Warwick Medical Schools, UK, which provide parallel courses for graduate entrants and school-leaver entrants, found that in Phase 1 (applied basic sciences, 2.5-years long for school-leavers, and accelerated to 1.5-years long for graduate students) no significant difference between the performance of the two groups was identified. However, in the midpoint intermediate clinical examination, school-leaver entrants performed significantly better than graduate entrants, but there was no significant difference in the final professional examination (Shehman et al. 2010). Research at the University of Nottingham comparing the full-time clinical summative assessment results of GEP and SEP students found them to be very similar in terms of their overall competence, with similarly high proportions completing their medical degree (Manning and Garrud 2009). However, the two groups showed different patterns of ability: in clinical Phase 1, GEP students did better in their assessments, but subsequently they performed less well in clinical Phases 2 and 3 than their SEP colleagues.

In contrast, a comparison of bioscience knowledge and the clinical skills assessments by Objective Structured Clinical Examination (OSCE) for GEP and SEP students at the University of Melbourne showed marginally better results for the GEP students during the early years, which were attributed to prior bioscience knowledge. However they also performed better in clinical skills that could not be attributed to prior learning (Dodds et al. 2010). Other studies from the University of Queensland (Groves et al. 2003) and the University of Melbourne (Reid et al. 2012) also indicated that GEP students performed better than SEP students in their early years, but the difference seemed to disappear by the final years.

Taken overall, these studies seem indicate some advantages of GEP, especially in the earlier stages of medical education, but these advantages seem to be lost in the later, more clinical parts of the course.

Career choice of the GEP graduates

A final area of interest relates to whether there are any differences in the final outcome of GEP and SEP students in terms of the career choices they make. Research at Osaka University Medical School on the career choice of 405 GEP students from 1975 to 2004 revealed that GEP students were less likely to work as academics in medical schools; however, they were more likely to work in departments of basic medical science. Full professors and hospital directors were more likely to come from GEP and a higher percentage of private clinical practitioners were from GEP (Kiyohara et al. 2005). The principal aims of GEP in Osaka University Medical School are the integration of medicine and science, nurture of leaders in medical science, medical education and clinical medicine, and they concluded their GEP to be successful. Flinders University in Australia offered a 1-year elective Parallel Rural Community Curriculum (PRCC) and Northern Territory Clinical School (NTCS) to the entire SEP Year 3 in addition to GEP students (Worley et al. 2008). They studied subsequent preference for a rural medical career in 150 eligible graduates. The results showed a higher percentage of PRCC and NTCS graduates choosing general practice, but no association between specialty choice, gender or rural background of the students. Interestingly, they found that for each 1-year increase in age at admission, there was a 15 per cent increase in the likelihood of choosing general practice.

Origins of initiative

One clear influence on the success of GEPs may concern the reasons why the programmes are being developed. The case studies from the Saudi Arabia and UK suggest that their programmes developed out of a demand from graduates to retrain and fulfil ambitions. In these case studies the motivation for and perceived success of GEPs are high. In contrast, the case studies from Japan and South Korea suggest that GEPs are less popular. In the South Korean case study in particular, changing political decisions appear to have reduced the enthusiasm for such programmes within medical schools.

Summary and suggestions for future studies

The findings outlined in the studies highlighted above are not uniform or extensive enough to conclude that graduate entrants are superior to school-leavers. Comparisons of SEP and GEP students in the same curriculum showed no consistent evidence of the advantages of GEP, although some advantages associated with age were indicated. However, in these studies numbers of GEP students were consistently lower than numbers of SEP students and in some of the reports the students did not study the same curriculum simultaneously.

The possibility of GEP programmes increasing the diversity of background of medical students was repeatedly emphasised. However, with the cost of higher education having increased dramatically in countries such as the UK, the cost of studying on a GEP programme will increase the debt burden for these students and there is no guarantee that any increase in the diversity of students, particularly around social class, will continue. What is needed is large-scale, well-designed longitudinal tracking of both SEPs and GEPs to finally answer the questions of academic performance, stress management and influence on career choice. Overall therefore, at the present time, the published literature does not demonstrate any clear advantage for schools to move from SEP to GEP.

Take-home messages

- With the exception of North America, entry to study medicine has traditionally been on leaving high school.
- Changes to curricula and teaching methods that promote greater independent and active learning have raised questions about whether school-leavers have the appropriate maturity, life and study skills to benefit fully from a demanding learning experience.
- A variety of challenges have been identified to running graduate-entry programmes, both administratively and with regard to student knowledge and ability. Arguments have been raised as to whether the additional time and resources required are a worthwhile investment.
- Differences exist in relation to evidence of the relative performance of SEP and GEP students. However, most studies conclude that, where differences in levels of performance exist, these lessen over time.
- The case studies reveal a range of practical strategies that have been employed to minimise any disadvantages experienced by SEP and GEP, including pre-entry or access courses, and PBL.
- Graduate entry remains a contentious issue in some areas, particularly where it has been forcefully administered.

Bibliography

Australian Qualification Framework Council (2013) *Australian qualification framework (second edition)*. Available HTTP: http://www.aqf.edu.au/wp-content/uploads/2013/05/AQF (accessed 15 November 2013).

Barrows, H.S. and Tamblyn, R.M. (1980) *Problem-based learning*, New York, NY: Springer.

Calvert, M.J., Ross, N.M., Freemantle, N., Xu, Y., Zvauya, R. and Parle, J.V. (2009) 'Examination performance of graduate entry medical students compared with mainstream students', *Journal of the Royal Society of Medicine*, 102(10): 425–30.

Chan, K. *Course description: 2500MED – Human skills for medicine*, Griffith University. Online. Available HTTP: https://www.148.griffith.edu.au/programs-courses (accessed 15 November 2013).

Charton, R. and Sihota, J. (2011) 'Challenges and opportunities: Graduate Entry Medicine (GEM)', *Irish Medical Journal*, 104(1): 25–6.

Craig, P.L., Gordon, J.J., Clark, R.M. and Langendyk, V. (2004) 'Prior academic background and student performance in assessment in a graduate entry programme', *Medical Education*, 38(11): 1164–8.

Cullen, W., Power, D. and Bury, G. (2007) 'The introduction of graduate entry medical programmes: Potential benefits and likely challenges', *Irish Medical Journal*, 100(6): 500–4.

De Clercq, L., Pearson, S.A. and Rolfe, I.E. (2001) 'The relationship between previous tertiary education and course performance in first year medical students at Newcastle University, Australia', *Education for Health*, 14(3): 417–26.

Dickman, R.L., Sarnacki, R.E., Schimphauser, F.T. and Katz, L.A. (1980) 'Medical students from natural science and non-science undergraduate backgrounds. Similar academic performance and residency selection', *Journal of American Medical Association*, 27(243): 2506–9.

Dodds, A.F., Reid, K.J., Conn, J.J., Elliott, S.L. and McColl, G.J. (2010) 'Comparing the academic performance of graduate- and undergraduate-entry medical students', *Medical Education*, 44(2): 197–204.

Finucane, P., Arnett, R., Johnson, A. and Waters, M. (2008) 'Graduate medical education in Ireland: A profile of the first cohort of students', *Irish Journal of Medical Science*, 177(1): 19–22.

Flexner, A. (1910) *Medical education in the United States and Canada: A report to the Carnegie Foundation for the Advancement of Teaching. Bulletin no. 4*, Boston, MA: Updyke.

Garrud, P. (2011) 'Who applies and who gets admitted to UK graduate entry medicine? An analysis of UK admission statistics', *BMC Medical Education*, 26(11): 71.

Geffen, L.B. (1991) 'The case for graduate schools of medicine in Australia', *Medical Journal of Australia*, 155(11–12): 737–40.

Groves, M., O'Rourke, P. and Alexander, H. (2003) 'The association between student characteristics and the development of clinical reasoning in a graduate-entry, PBL medical programme', *Medical Teacher*, 25(6): 626–31.

Harth, S.C., Biggs, S.G. and Thong, .H. (1990) 'Mature-age entrants to medical school: A controlled study of socio-demographic characteristics, career choice and job satisfaction', *Medical Education*, 24(6): 488–98.

Hawthorne, L. and Birrell, B. (2002) 'Doctor shortages and their impact on the quality of medical care in Australia', *People and Place*, 10(3): 55–67.

Hayes, K., Feather, A., Hall, A., Sedgwick, P., Wannan, G., Wessier-Smith, A., Green, T. and McCrorie, P. (2004) 'Anxiety in medical students: Is preparation for full-time clinical attachments more dependent upon differences in maturity or on educational programmes for undergraduate and graduate entry students?', *Medical Education*, 38(11): 1154–63.

Horton, R. (1998) 'Why graduate medical schools make sense', *The Lancet*, 351(9105): 826–8.

James, D., Ferguson, E., Powis, D., Symonds, I. and Yates, J. (2008) 'Graduate entry to medicine: Widening academic and socio-demographic access', *Medical Education*, 42(3): 294–300.

Kiyohara, T., Watabe, K., Noguchi, S. and Aozasa, K. (2005) 'Summary of a 30-year-old system of graduate entry at Osaka University Medical School', *Medical Education* (Japan), 36(4): 259–64 (in Japanese with English abstract).

Kronqvist, P., Mäkinen, J., Ranne, S., Kääpä, P. and Vainio, O. (2007) 'Study orientations of graduate entry medical students', *Medical Teacher*, 29(8): 836–8.

Majdzadeh, R., Nedjat, S., Keshhavarz, H., Rashidian, A. Eynollahi, B., Larijani, B. and Lankarani, K.B. (2009) 'A new experience in medical student admission in Iran', *Iranian Journal of Public Health*, 38(Supp 1): 36–9.

Manning, G. and Garrud, P. (2009) 'Comparative attainment of 5-year undergraduate and 4-year graduate entry medical students moving into foundation training', *BMC Medical Education*, 9(76): 1–5.

Martin, S. (2003) 'Impact of a graduate entry programme on a medical school library service', *Health Information and Libraries Journal*, 20(1): 42–9.

McCrorie, P. (2001) 'Tales from Tooting: Reflections on the first year of the MBBS Graduate Entry Programme at St George's Medical School', *Medical Education*, 35(12): 1144–9.

Medical Schools Council (2014) *Graduate entry*. Online. Available HTTP: http://www.medschools.ac.uk/students/courses/pages/graduate.aspx (accessed 13 June 2014).

Nara, N., Suzuki, T. and Nitta, Y. (2011) 'The present state and problems of Graduate-Entry Programs (GEP) in national medical schools in Japan', *Journal of Medical and Dental Science*, 58(2): 23–7.

Powis, D., Hamilton, J. and Gordon, J. (2004) 'Are graduate entry programmes the answer to recruiting and selecting tomorrow's doctors?', *Medical Education*, 38(11): 1147–53.

Price, R. and Wright, S.R. (2010) 'Comparisons of examination performance between conventional and graduate entry programme students: The Newcastle experience', *Medical Teacher*, 32(1): 80–2.

Prideaux, D. (2009) 'Medical education in Australia: Much has changed but what remains?', *Medical Teacher*, 31(2): 96–100.

Prideaux, D., Teubner, J., Sefton, A., Field, M., Gordon, J. and Price, D. (2000) 'The consortium of graduate medical schools in Australia: Formal and informal collaboration in medical education', *Medical Education*, 34(6): 449–54.

Radcliffe, C. and Lester, H. (2003) 'Perceived stress during undergraduate medical training: A qualitative study', *Medical Education*, 37(1): 32–8.

Reid, K.J., Dodds, A.E. and McColl, G.J. (2012) 'Clinical assessment performance of graduate- and undergraduate-entry medical students', *Medical Teacher*, 34(2): 168–71.

Rolfe, I.E., Ringland, C. and Pearson, S-A. (2004) 'Graduate entry to medical school? Testing some assumptions', *Medical Education*, 38(7): 778–86.

Searle, J. (2004) 'Graduate entry medicine: What it is and what it isn't', *Medical Education*, 38(11): 1130–2.

Sefton, A.J. (1995) 'Australian medical education in a time of change: A view from the University of Sydney', *Medical Education*, 29(3): 181–6.

Shehman, M., Haldane, T., Price-Forbes, A., Macdougall, C., Fraser, I., Peterson, S. and Peile, E. (2010) 'Comparing the performance of graduate-entry and school-leaver medical students', *Medical Education*, 44(7): 699–705.

Simpson, D. (2000) *The Adelaide medical school, 1885–1914: A study of Anglo-Australian synergies in medical education*. Doctor of Medicine thesis. University of Adelaide. Online. Available HTTP: http://hdl.handle.net/2440/38422 (accessed 15 November 2013).

Wilkinson, T.J., Wells, J.E. and Bushnell, J.A. (2004) 'Are differences between graduates and undergraduates in a medical course due to age or prior degree?', *Medical Education*, 38(11): 1141–6.

Worley, P., Martin, A, Prideaux, D., Woodman, R., Worley, E. and Lowe, M. (2008) 'Vocational career paths of graduate entry medical students at Flinders University: A comparison of rural, remote and tertiary tracks', *Medical Journal of Australia*, 188(3): 177–8.

6

HOW DO WE SELECT STUDENTS WITH THE NECESSARY ABILITIES?

Jon Dowell

The last two decades have witnessed dramatic changes in how we view the science and art of selecting students for admission to medical studies.

Recent decades have witnessed dramatic changes in how we view the art of selecting medical students as the evidence evolves (Cleland et al. 2013). High academic ability alone is no longer considered sufficient and sound interpersonal skills and attitudes are increasingly considered fundamental. Although it is sometimes argued communication skills or even professional behaviour can be taught, it is logical to select the best in multiple domains where we have opportunity, as it makes teaching easier and higher competence achievable. In this chapter we shall briefly consider why selection matters and what it seeks to achieve before examining some of the available tools and exploring practical issues such as resources, legal frameworks and context.

So why does selection matter? Firstly, medical training universally recruits academically elite students with great potential and then invests hugely in them. Typically at least 90 per cent of entrants graduate, so selection plays a key role in determining this human and financial 'resource' use. Medicine also plays a significant societal role; it is highly competitive, very influential and carries high status. We all want 'good doctors' and not 'bad doctors', two dimensions of selection we shall return to later.

In practice, a wide range of approaches to selection have been adopted around the world, reflecting the lack of clear evidence. Countries such as France allow any student to enter a medical course and then robustly select after the first year of studies. The Dutch have historically used a lottery allocation for those of high academic ability but are increasingly moving to a more selective system like those operated by most Western countries. The latter generally operate systems that include a range of applicant attributes, albeit in very different ways. Academic achievement is a universal element but increasingly this is supplemented with aptitude tests such as: (1) Medical College Admissions Test (MCAT) in the USA; (2) United Kingdom Clinical Aptitude Test (UKCAT); (3) Graduate Medical Schools Admissions Test (GAMSAT) in Australia; (4) Biomedical Admissions Test (BMAT) in the UK; and (5) Health Professions Admissions Test (HPAT) in Eire, and there is new interest in interviews based on a highly structured approach, the Multiple Mini-Interview (MMI). In addition, disappointing evidence has emerged from evaluations of personality measures as well as some longstanding tools such as personal statements and references (that may be particularly vulnerable to 'gaming', cheating and other influences such as applicant's background). So the weight placed on these traditional measures is being challenged.

Selection never exists in a vacuum and local workforce issues as well as those of gender, ethnic and socio-economic equity are always at play. The local nature and complexity of these require local resolutions and the first case study from Pakistan illustrates how Aga Khan University addresses equal opportunity through a 'needs-blind' policy.

Case study 6.1 Selecting students with the necessary abilities, Aga Khan University, Pakistan

Rukhsana W. Zuberi and Laila Akbarali

Aga Khan University (AKU), chartered in 1983, was Pakistan's first private university and, according to the country's Higher Education Commission, is one of its premier institutions. It is a not-for-profit international university with campuses in south-central Asia, East Africa and the UK. The university's Medical College admits 100 students annually to a 5-year undergraduate medical (MBBS) degree programme. The Registrar's Office is responsible for admissions. Student selection is aligned to AKU's vision and mission and the underpinning philosophy of quality, accessibility, relevance and impact. It is not only essential to select students with the right abilities; it is also essential to be accessible to such students.

AKU admissions are responsive to social accountability. To ensure that distance or travel-related costs do not preclude applicants, either from less-privileged areas of Pakistan or from international sites, the University Admission Test (UAT) is conducted in several cities in Pakistan and in seven centres around the world (London, Dar-es-Salaam, Toronto, Nairobi, Kampala, New York, Dubai), and, more recently, in Bangladesh, Singapore and Malaysia. The university makes every effort to accommodate a candidate's request to conduct the test close to his or her home town.

Although not the first language in Pakistan, English is the language of instruction at AKU. To improve accessibility from underprivileged areas, English scores are reported separately when shortlisting candidates. Thus, students with high cumulative scores in UAT's science component (mathematical reasoning, science reasoning, science achievement based on assimilation of knowledge) but less than average English scores can be identified and coached in English if admitted.

Approximately 4,000 candidates apply each year, with roughly the top 10 per cent selected for interviews. The interviews are also scheduled close to candidates' home towns. Within Pakistan, faculty members travel to seven different cities to carry out the interviews; for interviews conducted outside Pakistan, wherever possible, Medical College alumni are utilised.

The Medical College's interview form has been designed to assess 11 attributes that also keep in mind the opportunities available to the candidates. These attributes are responsibility; maturity; independent and critical thinking; honesty and integrity; adaptability and tolerance for others; socio-cultural awareness; health awareness; communication skills; motivation, interest and commitment to the medical profession; teamwork and leadership potential; and their aspirations in life.

Faculty training workshops for student selection are held to increase inter-rater reliability, and to hone faculty interviewing and narrative-writing skills. The interviews are conducted by two faculty members: either a basic scientist or a community health scientist and a clinician. Each interview is conducted separately and lasts about half an hour. Interviewers are not privy to test scores or

(continued)

> *(continued)*
> scholastic achievements of the candidate. They are required to provide a narrative for each of the 11 characteristics, and an overall assessment regarding the suitability of the candidate for AKU.
>
> The Admissions Committee is chaired by the Dean and consists of seven members from within AKU (including the Chair of the Examinations and Promotions Committee; Associate Dean Education and the University Registrar), an AKU alumna/alumnus, a non-AKU educationist and four eminent citizens of Karachi.
>
> In making its decisions, the Admissions Committee has access to the candidates' secondary school certificate scores (or British and American school system equivalents), the UAT scores (or SAT scores for international candidates). Group percentiles of the test scores are also available to members of the Admissions Committee.
>
> Each candidate's profile is presented anonymously to the Admissions Committee for consideration. The profile includes the candidate's application and personal statement, certificates from school, the two complete interview reports and two school recommendations. Committee members use a scale from one to four to provide their feedback on each candidate; the top hundred are selected.
>
> ### *Needs-blind admission policy*
>
> Once admitted, a student's ability to pay is determined. Interest-free financial assistance is available for tuition, fees, hostel accommodation and a subsistence allowance, as needed. No student is denied admission on the basis of financial constraints.
>
> Candidates are short-listed based on knowledge and reasoning ability, and selected based on humanistic, extracurricular and leadership abilities. The 11-member Admissions Committee ensures reliability and validity of decisions made.

Studying medicine is a high-status activity subject to competitive selection. Thus, attention to the process is important and is often contentious. Ideally a clear legal framework would support open, fair and transparent selection processes, which would in turn result in a diverse population of students broadly representative of inhabitants. Demonstrably reliable and valid measures of academic and non-academic attributes would be used and these would then show meaningful predictive validity, both during training and beyond. All this would be done at reasonable cost and in a manner acceptable to candidates and others. Unfortunately, we are not there yet but it is likely we shall take some significant steps forward in the coming decade. We should not forget though that each individual's decision to apply is the primary determinant of who enters, not our selection methods.

Context

Globally there is interest in who gains access to study medicine, partly because it reflects our societies' particular racial, gender, religious or other issues interacting with what is generally portrayed as a 'fair' process. For instance, efforts are made to increase black and Hispanic entrants in the USA, and native Aboriginal entrants in Canada and Australia. In the UK context (known best to the author) there is longstanding evidence that those from lower socio-economic classes rarely apply for medical school and fare a little less well when they do (Cleland et al. 2013: 49). This is despite numerous initiatives and considerable investment in outreach, bespoke supported and extended courses and some positive discrimination within selection. A number of studies have shown how strong cultural factors influence potential applicants' choices, with medicine in the UK being viewed as a 'posh club'. Whatever the contextual issue, they can usefully be separated into distinct elements that can be considered and addressed individually. Namely:

- getting ready;
- getting in;
- staying in;
- getting on.

There are four core reasons why it is important to consider how local context influences the individuals who study medicine: equity, optimising potential, impact on learning and impact on workforce. First, as a highly competitive, high-profile subject medicine is a barometer of opportunity within societies. Second, to identify the best it is necessary to seek those with most potential from the broadest base available. Unless the necessary attributes required are absent from some applicant groups all individuals with suitable potential should be encouraged. Third is the influence a broad mix of students can have within a school and the learning that occurs there, for instance towards ethnicity, sexuality or disability. Last, there is emerging evidence that career choice depends to some extent on origin, with doctors more likely to return to and serve rural or deprived home communities.

This UK case study demonstrates how some medical schools have sought to broaden selection more robustly to include non-cognitive attributes.

Case study 6.2 Assessing non-academic attributes for medical and dental school admissions using a situational judgement test, United Kingdom

Fiona Patterson, Emma Rowett, Máire Kerrin and Stuart Martin

Applicants to UK university medical and dental schools are of a consistently high calibre with regard to their academic qualifications; the UKCAT (UKCAT 2014) is used by a consortium of universities to help them make more informed choices from among the many highly qualified applicants who apply for the medical and dental degree programmes. Until 2013, the UKCAT consisted of tests of verbal, quantitative, abstract reasoning and decision-making analysis.

Role analyses of numerous specialties in the medical and dental arena have indicated that non-academic or professional attributes (such as integrity and team working) are essential requirements for a clinician. Situational judgement tests (SJTs) are an increasingly popular and well-established selection method for assessing these non-academic attributes. SJTs are a measurement method and, in an SJT, candidates are presented with challenging hypothetical situations which are likely to be encountered in the target role, where candidates are required to make a judgement on the effectiveness of various response options. The responses of candidates are scored against a pre-determined key agreed by subject matter experts. Once designed, SJTs are cost-effective to score and administer, and research indicates that SJTs have significant validity in predicting role performance over and above both IQ tests and personality tests (McDaniel et al. 2001; McDaniel and Whetzel, 2007; Patterson et al. 2009, 2012). Other benefits of SJTs

(continued)

(continued)

are that they generally have smaller subgroup differences than cognitive ability tests (Lievens et al. 2005), favourable candidate reactions and high face validity. In addition, certain response formats can minimise susceptibility to coaching, which is an important consideration in selection for medicine.

In order to assess non-academic attributes in applicants to medical and dental schools, a newly designed SJT was piloted in 2011–12 and since 2013 has been used for live medical and dental school admissions. The SJT scenarios used in the UKCAT are based on analyses of medical/dental roles but do not require any clinical knowledge as it is important that the test is fair and appropriate for a novice population.

The UKCAT SJT targets three domains: integrity, perspective taking and team involvement. The 2012 pilot test content was developed by subject matter experts ($n = 38$) and experienced psychometricians ($n = 5$). The SJT presents candidates with a set of hypothetical scenarios which are based in either a clinical setting or during educational training as a student. Scenarios may involve a student,

---

A consultation is taking place between a senior doctor and a patient. A medical student, Lucas, is observing. The senior doctor tells the patient that he requires some blood tests to rule out a terminal disease. The senior doctor is called away urgently, leaving Lucas alone with the patient. The patient tells Lucas that he is worried that he is going to die and asks the student what the blood tests will show.

How **appropriate** are each of the following responses by **Lucas** in this situation?

A   Explain to the patient that he is unable to comment on what the tests will show as he is a medical student

- ☐ A very appropriate thing to do
- ☐ Appropriate, but not ideal
- ☐ Inappropriate, but not awful
- ☐ A very inappropriate thing to do

B   Acknowledge the patient's concerns and ask whether he would like them to be raised with the senior doctor

- ☐ A very appropriate thing to do
- ☐ Appropriate, but not ideal
- ☐ Inappropriate, but not awful
- ☐ A very inappropriate thing to do

C   Suggest to the patient that he poses these questions to the senior doctor when he returns

- ☐ A very appropriate thing to do
- ☐ Appropriate, but not ideal
- ☐ Inappropriate, but not awful
- ☐ A very inappropriate thing to do

D   Tell the patient that he should not worry and that it is unlikely that he will die

- ☐ A very appropriate thing to do
- ☐ Appropriate, but not ideal
- ☐ Inappropriate, but not awful
- ☐ A very inappropriate thing to do

Figure 6.1 Example SJT item.

patient or clinician, and each targets one of the three domains which has been identified as being important to the role of a medical or dental student.

In 2012, 18 test forms were piloted online alongside the other UKCAT subtests. A total of 25,431 applicants sat the pilot. Each SJT scenario asked applicants to rate between four and six response options and two formats of rating scales (1 to 4 scale) were used: very appropriate to not appropriate at all and very important to not important at all. An example SJT item is provided in Figure 6.1.

Candidates' responses to SJT items were evaluated against a pre-determined scoring key to provide a picture of their situational judgement and marks were assigned dependent on response proximity by the candidate to the correct answers. Full marks for an item were awarded if a candidate's response matched the agreed expert key and partial marks were awarded if the response was close to the agreed correct answer.

Psychometric analysis of the pilot SJT demonstrated good levels of reliability ($\alpha = 0.75–0.85$). Initial evidence of criterion-related validity was established as applicant scores on the SJT correlated significantly with the other UKCAT subtests. On average, the SJT correlated more strongly with the verbal and decision-making analysis test than with the numerical and abstract tests. However, the sizes of the correlations were moderate (as expected), as the SJT is designed to measure non-academic attributes that are important for anyone embarking on a career within medicine and dentistry. Unlike academic indicators used in selection (such as A levels), early results show that performance on the SJT is not related to socio-economic status, which is an important finding in relation to a broader widening participation agenda.

SJTs offer a standardised method of objectively assessing a broad range of professional role-related attributes in large numbers of applicants, and demonstrate face validity to candidates because the scenarios used in SJTs are based on relevant situations (Patterson et al. 2012). Outcomes from the UKCAT SJT demonstrated that an SJT is a reliable and valid selection methodology for testing important non-academic attributes for entry to medical and dental school.

Medical school selection needs to be fit for purpose in the local context. To achieve a desirable mix within the final workforce and deliver a fair and open process may require quite different systems in different countries or regions. The same principles, however, are likely to apply.

Academic ability

Academic ability, or more specifically, academic achievement in terms of exam performance at school or university, has been the mainstay of medical school selection for generations. It remains the most obviously justifiable way of separating candidates and has the best evidence base in terms of predicting future exam performance, and to a lesser extent in postgraduate assessments. However, there are also a number of concerns about utilising measures of achievement too heavily and an awareness that exam grades are not the only outcome of importance.

Generally measures of achievement are freely available and quantified reliably because they result from quality-assured assessment at school or university. There is clear face validity in requiring medical students to be high performers, which is supported by moderate levels of predictive validity. Because medicine is oversubscribed, one option is simply to select the very best academically. However this risks two things. First, achievement may often not be easily compared or reflect true potential because educational opportunity is not equal. Even in countries with little variation in the quality of education, applicants will receive widely different levels of home support and encouragement.

One approach to moderating this is universal testing, which tries to compare applicants more fairly, at least partly by measuring stable aspects of so-called 'fluid intelligence', known to be less dependent on education and background. A number of such tests have now been developed which vary in their format and content, reflecting the context in which they were developed. Availability, cost and content all require consideration. For instance, although research on MCAT 2013 shows it is the science component that best predicts performance, the UKCAT 2103 chose a pure aptitude test format. This was because a key aspiration was to help 'widen access' in the UK and a lower level of predictive validity was traded against a test focused on 'potential'.

So, prior achievement should be viewed in local context. Though tempting simply to select the highest achievers, it may be more logical to consider 'how good is good enough'. This opens the door to consider what other attributes educators require from entrants.

There are a number of reasons why other attributes may be worth considering. First, there is an argument that those presenting with broader talents have some 'reserve in the tank' for when the going gets tough. More importantly, it is clear that patients require clinicians to offer more than academic brilliance alone. In modern healthcare settings, high value is placed upon interpersonal communication skills, attitudes, integrity and an ability to work effectively within multidisciplinary teams. Medical schools are increasingly seeking to ensure that assessments of such aptitudes are included in selection, as demonstrated in the UK case study. The problem is that validated and justifiable measures of these attributes are only just emerging.

Non-academic attributes

Despite long-term interest in the non-academic attributes of doctors, the evidence base remains weak. Even the terminology, non-academic versus non-cognitive, remains disputed. This is not good news for high-stakes selection systems where a sound evidence base justifies use of academic grades while primarily strong beliefs support the inclusion of 'softer skills'.

Despite the lack of convincing evidence, non-academic attributes have often been applied, including personal statements, character references, personality tests and various forms of interviews. Unfortunately none has stood up to rigorous scrutiny and, as a result, a range of alternative approaches is being developed and tested.

Foremost among these is now the structured interview and in particular the MMI. This system, based upon the Objective Structured Clinical Examination (OSCE), has consistently demonstrated satisfactory reliability and its use is spreading rapidly based on evolving evidence of predictive validity within medical school and even beyond. The Canadian case study discusses the introduction of the MMI into medical school admissions. As selection science develops further it seems likely that selection centres will evolve, as is the case in Israel (Gafni et al. 2012: 277).

Case study 6.3 The true fairy tale of the Multiple Mini-Interview, McMaster University, Canada

Harold I. Reiter and Kevin W. Eva

The apocryphal story held that the daughter of a neighbour to a dean or associate dean, having clearly demonstrated to all who knew her that she was the fairest medical school applicant in the land, nevertheless failed to secure an offer of admission to her local medical school. A retreat was called to review the admissions processes of all schools in McMaster University's health science kingdom. By this time, the process of medical school admissions had devolved into a labyrinthine path, as one well-intended process correction followed another, each correction solving one perceived problem while creating new difficulties. Concerned with the defensibility of his realm, the Earl of Admissions sought support from a neighbouring village of faculty with broader experience in assessment.

At a meeting to discuss possible research on OSCE feedback, 5 minutes were set aside to consider a response to the plea from the Earl of Admissions. Ideas were batted about, including the concept of an 'admissions OSCE', but the concept was immediately discarded (with much laughter) due to the perception of overwhelming resource requirements. There the idea would have died had not one member, that weekend, put quill to parchment and realised that less gold would be needed to run an admissions OSCE than to continue with the traditional interview system (Rosenfeld et al. 2008). At the kingdom's retreat the idea garnered sufficient support to merit $5,000 (CAD) in seed funding from the faculty. A small 2001 pilot study of 18 graduate students and a six-station MMI yielded sufficient promise to lead our protagonists to continue their quest (Eva et al. 2004).

As supportive evidence in the form of improved test–retest reliability, feasibility and acceptability rolled in over subsequent studies with real applicants, the parry and thrust that ultimately won the argument was that the absence of evidence regarding predictive validity of the MMI was better than evidence of the absence of predictive validity that was available for any of the measures of personal characteristics in traditional use (Kulatunga-Moruzi and Norman 2002). At least the MMI had the potential for validity, which was only later realised (Reiter et al. 2007; Eva et al. 2009, 2012).

The process of ridding the kingdom of dragons, however, was not entirely painless as many knights of the Admissions Committee were resistant, having invested immeasurably in the traditional practices. For those knights, the MMI was anathema to all that they knew to be good and true in the world and intellectual arguments could not sway their emotional attachments. The new Earl of Admissions, committed to sweeping changes of which the MMI was an integral part, faced the dual tasks of fighting a rearguard action and supporting innovative development. After initial raucous committee meetings, it was necessary to reorganise the committee and terms of reference were written that required, henceforth, all knights to prove their mettle with an assigned 'portfolio' (e.g. the MMI, the autobiographical submission, research of newer tools) or relinquish their knighthood. Each portfolio required a specific skill set that included a willingness to look beyond convictions that one 'knew' who would become good doctors.

Community buy-in from the villagers proved the easiest to achieve as the Earl of Admissions sought out to draw upon the broad and variable expertise present in the land. To mount an MMI well with structured interview stations requires an assessment blueprint, so a paired comparison survey was sent throughout the realm to enable many stakeholders from across the kingdom to define the relative importance to be placed on various applicant characteristics (Reiter and Eva 2005). Villagers were also recruited as MMI station writers and interviewers, lending an additional medieval faire-like air to the MMI dates.

While there remain questions to be answered, the proverbial genie that is the MMI is now out of the bottle. Based upon research diligently conducted within a culture of evidence-based decision making and with the support of the Deanery, the MMI was implemented in 2004. In hindsight, each of these factors, scientific and political, were necessary components for its coming to fruition. Since then, at least 80 papers have been published on the MMI (www.tinyurl.com/mmiresearch), most emanating from outside of McMaster. At last count, close to a quarter of Canadian and American medical schools are using the MMI, along with countless other health professional schools worldwide (Eva et al. 2012). As the MMI is a process rather than an instrument, its use will vary from place to place. Our experience would lead us to believe, however, that universal factors enabling successful implementation include: (1) recognition of a problem; (2) collaboration between individuals with complementary expertise; (3) a spirit of innovation; (4) dedicated scholarship; (5) strong leadership; and of course, (6) a healthy dose of serendipity.

Although interviews appear to be the method of choice for assessing interpersonal skills, they typically also include assessments of critical thinking, integrity or moral reasoning, which make less sense. In a face-to-face format it is very costly to present a satisfactory number of situations to candidates and is difficult to grade them consistently enough. By contrast, SJTs, as described in the UK case study above, appear to offer this potential (Cleland et al. 2013: 29). These tests, which present candidates with a series of dilemmas and require them to rank a range of responses, have been shown to be reliable and offer an interesting new tool with high face validity.

By contrast, personality tests have now been extensively assessed without finding favour, perhaps because of fears over 'faking' in high-stakes situations and, although reliability is high, predictive validity has been very limited (Cleland et al. 2013: 34).

So it seems quite feasible that within the next 5–10 years a valid system for evaluating non-academic skills will develop and, as the evidence base emerges, the currently diverse range of practices will converge around those techniques known to be cost-effective. Of course the competitive nature of medical selection will continue and it remains to be seen how immune these approaches will be from coaching effects.

The bigger picture

Medical practice varies around the globe and, although a need for high academic ability may be universal, there may be great local variation in the non-academic qualities required. For instance, different weight may be put upon communication skills or patient-centred attitudes within different healthcare systems. Others may prioritise resilience or personal motivation, and others select for those with a particular focus on rural service. Each will require and want a somewhat different emphasis within its selection system. So the question of how different elements are used and combined emerges. For instance, different scores can be used as hurdles or combined into a summary rank. Some or even all elements may be multiplied to introduce an adjustment for educational or personal adversity (so-called contextual assessment). Selectors may wish to include systems capable of deselecting otherwise promising individuals for reasons not explicitly included within the scoring algorithm, such as deception within the application process or even unacceptable attitudes (e.g. racism). All of this must be considered with an awareness of the strengths and weaknesses of the information available. For instance, professional references may be valuable in some cultures but not in all. However, beyond any direct impact on selection, the system chosen will have a potentially far larger effect by influencing who applies.

Hence, it is necessary to consider what you wish to prioritise and whether the process suits the mission of the institution. In addition, it is important to ensure that the decision-making process has balance and is not dominated by any particular perspective. The constitution of the relevant guiding body or committee should include broad representation, including patient or lay members to counter the narrow focus of academic staff.

A framework for selection

Figure 6.2 demonstrates an integrated framework for selection of medical students.

The way such a schema might be operated is outlined below. Assessments on each domain may be used to identify concerning individuals whose progress will be barred ('hurdles-based') as well as contributing to a rank for those remaining.

Jon Dowell

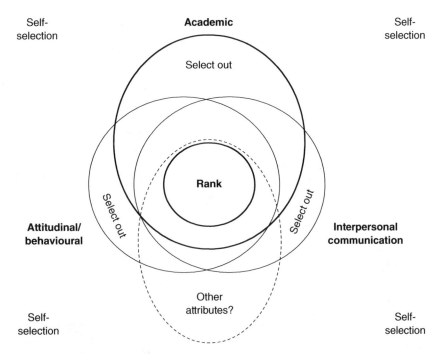

Figure 6.2 A framework for selection.

Academic

Academic achievement, with or without the addition of aptitude testing, will continue to form the backbone of selection systems. Because academic assessments are widely accepted, cheap and reasonably reliable and valid it is clearly appropriate to continue using these as a primary filter or screening tool.

Attitudinal/behavioural

Attitudinal or behavioural attributes may be measured through SJTs or at interview or even personality inventories (Goldberg 'Big 5' Personality Test, Personal Qualities Assessment). They may then be used in conjunction with some or all of the other scores available or in their own right, for instance, to exclude those with highly aberrant views. It may be possible and appropriate to include other sorts of evidence here, such as previous legal convictions or references, if a robust system exists.

Interpersonal communication

Broad consensus over the importance of interpersonal communication skills has led to the widespread use of interviews. Often, however, the elements of communication being assessed are ill defined. They will include an assessment of the ability to interact effectively on a one-to-one basis but increasingly, more refined and sophisticated challenges are presented (for example, the ability to convey empathy within role-play situations). The MMI is clearly emerging as a leading methodology.

Other attributes?

There are a number of other attributes that schools might consider depending on their circumstances. Examples include: motivation to study medicine or at that specific school, career awareness, language abilities or an interest in serving a particular community. Specifically, an assessment of 'fitness to practise' as a clinician may sometimes be required due to individual circumstances such as disability (Higher Educational Occupational Physicians 2011) or probity. The Dutch case study offers an example of how satisfactory performance in multiple areas can be used to 'select out'.

Case study 6.4   Consequences of 'selecting out' in the Netherlands

Fred Tromp and Margit I. Vermeulen

The Dutch postgraduate training for general practice (GP) has a nationally endorsed curriculum. The Departments of General Practice of the eight university medical centres are responsible for the organisation of the 3-year postgraduate training.

The Dutch selection procedure of GP training was studied by Vermeulen et al. (2012). This procedure, which consists of selection on the basis of a letter of application and a semi-structured interview, is nationally legislated but locally conducted. It was found that, despite legislation, different standards were used across different institutes and that the department itself was a strong predictor of being admitted. Viewing the results of their study, the authors expressed their concerns regarding the fairness of the selection procedure and pleaded for a rethink of the current approach.

Since 2010, a fair, standardised selection procedure has been developed. Because of the decreasing number of candidates in relation to available vacancies and the societal responsibility to ensure qualified GPs, a selecting-out approach was chosen. The new procedure aimed to identify unsuitable candidates who are likely to encounter difficulties and will not finish the training successfully. Despite the fact that most candidates finish the training successfully in the Netherlands, drop-outs and poor performers cost the departments a large amount of effort and money. In addition, their places cannot be reallocated, which is a waste of capacity.

The first step in the development of the procedure was a content analysis to establish the required level of competence. The curriculum of GP training in the Netherlands is based on the Canadian Physician Competency Framework (CanMEDS) competencies. To determine which of these competencies should be targeted for the selection procedure for GP training, we invited a panel of 16 experts. In a Delphi procedure the panellists determined 'which of the CanMEDS-competencies should already be present before entering GP training in order to finish the training successfully'. The second step was to determine which assessment instruments to use. In a high-stake situation, no single assessment instrument can provide the necessary information for judgement (van der Vleuten and Schuwirth 2005; Prideaux et al. 2011). Therefore, four instruments were included to assess competencies needed to start the training: the Knowledge Test for General Practice; an SJT; three mini-simulations (SIMs); and a Patterned Behaviour Descriptive Interview (PBDI).

After the candidates completed all instruments, the assessments were aggregated and substantiated by the assessors involved. As the instruments provided incremental information of the candidates' competencies, appropriate recommendations could be made. Candidates were accepted after establishing whether all targeted competencies were present to a certain extent. This means that if one competency could not be shown by the candidates, they were rejected no matter how high the other scores were (see examples below).

Example 1

A female candidate, 25 years old, applied for the first time. She graduated with honours and started 6 months ago as an MD in an emergency room. She scored high on all instruments, except on one competency in the PBDI – self-care. Lack of self-care is a well-known cause of problems during the GP training.

Example 2

A male candidate, 33 years old, applied for the first time. He already had a lot of different working experience as an MD. He scored high on all instruments, except on one competency in the SIM: showing respect to the patient. He patronised the patient and was very judgemental towards the patient. Afterwards he did not show any reflection on his behaviour.

We realise rejection is hard to comprehend for these particular candidates, as they performed well in general. Therefore, formulating the required level of competency unambiguously and clearly is of utmost importance. Our new procedure is transparent, and the candidates are informed which competencies will be assessed and that a deficiency cannot be compensated for. Extensive feedback was provided to the rejected candidates, which is important because this enables candidates to remedy their deficiencies so that they can reapply. Feedback to admitted candidates can be used at the start of the training.

Ranking and selecting out

Once applicants have survived the initial screening process, progressed through whatever subsequent assessments are required and made it into the final cohort, some form of final selection is required. In theory this entire group should be very suitable entrants to study medicine and many would argue that a random allocation system would be fairest at this point. Historically, however, it is more common to rank applicants and invite the 'best'. Ideally this is based upon an analysis of the way in which the respective components of the selection system operates locally, for instance, how strongly different components predict performance on the course. Often, however, this level of evidence is lacking and a decision must be based upon the views of an admissions committee, preferably with intimate knowledge of the system in practice.

Assessing success

A recurrent theme of this chapter has been the challenge of validating admissions tools without a suitable range of outcome measures. We know that patients highly value clinicians' interpersonal skills and there is a consensus that teamwork is important for patient safety. However medical schools do not typically measure these attributes distinctly. As more reliable and valid means of selecting students emerge it is increasingly important to ensure these are benchmarked against appropriate outcome markers and not simply knowledge-based tests. And although we will never identify and avoid all unsuitable entrants, it is important to study rare events such as fitness-to-practise concerns. We are at an interesting stage in the evolution of selection techniques with the advent of new tools such as SJTs and MMIs. To make significant progress with this agenda, long-term follow-up studies are required which include issues such as career choice and satisfaction as well as undergraduate performance.

Take-home messages

- Selection for medical school is a complex and contentious task which is currently based on an inadequate evidence base.
- There are a number of promising initiatives arising, in particular the advent of the MMI and greater use of aptitude testing in addition to prior academic achievement and the development of tools such as the SJTs.
- It must be recognised that medical education exists in widely varied contexts, educational institutions and societies, with different expectations and different workforce requirements. All of these will have a local effect in determining what approach is appropriate.
- It certainly seems desirable to use an approach which balances achievements in both academic and non-academic areas and which is capable of selecting out the minority of unsuitable applicants as effectively as it ranks the high achievers.
- In a perfect world, markers of both academic and non-academic attributes would be both reliable and valid predictors of future performance. At present though we are some way off this ideal and require some sophisticated long-term studies to achieve it. However this is an area of medical education worth watching over the coming years.

Bibliography

Admission Testing Service (2014) *About the Biomedical Admission Test (BMAT)*. Online. Available HTTP: www.admissiontestingservice.org/our-services/medicine-and-healthcare/bmat/about-bmat (accessed 22 May 2014).

Association of American Medical Colleges (2013) *Medical college admission test*. Online. Available HTTP: https://www.aamc.org/students/applying/mcat/about/ (accessed 22 June 2013).

Australian Council for Educational Research (2013a) *Graduate medical schools admissions test*. Online. Available HTTP: http://gamsat.acer.edu.au/about-gamsat (accessed 22 June 2013).

Australian Council for Educational Research (2013b) *Health professions admissions test: Ireland*. Online. Available HTTP: http://www.hpat-ireland.acer.edu.au (accessed 22 June 2013).

Cleland, J., Dowell, J., McLachlan, J., Nicholson, S. and Patterson, F. (2013) *Identifying best practice in the selection of medical students*, London: GMC. Online. Available HTTP: http://www.gmc-uk.org/Identifying_best_practice_in_the_selection_of_medical_students.pdf_51119804.pdf (accessed 22 June 2013).

Eva, K.W., Rosenfeld, J., Reiter, H.I. and Norman, G.R. (2004) 'An admissions OSCE: The Multiple Mini-Interview', *Medical Education*, 38: 314–26.

Eva, K.W., Reiter, H.I., Trinh, K., Wasi, P., Rosenfeld, J. and Norman, G. (2009) 'Predictive validity of the Multiple Mini-Interview for selecting medical trainees', *Medical Education*, 43: 767–85.

Eva, K.W., Reiter, H.I., Rosenfeld, J., Trinh, K., Wood, T.J. and Norman, G.R. (2012) 'Association between a medical school admission process using the Multiple Mini-Interview and national licensing examination scores', *Journal of the American Medical Association*, 308: 2233–40.

Gafni, N., Moshinsky, A., Eisenberg, O., Zeigler, D. and Ziv, A. (2012) 'Reliability estimates: Behavioural stations and questionnaires in medical school admissions', *Medical Education*, 46(3): 277–88.

Higher Educational Occupational Physicians (2011) *Medical students – Standards of medical fitness to train*. Online. Available HTTP: http://www.heops.org.uk/HEOPS_Medical_Students_fitness_standards_2013_v10.pdf (accessed 23 March 2105).

Kulatunga-Moruzi, C. and Norman, G.R. (2002) 'Validity of admissions measures in predicting performance outcomes: A comparison of those who were and were not accepted at McMaster', *Teaching and Learning Medicine*, 14: 43–8.

Lievens, F., Buyse, T. and Sackett, P. (2005) 'The operational validity of a video-based situational judgement test for medical college admissions: Illustrating the importance of matching predictor and criterion construct domains', *Journal of Applied Psychology*, 90(3): 442–52.

McDaniel, M. and Whetzel, D. (2007) 'Situational judgement tests', In G.R. Wheaton and D.L. Whetzel (eds) *Applied measurement: Industrial psychology in human resources management*, Mahwah, NJ: Lawrence Erlbaum Associates.

McDaniel, M., Morgeson, F.P., Finnegan, E.B., Campion, M.A. and Braverman, E.P. (2001) 'Use of situational judgement tests to predict job performance: A clarification of the literature', *Journal of Applied Psychology*, 86(4): 730–40.

Patterson, F., Carr, V., Zibarras, L., Burr, B., Berkin, L., Plint, S., Irish, B. and Gregory, S. (2009) 'New machine-marked tests for selection into core medical training: Evidence from two validation studies', *Clinical Medicine*, 9(5): 417–20.

Patterson, F., Ashworth, V., Zibarras, L., Coan, P., Kerrin, M. and O'Neill, P. (2012) 'Evaluating situational judgement tests to assess non-academic attributes in selection', *Medical Education*, 46: 850–65.

Prideaux, D., Roberts, C., Eva, K., Centeno, Aa, McCrorie, P., McManus, C., Patterson, F., Pavis, D., Tekian, A. and Wilkinson, D. (2011) 'Assessment for selection for the health care professions and specialty training: Consensus statement and recommendations from the Ottawa 2010 Conference'. *Medical Teacher*, 33: 215–23.

Reiter, H.I. and Eva, K.W. (2005) 'Reflecting the relative values of community, faculty, and students in the admissions tools of medical school', *Teaching and Learning in Medicine*, 17: 4–8.

Reiter, H.I., Eva, K.W., Rosenfeld, J. and Norman, G.R. (2007) 'Multiple mini-interview predicts clerkship and licensing exam performance', *Medical Education*, 41: 378–84.

Rosenfeld, J., Reiter, H.I., Trinh, K. and Eva, K.W. (2008) 'A cost efficiency comparison between the multiple mini-interview and traditional admissions interviews', *Advances in Health Sciences Education*, 13: 43–58.

UK Clinical Aptitude Test (2014) *UK Clinical Aptitude Test*. Online. Available HTTP: http://www.ukcat.ac.uk/ (accessed 23 March 2015).

van der Vleuten, C.P.M. and Schuwirth, L.W. (2005) 'Assessing professional competence: From methods to programmes', *Medical Education*, 39: 309–17.

Vermeulen, M.I., Kuyvenhoven, M.M., Zuithoff, N.P.A., Tromp, F., Graaf van der, Y. and Pieters, H.M. (2012) 'Selection for Dutch postgraduate GP training: Time for improvement', *European Journal of General Practice*, 18: 201–5.

7

THE SECRET INGREDIENT

The students' role and how they can be engaged with the curriculum

*Khalid A. Bin Abdulrahman and
Catherine Kennedy*

> *The benefits to be gained from significant student engagement in medical school activities are now widely appreciated.*

Relationships between students, teachers and their educational institutions have changed dramatically over recent decades. What had been seen as unidirectional learning from teacher to student is now increasingly seen as more symbiotic. In some countries the model of financing education has changed, with a corresponding shift from seeing students as the recipients of education to that of consumers. In addition, changing emphases in delivery and modes of learning have promoted the requirement of 'active' and 'engaged' learning while at the same time increasing the opportunities for students to learn remotely and at a distance. Combined together, these and other changes have increased the significance of student engagement in medical education. In this chapter we will explore the differing perspectives of what student engagement is and how it can be promoted and explore the experiences at a number of case study institutions.

What is 'student engagement'?

In higher education there is growing interest in student engagement, in the 'student voice' and in staff working in partnership with students to deliver the education programme and to facilitate change (Baron and Corbin 2012). Many perceived benefits are often highlighted for students, such as improving student experience and achievement, and for institutions as an indicator of success, quality assurance and competitive advantage. However, understandings of what 'student engagement' is vary between individuals, their disciplines, institutions and countries.

The term 'student engagement' can be traced to debates about student involvement, and is a term in common use, particularly in North America and Australasia, where annual large-scale student engagement surveys have been conducted for a number of years (Trowler 2010). These surveys, the US National Survey of Student Engagement (NSSE) and the Australian Survey of Student Engagement (AUSSE), comprise self-rating questionnaires completed by students based on indicators of best practice: academic challenge; active and collaborative learning; student–faculty interaction; enriching educational experiences; supportive campus environment; and work-integrated learning (AUSSE only). However in this approach, using a survey method, the issue has become focused on what students are doing, and any assessment of students' perceptions or expectations of their experience has been lost (Hand and Bryson 2008).

The term has traditionally been used less commonly in Europe and has been associated more with debates regarding student feedback, student representation and student approaches to learning (Trowler 2010). However, student engagement has been a significant part of education policy for a number of years. For example, student-centred learning in higher education 'characterised by innovative methods of teaching that involve students as active participants in their own learning' is a commitment of the European Higher Education Area (EHEA) Bologna Process (2012: 2). Indeed, one of the Bologna Process priorities for 2012–15 is to 'Establish conditions that foster student-centred learning, innovative teaching methods and a supportive and inspiring working and learning environment, while continuing to involve students and staff in governance structures at all levels' (EHEA 2012: 5).

In addition, recent research conducted into curriculum trends as part of the Medical Education in Europe (MEDINE2) project identified the empowerment of students to take responsibility for their own learning and student involvement in curriculum-planning committees as major current trends that it was hoped would develop further in the future (Kennedy et al. 2013).

While all agree that student engagement is important, there is considerable disagreement about what it means. As Kahu (2013) notes, 'A key problem is a lack of distinction between the state of engagement, its antecedents and its consequences' (2013: 758).

She identifies four relatively distinct approaches to engagement:

1. behavioural, which focuses on student behaviour and effective teaching practice;
2. psychological, which concerns the internal individual process of engagement, including behaviour, cognition, emotion and conation;
3. social-cultural, acknowledging the impact of the broader social, cultural and political context;
4. holistic, an approach which attempts to combine the strands together.

Others have drawn a distinction between market and developmental approaches to student engagement. The market model is based on neo-liberal thinking, identifies students as consumers and approaches engagement from a consumer rights and institutional market position. In contrast, the developmental model is based on a constructivist concept of learning and identifies students as partners in a learning community, emphasising student development and quality of learning (Higher Education Academy 2010: 3).

Each of the approaches to student engagement has strengths and limitations and Kahu (2013) presents a conceptual framework which seeks to combine all elements and present student engagement as, 'A psycho-social process, influenced by institutional and personal factors, and embedded within a wider social context, [that] integrates the social-cultural perspective with the psychological and behavioural' (2013: 768).

Benefits of student engagement

Engagement has been argued to hold many benefits for students, including a greater sense of 'connectedness, affiliation and belonging' (Bensimon 2009: xxii–xxiii); satisfaction with studies (Kuh et al. 2005); improvements in learning, cognitive development and critical thinking (Kuh

1995; Kuh et al. 2005); and improved grades (Tross et al. 2000). Research has suggested a strong link between academic and social engagement, with a sense of belonging aiding student learning (Bok 2006). There are many potential benefits to be gained by institutions, such as increased student retention (Kuh et al. 2008), reputational and quality assurance (Coates 2005). Medical education itself is also a potential beneficiary if student engagement in academic research and teaching is encouraged (McLean et al. 2013)

Challenges and constraints

The rapidly changing nature of higher education and of students' lives has led several authors to highlight the importance of the broader social, cultural and political context. Baron and Corbin (2012) note that, despite the policy push to adopt practices that enhance engagement, what is implemented is often fragmented and contradictory. They argue that, while student engagement is seen as positive by governments, universities and individual academics, many of their practices may have had the opposite effect. They highlight reduced support for student social activities, performance-oriented university cultures, larger class sizes and reduced contact time, in addition to the increasing marketisation of higher education and the shift in the perception of students to being consumers and commodities. Fundamental change in the relationship between students and institutions has led to renewed efforts by institutions to ensure students' voices are heard and acted upon (Little et al. 2009).

The importance of student engagement in extracurricular activities and voluntary service has been highlighted. However, the demanding and intensive nature of medical school curricula can often leave little space for personal development and engagement within the academic community, and social isolation, burnout and depression are common among medical students (Bicket et al. 2010). In addition, the demands placed on students in their lives outside of studying have also been increasing. For example, James et al. (2010) reporting on research conducted in Australia note that, in 2009, 61 per cent of first-year full-time students were in paid employment of around 13 hours a week. The need to balance work and study is leading students to adopt a 'time-savvy' approach to learning, making calculated decisions about how best to use their time (Tarrant 2006).

Frameworks for engagement

Hand and Bryson (2008), following their review of student engagement, identified four important considerations for those wishing to enhance the student experience: the gap between staff and student expectations of who is responsible for engagement; the importance of establishing engagement (social and academic) early in university life; for significant gains it is important that an institutional approach is adopted; and engagement needs purpose: learning experiences that provide opportunities for autonomy, personal growth and change (Hand and Bryson 2008: 31).

A range of frameworks for measuring student engagement exist. The UK Quality Assurance Agency for Higher Education (QAA) highlights student engagement as relating to two core areas: improving student motivation to engage in learning and independent learning; and promoting student participation in quality assurance and enhancement processes (QAA 2012: 2). They note the positive influence student involvement can have on the development and delivery of all aspects of educational experience, from admissions and induction, through curriculum design and teaching delivery, to learning opportunities and assessment. The *Quality Code* (QAA 2012) highlights the requirement of higher-education providers to: 'take deliberate steps to engage all students, individually and collectively, as partners in the assurance and enhancement of their educational experience' (QAA 2012:12).

Seven indicators of sound practice are also identified: defining and promoting opportunities for any student to engage in educational enhancement and quality assurance; creating and maintaining an environment within which students and staff engage in discussions about demonstrable enhancement of the educational experience; arrangements for the effective representation of the collective student voice at all organisational levels; student representatives and staff having access to training and ongoing support to equip them to fulfil their roles in educational enhancement and quality assurance effectively; students and staff engaging in evidence-based discussions based on the mutual sharing of information; staff and students disseminating and jointly recognising the enhancements made to the student educational experience; and the effectiveness of student engagement being monitored and reviewed at least annually.

Student Participation in Quality Scotland (SPARQS), along with the key higher-education agencies in Scotland, have developed a framework for Scotland based on five key elements: students feeling part of a supportive institution; students engaging in their own learning; students working with their institution in shaping the direction of learning; formal mechanisms for quality and governance; and influencing the student experience at a national level. The framework also identifies six features of effective student engagement: a culture of engagement; students as partners; responding to diversity; valuing the student contribution; focus on enhancement and change; and appropriate resources and support (SPARQS 2012).

Operationalising student engagement

It is clear from the preceding discussion that student engagement can exist or be promoted at a number of levels. While ultimately it will occur at the level of the individual motivation to learn and engage in personal and professional development, there are a range of spheres in which universities and medical schools can seek to enhance the development of student engagement. The ASPIRE-to-Excellence in Medical Education initiative (www.aspire-to-excellence.org), in developing a set of assessment criteria for student engagement in medical schools, identified four spheres of student engagement: management of the medical school; provision of the medical school; research and the academic community; and local community and service delivery.

Each of these spheres represents a different context in which medical schools can support and promote social engagement. For example, student engagement in the management of a medical school could take the form of formal student involvement in the development of institutional or school mission or policy statements, accreditation processes or faculty development. The inclusion of the findings of student evaluations into teaching, learning and curriculum development, and the encouragement of students to engage in active learning, peer teaching and self and peer assessment are ways in which student engagement can be developed within medical school provision.

It is important to note that there is no blueprint for student engagement or threshold that must be attained before engagement can be said to be taking place. Rather, the format and extent of student engagement will differ within and between institutions. A more instructive way for assessing the development of student engagement is to see it as occurring along a spectrum, from a 'traditional school' characterised by low engagement to an 'innovative school' where engagement is high.

Table 7.1 Student engagement with the management of the medical school in traditional and innovative schools

	Traditional school	Innovative school
1	Students not involved in the development of the school's vision and mission	Students have been involved in the development of the school's vision and mission
2	Students are not represented on medical school committees	Students are represented on medical school committees
3	Students are not involved in the establishment of policy statements or guidelines	Students are involved in the establishment of policy statements or guidelines
4	Students are not involved in the accreditation process for the medical school	Students are involved in the accreditation process for the medical school
5	Students do not have any management/ leadership role in relation to elements of the curriculum	Students have a management/ leadership role in relation to elements of the curriculum
6	Students' views are not taken into account in decisions about faculty (teaching staff) promotion	Students' views are taken into account in decisions about faculty (teaching staff) promotion
7	Students play a passive part in faculty (staff) development activities	Students play an active part in faculty (staff) development activities

Student engagement in the management of a medical school

As Baron and Corbin (2012) have argued,

> Student engagement cannot be successfully pursued at the level of the individual teacher, school or faculty but must be pursued holistically in a 'whole-of-university' approach and with a common understanding of what it is the institution seeks to achieve.
>
> *(Baron and Corbin 2012: 760)*

This could include involving students in the development of school mission and vision statements or any subsequent revisions that are made to underpinning values and commitments. Table 7.1 summarises a range of criteria for identifying student engagement in the management of a medical school, and how this would differ within a traditional and an innovative school.

While many schools have moved a long way from the 'traditional' end of this spectrum, with student representation on committees fairly common, some have suggested that student involvement can be tokenistic. The key to engagement is to ensure that involvement leads to action; that student voices are heard within mission statements and policy guidance, and that their views and experiences feed into faculty development and promotion. The case study from the University of Helsinki Medical Faculty, Finland demonstrates the widespread involvement of students in decision making at the institution, including within faculty promotion procedures.

Case study 7.1   Student engagement at the Faculty of Medicine in Helsinki

Minna Kaila, Anna T. Heino, Kari Heinonen and Anne Pitkäranta

At the University of Helsinki Medical Faculty students are consistently engaged at all levels of development and decision making. There are about 40 student representative positions in more than ten different university bodies, ranging from the Student Selection Committee to the Committee for Evaluation of Teaching Skills, the Medical Library and the University Restaurant's Committee. There are even student representatives at the highest level, with four of 18 members of the Faculty Council being students.

Student-centred learning methods dominate the learning encounters, most of which are organised in small groups, where interactions with both the teacher and peers are important. Within the Growing to be a Physician (GBP) studies spanning the 6 years of medical school, learning communication skills is supported by receiving and learning to give constructive feedback by teachers and peers. The ethics studies focus on hands-on ethical questions. The GBP track is a path to becoming a physician, a colleague and fellow learner in the world of continuous professional development.

During the first 2 years of medical school the primary method is problem-based learning (PBL), where also older students tutor younger ones. PBL evolves into case-based learning (CBL) during the clinical years. Starting from the third year students take histories and examine patients, presenting their findings to the clinical teacher and each other in a small group, learning together, and learning by doing, under close supervision by the clinician. Students have promoted active-learning environments such as skills labs, and self-directed learning by virtual patient pool (VPP), developed to enable students to practise diagnostic and treatment skills autonomously.

(continued)

(continued)

The students can start their practical training in the service system after the third year in specific training positions (junior amanuensis) under licensed physician supervision. After the fourth year they can practise as stand-in physicians during vacations, but only after having passed all courses of the first 4 years, and after the fifth year they can work in primary healthcare practices. The students get experience as practising physicians, responsible for the care of their own patients under senior physician supervision.

Professor applicants have their teaching portfolios reviewed by the Committee for the Evaluation of Teaching Skills, using an evaluation matrix. The University of Helsinki founded a Teachers' Academy in 2013. Three teachers of the Faculty of Medicine were selected into the group of 30 founding members of the Academy. The applicants had to include a supportive statement from students in their application. The Academy will aim to improve the status of teaching in the academic community. By rewarding teachers, the university invests in students and the quality of learning.

A working group of the Medical Faculty is charged with the task of critically evaluating the present curriculum's actual emphasis and volume. There are seven members, two of whom are students. The next step will be to update and improve the curriculum based on the evidence from the evaluation. Another group works on improving the 4-month real-life practising (amanuensis) processes and content. There are another two students involved, together with clinical teachers, primary care and local hospital workplace representatives.

It is important to engage students systematically, in the structures and in all improvement projects. There is always room to do things better. Students could become more actively involved also in provision of teaching, peer teaching and peer tutoring. Provision of iPads to all first-year students may pave the way to join forces in teaching and learning in the e-world, building on the real-world work that has been done.

Student engagement in medical school educational provision

It is commonplace for students to fill in evaluation forms and surveys at the end of modules or years of study, but to what extent do schools act on the lessons held within them and adapt teaching and learning processes or revise the curriculum? Being able to see that their experiences and opinions are taken on board is essential to supporting student engagement. Engagement can also be fostered within a school's teaching, learning and assessment processes through the development of active and self-directed learning initiatives and the skills for self-assessment. The involvement of students in peer mentoring, teaching and assessment has been shown to be highly beneficial for students' own learning skills and development as well as increasing feelings of engagement (Yu et al. 2011; Nelson et al. 2013). Table 7.2 summarises a range of criteria for identifying student engagement in the educational provision of a medical school, and how this would differ within a traditional and an innovative school.

The case study from the University of Helsinki outlines a range of student-centred learning encounters, while the following case study from Slovenia demonstrates a success story of student-led initiative in peer tutoring.

Table 7.2 Student engagement in the provision of medical school education in traditional and innovative schools

	Traditional school	Innovative school
1	Students were not engaged in the evaluation of the curriculum, teaching and learning processes	Students evaluate the curriculum and teaching and learning processes
2	Feedback from the student body is not taken into account in curriculum development	Feedback from the student body is taken into account in curriculum development
3	Students participate as passive learners	Students participate as active learners with responsibility for their own learning
4	Students are not involved formally and rarely informally in peer teaching	Students are involved formally and/or informally in peer teaching
5	Students are not engaged in the development of learning resources for use by other students	Students are engaged in the development of learning resources for use by other students
6	Students have no role in providing a supportive or mentor role for other students	Students provide a supportive or mentor role for other students
7	Students are not encouraged to assess their own competence	Students are encouraged to assess their own competence
8	Students are not engaged in peer assessment	Students engage in peer assessment

Case study 7.2   Student involvement – from scratch, over self-sustainability, to the future, University of Maribor, Slovenia

Marko Zdravkovic, Kristijan Jejcic and Ivan Krajnc

In 2008 our medical school implemented a peer tutorial system (TS) initiative that had been developed by students. The student-driven project was associated with improved academic performance (Zdravkovic and Krajnc 2010) and its great success was further depicted in 2010 Senate conclusion: 'We recommend our students to attend complementary education under peer tutors' (PT) guidance' (Krajnc and Kriz 2010).

We built on Topping's (1996: 322) definition of peer-assisted learning (PAL), as 'people from similar social groupings who are not professional teachers helping each other to learn and learning themselves by teaching' and added an important 'General' component (G-PAL). This means that our PTs are not dedicated to a specific subject area but they give support for all subjects in Year 1 and Year 2 of studies. Moreover, they also offer general guidance about student life.

The non-compulsory G-PAL initiative began in 2008–9 with meetings based on three pillars: general guidance, core medical topic reinforcement and exam preparations. The implementation of these three pillars into practice was sequential and varied across tutoring groups. Initially, most groups focused on general guidance and core medical topics, for example, addressing the initial confusion in transition from secondary school to university, and motivating tutees for their learning.

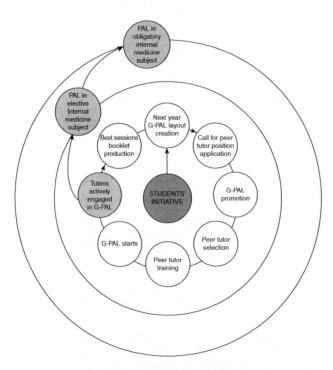

Figure 7.1 The process of self-sustainable general peer-assisted learning (G-PAL) evolution and two spin-offs continuing circular evolution similar to G-PAL.

Since 2010 our G-PAL has evolved to a more objective-based programme with exam preparations central to sessions. As shown in Figure 7.1, G-PAL evolution is linked to a vigorous PT selection process and intensive training before they start, i.e. PT development. Evidently, we implemented a self-sustainable system, as tutees engaged in G-PAL sessions were successfully recruited to become PT. Positive experiences were preserved in the G-PAL session booklet, containing remarks on session structure, content and teaching methodology.

A tripartite approach was used for G-PAL evaluation: the number of sessions and tutees' attendance, next year's advancement rates, and students' feedback collected by a special student taskforce. Looking at some results in Year 1, there has been a shift in median number of session visits from three to nine in 1 year (despite G-PAL being non-obligatory), we observed an increase in students' advancement rates to Year 2, and tutees increasingly reported being academically more successful due to G-PAL, from 46 to 73 per cent in a year (Zdravkovic and Krajnc 2010). In addition, student satisfaction with the peer tutor experience is demonstrated in the following examples of student feedback:

> First-hand information about literature and exam experience have strongly affected my learning and improved my academic performance.
>
> I find discussing learnt topics the best way to really master them.

An elective subject on propaedeutics was launched in 2010 based on PAL and utilising our simulation equipment, including the first undergraduate Objective Structured Clinical Examination (OSCE) in Slovenia (Zdravkovic et al. 2012). By including PT in the OSCE scoring, we foster peer assessment as an integral part of physician lifelong learning (Todorovic et al. 2012b). Finally, in 2012 we included PAL of clinical skills as an obligatory part of internal medicine with an OSCE before admitting students to clinical environment (Todorovic et al. 2012c).

As medical graduates should be able to 'function effectively as a mentor and teacher' (General Medical Council 2009: 27), emphasis should be given to peer teaching results and tutee benefits (Todorovic et al. 2012a; Zdravkovic and Zdravkovic 2012). In our experience, this positive feedback stemming from outcome-based teaching is the ultimate factor for continuous involvement in medical education, leading to state-of-the-art future medical educators.

For more information and our final report on TS implementation, visit the Center for Medical Education website at www.mf.uni-mb.si.

Student involvement in the academic community

Traditionally engagement in research and its dissemination, and participation in learned societies have been the preserve of faculty. However, the reduction in the number of doctors moving into academic medicine and medical education has become an area of concern. McLean et al. (2013) have suggested that providing students with opportunities to participate in research, become involved with the academic research community and present and publish their research has the potential to inspire student interest and reverse this trend. Additional benefits through involvement of students in these activities include communication and skills for lifelong learning. Table 7.3 summarises differences in student engagement in the academic community between traditional and innovative schools.

Table 7.3 Student engagement in the academic community in traditional and innovative schools

	Traditional school	Innovative school
1	Students are not engaged in school research projects carried out by faculty members	Students are engaged in school research projects carried out by faculty members
2	Students are not supported in their participation at local, regional or international medical and medical education meetings	Students are supported in their participation at local, regional or international medical and medical education meetings

Examples of the range of activities that can be promoted include involvement in the research work of faculty members, the development of student journals and conferences for disseminating their research findings.

Student engagement in the local community and service delivery

Student engagement activities can extend beyond the direct academic curriculum and be encouraged in relation to local communities and service delivery as well as extracurricular activities (Krause 2011). Students may become involved in local community projects or health services on a voluntary basis, as part of their studies or as employees. Extracurricular activities can provide an important means of integrating students into university life and fostering a sense of belonging, while the increasing globalisation of medicine means that students often desire and are encouraged to experience healthcare delivery in overseas electives. Table 7.4 summarises the differences in student engagement in local communities and service delivery between traditional and innovative schools.

The two following case studies demonstrate differing ways in which student engagement in the local community and understanding of social contexts can be developed. The College of Medicine, United Arab Emirates has introduced a team-based health promotion project for first-year medical students on a range of health topics to aid students' understanding of local health issues and their impact on the community. The School of Medicine at Trinity College Dublin has sought to promote students' awareness of global determinants of health through the curriculum, learning styles and opportunities for electives in developing countries.

Table 7.4 Student engagement in the local community and the service delivery in traditional and innovative schools

	Traditional school	Innovative school
1	Students are not involved in local community projects	Students are involved in local community projects
2	Students are not participating in the delivery of local healthcare services	Students participate in the delivery of local healthcare services
3	Students are not participating in healthcare delivery during electives/attachments overseas	Students participate in healthcare delivery during electives/attachments overseas
4	Students are not engaging with arranged extracurricular activities	Students engage with arranged extracurricular activities

Case study 7.3 Student mini-projects – celebrating World Health Day, United Arab Emirates

Venkatramana Manda, Ishtiyaq A. Shaafie and Kadayam G. Gomathi

The College of Medicine at Gulf Medical University, Ajman, United Arab Emirates has adopted the organ system-based integrated curriculum for its MBBS programme since September 2008; this has provided the opportunity to introduce innovative trends in medical education, including teaching/learning methods. The programme has three phases: Phase I provides the foundation of the basic medical sciences and prepares the students for integrated learning during Phase II (organ systems) and Phase III (clerkships) of the curriculum. Multiple teaching/learning strategies and modes of assessment are employed in each phase. Mini-projects based on the themes of important world and international health days recognised by the World Health Organization are conducted during Phase I, or the first year in medical school.

The mini-project, an activity that is entirely a student initiative, seeks to maximise student engagement by combining fun with learning during the first year of medical school. At the start of each academic year, all 70 newly admitted medical students in groups of five are allotted mini-projects by draw of lots. Each group is assigned a faculty supervisor to monitor their progress. The theme of each project signifies a world health or international health day. The aim of the mini-project is to make students understand the clinical, social, psychological and preventive aspects of a health day, make them work in teams and improve their communication and presentation skills. Each group elects a leader who guides and coordinates the group activities. Enough time is given to students to prepare the projects. Frequent meetings are held by the groups towards preparation of the project. The minutes of all meetings are recorded and submitted to the faculty supervisor for guidance and advice.

The projects are presented by the group on the specific world or international health day in two parts to all other students, faculty and invited guests. The first part is conducted in the college foyer and activities include quizzes, skits, role playing and games to convey the message of the health day. Brochures containing general information about the health day are distributed to the other students and staff of the college as part of health education. The second part is usually an interactive session conducted in the college auditorium using PowerPoint slides with activities such as games, models, charts and images.

The students are assessed for the content of the project and their presentation skills. A faculty supervisor assesses the group for the teamwork. Peer and self-evaluation and reflections form part of the assessment. The knowledge and awareness about the psychosocial and preventive aspects of major health problems covered in the mini-projects are assessed in the summative examinations.

The major health days covered in an academic year include World Elder's Day, World Mental Health Day and World Arthritis Day in October; World Diabetes Day and Universal Children's Day in November; World AIDS Day and International Day of Persons with Disabilities in December; World Kidney Day in March; World Haemophilia Day and World Malaria Day in April; Thalassaemia Day and World 'No Smoking' Day in the month of May.

Carrying out these mini-projects has provided first-year medical students with an important and early experience of common diseases in the community and their impact on health and society, and given them an opportunity to learn about prevention, combining fun with learning. Analyses of peer, self and faculty evaluations show that the mini-projects have helped students in gaining knowledge about common diseases, encouraged them to work as teams and prepared them to conduct research projects in subsequent phases.

Case study 7.4 Engaging students to take a global view of healthcare through the global determinants of health and development course in Trinity College Dublin

Katherine T. Gavin and Orla Hanratty

The School of Medicine, Trinity College Dublin, Ireland was founded in 1711. In the academic year 2012–13 there were 756 students registered in the 5-year undergraduate programme. The School aims to educate graduates recognisable by their unique qualities of scholarship, engagement and innovation that are responsive to the needs and health problems of society nationally and internationally. A need for global health education was acknowledged and resulted in the introduction of the Global Determinants of Health and Development (GDH&D) course in the medical curriculum in 2009. This course aims to develop students' understanding of emerging health issues in Ireland and their relationship with global health issues and international development (Skillshare International Ireland 2013).

The course is a compulsory component of the advanced clinical and professional practice module in Year 3. Students build on their existing knowledge and experience within this intensive course which is scheduled to enable ongoing engagement. The week-long conference-style format incorporates a series of keynote, plenary speeches and small-group workshops that facilitate discussion, debate and active participation. Experts with practical field experience lead sessions based on a theme exploring the cultural, social, legal, political and economic dimensions of complex healthcare systems.

Assessment methods include an individual reflective essay and group poster presentation. A pre-course attitudinal questionnaire captures student attitudes to various issues and changes in attitudes are recorded in post-course questionnaires. Evidence of changes in student attitudes as a result of attending this course has been indicated in areas such as health worker migration, education and climate change (Hastings et al. 2012).

Analysis of a sample of students' reflective essays in 2010 reveals a better understanding of the relationships between poverty, development and its impact on health by a large majority of students following the course. One-fifth expressed an intention to engage with healthcare actively in developing countries (Pardinaz-Solis et al. unpublished).

One-third of students in Years 3 and 4 choose to go to developing countries for summer elective with the Medical Overseas Voluntary Electives (MOVE) charity. This may indicate ongoing engagement with the course. MOVE is organised and managed by Year 4 students with the support of the school. In 2013, Year 3 students organised their own clinical skills workshops within Global Health Week to teach second-level students and raised funds for MOVE.

Short courses can have an impact far beyond initial student contact. Courses that encourage active participation and reflection and provide opportunities for further engagement can create a platform for students to take forward their learning into committed action. As curriculum designers and medical educators, we should endeavour to be responsive to emerging needs and flexible in the approach to course design, delivery and assessment. Such an approach models the attributes we encourage in our students.

Summary

Many changes have taken place within medical education globally in recent decades that have impacted on the role of students, their relationship to the curriculum and their institution. Student engagement is now widely seen as important at all levels, from the individual student, through the institution to the wider community. Increasingly, the focus of teaching and learning has shifted to become more student-centred, with an emphasis on promoting active and self-directed learning. In addition there has been a renewed focus on the ability of the student voice to be included within the management of organisations and the design of curriculum. A range of frameworks are available offering guidance on operationalising student engagement, including the work of the ASPIRE-to-Excellence Initiative (www.aspire-to-excellence.org).

Take-home messages

- Student engagement offers the potential of improvements to learning, cognitive development, student retention, quality assurance and a sense of belonging.
- Changes to students' role need to be reflected in all aspects of medical education.
- Student engagement requires a holistic approach, involving the whole of the university.
- Policy changes to support engagement need to be cohesive and consistent, not fragmented and contradictory.
- Initiatives require strong institutional and financial support.
- Peer-led initiatives, including in teaching and learning offer excellent opportunities for enhancing social engagement.
- Extracurricular, social and community initiatives are as important as academic ones in fostering a sense of belonging.

Bibliography

ASPIRE (2014). Online. Available HTTP: http:www.aspire-to-excellence.org (accessed 8 September 2014).

Baron, P. and Corbin, L. (2012) 'Student engagement: Rhetoric and reality', *Higher Education Research and Development,* 31(6): 759–72.

Bensimon, E.M. (2009) 'Forward'. In S.R. Harper and S.J. Quaye (eds) *Student engagement in higher education.* London: Routledge.

Bicket, M., Misra, S., Wright, S.M. and Shohet, R. (2010) 'Medical student engagement and leadership within a new learning community', *BMC Medical Education,* 10: 20.

Bok, D. (2006) *Our underachieving colleges: A candid look at how students learn and why they should be learning more,* Princeton, NJ: Princeton University Press.

Coates, H. (2005) 'The value of student engagement for higher education quality assurance', *Quality in Higher Education,* 11(1): 25–36.

EHEA Ministerial Conference (2012) *Making the most of our potential: Consolidating the European higher education area. Bucharest communique,* Bucharest: European Higher Education Area.

General Medical Council (2009) *Tomorrow's doctors: Outcomes and standards for undergraduate medical education.* London: General Medical Council. Online. Available HTTP: http://www.gmc-uk.org/Tomorrow_s_Doctors_0414.pdf_48905759.pdf, p. 27 (accessed 20 November 2014).

Hand, L. and Bryson, C. (2008) *Student engagement,* London: Staff and Educational Development Association (SEDA).

Hastings, A., Pardiñaz-Solis, R., Phillips, M. and Hennessy, M. (2012) 'Measuring attitude change in medical students: Lessons from a short course on global health', *Medical Education Development,* 2(1): 1–4.

Higher Education Academy (2010) *Framework for action: Enhancing student engagement at the institutional level,* York: Higher Education Academy (HEA).

James, R., Krause, K.-L. and Jennings, C. (2010) *The first-year experience in Australian universities: Findings from 1994–2009,* Melbourne, Australia: Centre for the Study of Higher Education.

Kahu, E.R. (2013) 'Framing student engagement in higher education', *Studies in Higher Education,* 38(5): 758–73.

Kennedy, C., Lilley, P., Kiss, L., Littvay, L. and Harden, R.M. (2013) *Curriculum trends in medical education in Europe in the 21st century,* Dundee: AMEE/MEDINE2.

Krajnc, I. and Kriz, B. (2010) *Minutes from the 15th Regular Senate meeting at Faculty of Medicine University of Maribor: Conclusion 52.* 19 April 2010.

Krause, K.L.D. (2011) 'Transforming the learning experience to engage students', in L. Thomas and M. Tight (eds) *Institutional transformation to engage a diverse student body. International perspectives on higher education research, volume 6*, Bingley: Emerald Group.

Kuh, G.D. (1995) 'The other curriculum: Out-of-class experiences associated with student learning and personal development', *Journal of Higher Education*, 66(2): 123–55.

Kuh, G.D., Kinzie, J., Schuh, J.H. and Whitt, E.J. (2005) 'Never let it rest: Lessons about student success from high-performing colleges and universities', *Change: The Magazine of Higher Learning*, 37(4): 44–51.

Kuh, G.D., Cruce, T.M., Shoup, R., Kinzie, J. and Gonyea, R.M. (2008) 'Unmasking the effects of student engagement on first year college grades and persistence', *Journal of Higher Education*, 79(5): 540–63.

Little, B., Locke, W., Scesca, A. and Williams, R. (2009) *Report to HEFCE on student engagement*, Centre for Higher Education Research and Information. http://www.open.ac.uk/cheri/documents/student-engagement-report.pdf (accessed 27 September 2013).

McLean, A.L., Saunders, C., Velu, P.P., Iredale, J., Hor, K. and Russell, C.D. (2013) 'Twelve tips for teachers to encourage student engagement in academic medicine', *Medical Teacher*, 35(7): 549–54.

Nelson, A.J., Nelson, S.V., Linn, A.M.J., Raw, L.E., Kildea, H.B. and Tonkin, A.L. (2013) 'Tomorrow's educators . . . today? Implementing near-peer teaching for medical students', *Medical Teacher*, 35(2): 156–9.

Pardinaz-Solis, R., Newell-Jones, K., Hastings, A. and Phillips, M. (Unpublished) Learning global health: Impact on student after a short course in global health and development.

Quality Assurance Agency for Higher Education (QAA) (2012) *UK quality code for higher education. Part B: Chapter B5: Student engagement*, Gloucester: QAA.

Skillshare International Ireland (2013) *Global determinants of health and development course*. Online. Available HTTP: http://www.skillshare.ie/developmentawareness/gdhd.html (accessed 22 March 2013).

Students Participation in Quality Scotland (SPARQS) (2012) *A student engagement framework for Scotland*, Edinburgh: SPARQS. Online. Available HTTP: http://www.sparqs.ac.uk/upfiles/SEFScotland.pdf (accessed 1 October 2013).

Tarrant, J. (2006) 'Teaching time-savvy law students', *James Cook University Law Review*, 13: 64–80.

Todorovic, T., Pivec, N., Fluher, J. and Bevc, S. (2012a) '*Long-term clinical skills retention rate in peer teaching*', short lecture given at VII. SkillsLab Symposium, Marburg, March.

Todorovic, T., Pivec, N., Hojs, N., Zorman, T. and Bevc, S. (2012b) '*Who should evaluate at OSCE stations?*', Poster presented at Society in Europe for Simulation Applied to Medicine Annual Conference, Stavanger, June.

Todorovic, T., Zdravkovic, M. and Zeme, K. (2012c) 'Peer tutors guide: Peer teaching in Simulation Centre at Faculty of Medicine University of Maribor: Academic year 2012/2013 (original Slovenian title: Priročnik za tutorje: tutorstvo v Simulacijskem centru Medicinske fakultete Univerze v Mariboru: študijsko leto 2012/2013.)', Maribor, September.

Topping, K.J. (1996) 'The effectiveness of peer tutoring in further and higher education: A typology and review of the literature', *Higher Education*, 32(3): 321–45.

Tross, S.A., Harper, J.P., Osherr, L.W. and Kneidinger, L.M. (2000) 'Not just the usual cast of characteristics: Using personality to predict college performance and retention', *Journal of College Student Development*, 41(3): 325–36.

Trowler, V. (2010) *Student engagement literature review*, York: HEA.

Yu, T.C., Wilson, N.C., Singh, P.P., Lemanu, D.P., Hawke, S.J. and Hill, A.G. (2011) 'Medical-students-as-teachers: A systematic review of peer-assisted teaching during medical school', *Advances in Medical Education Practice*, June 23(2): 157–72.

Zdravkovic, M. and Krajnc, I. (2010) '*Peer assisted learning improves academic success*', poster presented at International Association for Medical Education Annual Conference, Glasgow, September. Online. Available HTTP: http://amee.org/getattachment/Conferences/AMEE-Past-Conferences/AMEE-Conference-2010/AMEE-2010-Abstract-book.pdf, p. 180-1 (accessed 20 November 2014).

Zdravkovic, B. and Zdravkovic, M. (2012) 'DREEMing in Slovenia: Peer versus faculty teaching in light of average grade', short communication presented at International Association for Medical Education Annual Conference, Lyon, August. Online. Available HTTP: http://amee.org/getattachment/Conferences/AMEE-Past-Conferences/AMEE-Conference-2012/AMEE-2012-ABSTRACT-BOOK.pdf, p. 337-8 (accessed 20 November 2014).

Zdravkovic, M., Todorovic, T. and Bevc, S. (2012) 'Following global trends in medical education: Objective structured clinical examination (original Slovenian title: Na sledi svetovnim trendom izobraževanja v medicini: Objektivni strukturiran klinični izpit.)', *ISIS*, 21(11): 74–9. Online. Available HTTP: http://issuu.com/visart.studio/docs/isis2012-11-brezoglasov/74?mode=window&viewMode=doublePage (accessed 30 March 2013).

8
STUDENT MOBILITY
A problem and an opportunity

Athol Kent and Chivaugn Gordon

> *Student mobility is one of the features of the internationalisation of education and should be considered in the planning of an educational programme.*

Student mobility concerns learning about healthcare in an environment that is socially or physically removed from a student's usual situation. Examples of this are:

- a student relocating from a different home town in order to study. This has particular relevance when the move is from a rural to an urban environment or vice versa;
- coursework conducted in satellite sites distant from the main academic hospital complex (community-based education);
- students doing electives during the course in settings/countries different to where their base campus is situated;
- students doing their course in another country.

Learning 'elsewhere' is not a virtual experience, but is being present in a genuinely unfamiliar or foreign environment where the rules of engagement are new and the opportunities for learning are seen from a different perspective.

It could be argued that, because of globalisation, the earth is already 'flat' and that differences are no longer meaningful, with regional and national characteristics subsumed by multinational brands and franchises, and that information is freely available on the internet. It is true that extensive information transfer exists across geographic and political boundaries and that television, the internet and social media have allowed everyone access to world events. We have grown closer in that we *know more* about each other but that does not necessarily mean we *understand* each other better, and there can be no substitute for first-hand interaction in learning about diversity from all patients.

Major differences exist in standards of healthcare between developed and developing countries, between regions within countries and by socio-economic status within societies. Facilitating student mobility is one of the best ways to get students to understand these differences; in particular, the social determinants of health (Bozorgmehr et al. 2010). A student's personal growth towards becoming a more complete health professional depends much on experiential learning, which in turn depends on the personal interpretation of new encounters. The more unfamiliar such encounters, the fewer the 'comfort zones'; the more students have to rely on their own knowledge, skills and acquired responses, the greater their chances for genuine maturation and transformation.

There are naturally logistical, managerial and financial challenges in organising community stays, electives and entire courses being taught and assessed off-site and these demands do stretch administrative and regulatory capacity. Faculties are under pressure to give priority to the teaching of knowledge and skills rather than the enhancement of the interactive attributes of professionalism, compassion, non-judgemental attitudes and bio-psycho-social approaches, which are learnt and fostered 'in the field'. To ensure fair, equitable and meaningful student mobility requires courage and faith in the learners but, as this chapter contends, will yield an ultimately better healthcare professional.

Mobility and diversity

All countries are trying to match their spectrum of healthcare workers to the general populations they serve. There are mechanisms being put in place whereby all races, socio-economic groups and minorities now have access to medical schools. Policies of 'positive discrimination' are being pursued in the UK, Australia, USA, Canada and South Africa to ensure a more equitable mix of professionals to care for all members of their societies more empathetically. In addition, evidence exists that the recruitment of students from rural or underserved places will facilitate an increased medical workforce in these areas (Dhalla et al. 2002).

This upward mobility of previously disadvantaged medical school entrants is bringing a richer mix of students into contact with each other and coincidentally requiring educators to be more flexible, resourceful, sensitive and even-handed in their teaching attitudes. Collaborative learning, be it through problem-based or combined project team efforts, does demand social norms to be explored and defined within the student population, thus allowing the learners' diversity to be a microcosm of society and provide a practical learning opportunity of understanding differences.

The more mixed the student population, the greater the opportunities for 'mind mobility'. Mind mobility refers to broadening students' minds to different backgrounds and experiences, thus enabling them to be more empathetic. This socialisation may not occur spontaneously and it is common for subgroups within classes to 'stick together' with limited 'cross-pollination', so administrators deliberately allocate students randomly to study groups without allowing a choice of partners or groupings. This prevention of cliques within classes speaks to the need for early exposure to views and resources different from one's own, the intention of which is to broaden outlook and promote mind mobility.

Other attempts to expand students' personal growth have been the introduction of modules within the medical curriculum of topics that address student attitudes, judgements and pre-conceived ideas about clinical situations. These help to foster generic attributes such as compassion and a better understanding of patients' needs, so that students can be equipped to handle patients from many cultural backgrounds.

The University of Cape Town, South Africa, has therefore introduced three modules into the medical degree course to promote open-mindedness. They cover the topics of abuse awareness, understanding of sexual and gender minorities, and compassion. Each subject is woven into the clinical curriculum, which is taught over 3 years, and the students revisit each topic as they expand their patient contacts. The method of instruction is highly interactive, using skilled facilitators who have a passion for the bio-psycho-social approach to medical practice.

Case study 8.1 Humanity in the workplace – Department of Obstetrics and Gynaecology, University of Cape Town, South Africa

Veronica Mitchell, Alexandra Muller and Chivaugn Gordon

The richness of student learning is not based on the material available for assimilation but on the experiences they encounter during their tuition and training. This experience creates 'mind mobility' or personal growth, one of the tenets of the hidden curriculum. Examining the source of this personal growth took the Department of Obstetrics and Gynaecology at the University of Cape Town to two important conclusions:

- First, having students from different backgrounds (entry mobility) and allowing them geographically differing learning (situational mobility) adds to the quality of their education.
- Second, creating curriculum space to address their personal growth was rewarding for students and staff alike.

Students in Years 3, 4 and 5 in their rotations through the Department of Obstetrics and Gynaecology are told at the outset of their block that they will be presenting a workshop on their experience of 'Humanity in the Workplace' towards the end of their time in the department. Broadly these topics are 'Compassion' in Year 3, 'Human Rights and Abuse' in Year 4 and 'Lesbian, Gay, Bisexual and Transgender (LGBT) Rights' in Year 5. They are divided into subgroups of between five and 15 students and asked to choose an issue within the general subject to observe and research during the block. They are told to prepare an interactive presentation (to the entire group, with a facilitator present) based on what they personally experience during the block and what their research has uncovered.

Compassion tutorials are held with groups of ten students. These provide a safe space for students to reflect on difficult situations experienced in their rotations, and how to maintain compassion for patients and themselves under the stressful conditions that they will experience in future practice. Personal examples are voluntarily offered.

Medical students are allocated to physically differing venues during their rotations. These are (apart from the base campus) satellite urban hospitals, midwife obstetric units – where they deliver babies – community clinics and sometimes rural hospitals. This mobility exposes them to a gamut of socio-economic variables in the patients they see, the educators that they learn from and the facilities available. This mobility has much to offer in broadening student life experience but requires input, resources and, specifically, skilled staff time to be optimally utilised.

The groups meet with their facilitator for a morning workshop where each subgroup of students presents their topic-within-a-topic in an interactive manner. The students act out scenes, role play, present mock television interviews, make videos and generally present evocative vignettes of their personal experiences as neophyte health professionals.

Each subgroup presentation is opened to comment and discussion, which is inevitably challenging, revealing and instructive. It allows real feelings, beliefs, fears, misgivings and widely differing views to be expressed, always enriched by the entry mobility of the participants with their diversity of geographical, cultural, racial, religious and socio-economic status plus the situational mobility of their campus, community and rural immersion during their rotation.

(continued)

> *(continued)*
>
> The students formulate their attitudes according to their role models, peers' views and personal experience. This experience is expanded by the mobility of students between venues and healthcare workers.
>
> The workshops provide the platform for articulated student reflection and research into topics that profoundly affect their personal growth, which is a crucial part of the hidden curriculum.
>
> Through this case study we have concluded that entry mobility, situational mobility and reflection on personal experiences enrich learning.

The student response to these interactive sessions has been extremely positive as they feel they can express and share their practical and emotional experiences with each other and their facilitators. They can feed back joyous or joyless aspects of their training, which they have sometimes been unaware of, unable to handle or feel loath to express. By offering safe situations to reflect upon or share their encounters they experience less isolation or personal insecurity. Group mind mobility is a means of personal validation as well as a means of vicarious personal maturity.

Mobility from campus to community

Most medical schools have similar structures. They have a campus from which administration is handled and teaching is organised. Instruction usually centres on a medical degree course as well as nursing plus health and rehabilitation disciplines.

The medical school campus usually consists of a university attachment to basic science studies which is affiliated to a tertiary referral hospital where much of the clinical teaching takes place. In close proximity are teaching facilities such as lecture theatres, education units, clinical skills centres, student administration, deans' offices, exam venues with libraries and information technology venues. Student cafeterias and social gathering places provide some geographical social centre point and the whole complex forms the medical campus. It is precisely distant from these campuses that community-based or rural education is focused.

The dimension that off-campus mobility seeks to accentuate is the primary care approach with a patient-centred philosophy. A holistic view of the patient within her or his family, environment and society is best grasped off campus. Moving the student to another learning context requires motivation, organisation, planning, financing, monitoring and research – all of which take ongoing determination and resources.

The venues of off-campus learning can be general practitioners' rooms, clinics, which may or may not be doctor-led, local or district hospitals and regional or country hospitals – or even mobile clinics. These diverse sources of learning need to have a number of aspects in common if they are to be used to broaden the scope of undergraduate medical education successfully. They all need willing local participants who are equal partners in these initiatives, dedicated to the service they provide and prepared to share this endeavour with students. Without attention to and appreciation of the service provider's role, student mobility is counter-productive.

If correctly managed, off-campus teaching sites can add prestige and scholarship to otherwise purely service delivery facilities. Students bring fresh views and sometimes a welcome extra pair of hands to such venues and their long-term views of the resident healthcare providers and patients are usually positive. With the ever-increasing technology roll-out there can be internet connections with access to central campus lectures via podcasts, tutorials online and easy access to expert opinion if required.

Against the advantages have to be weighed the set-up and maintenance costs. Negotiations between the university and either self- or government-employed workers present unique challenges of time constraints, financial terms, monitoring mechanisms, student assessments, fees plus transport and residence costs.

Many faculties are establishing rural campuses attached to district, county or regional hospitals to provide longitudinal student exposure to underserved areas. These are potential solutions to the imbalances being created by the rural-to-urban migration. Student mobility to train in these campuses is said to sensitise and encourage them to locate to non-urban areas post qualification.

In South Africa the establishment of satellite campuses has shown promise both from the acceptance and academic points of view. Initial misgivings from regional doctors have turned to enthusiasm and pride, while extended-length stays by students (up to 1 year) have shown that summative assessments at the parent institution have yielded equivalent, and in most instances superior, grade results (Van Schalkwyk et al. 2014).

Whole-course mobility

The concept of sending cohorts of students to train in other countries for re-import is a vexed issue. Underdeveloped countries are those in greatest need of qualifying more healthcare workers, especially doctors, but sponsoring education in developed countries with excess educational capacity is not a practical solution.

The brightest and best students are selected for entry into places in the medical faculties of their home country. Sending lower-ranked learners to elite schools in developed countries would seem unfair, even if such options were available and affordable. If the less gifted were allocated to developing countries the quality of their tuition would come into question, let alone issues of language, appropriateness of the syllabus, retraining on return and major cost factors.

Case study 8.2 The Cuban controversy – training South African medical students in Cuba

Chivaugn Gordon

After the fall of apartheid in South Africa (SA) in 1994, the new government realised that many more doctors would be required to improve the inequitable healthcare system. However, the eight SA medical schools did not have the capacity to meet this need. Cuba has 25 medical schools with large training capacities, from which 11,000 local and foreign doctors graduate annually. Based partly on political ties between the African National Congress and Cuba, an agreement was made with the Cuban government where SA students would receive 5 years of foundational medical training in Cuba, which would be rounded off with some time spent in SA medical schools on the students' return. Cuban-trained SA students form 8 per cent of all medical graduates in SA, a figure set to increase dramatically in future. It is said that the programme goes at least a quarter of the way towards meeting South Africa's medium-term needs for another 20,000 doctors in less than a decade.

This programme provides opportunities for underprivileged school leavers. Further, it seeks to populate rural healthcare centres. Therefore, key features of the programme are:

(continued)

(continued)
- Students are recruited from disadvantaged rural communities countrywide.
- Students are recruited with significantly lower university entrance requirements than would be needed for SA schools.
- The SA and Cuban governments jointly sponsor the students in exchange for 5 years of service in the area from which they were recruited.

Challenges

- *Language* – On arrival in Cuba, students are required to learn Spanish, the language in which they will be taught. For most, this is at least their third language. On their return to SA, they must relearn medical terminology in English. This process requires a tremendous amount of mind mobility, and is often where students struggle most.
- *Culture* – In order to succeed in their studies, students must also be 'culturally mobile'. In Cuba, students find themselves in a culture which is entirely alien. The 'culture' of how students are taught and assessed in Cuba also differs substantially from local practice.
- *Burden of disease* – Cuba has a largely healthy population, and their focus is on disease prevention and health promotion. SA has a vastly different disease profile, and a failing healthcare system. Students trained in Cuba often struggle to adapt to the South African system, which focuses mainly on treatment, not prevention and health promotion.

Success of the programme

No research exists to show how well Cuban-trained students perform as doctors, nor whether they remain working in their regions of origin. The SA module failure rate of Cuban-trained students is nearly double that of locally trained students. This trend often creates the opinion that the Cuban training is inadequate. Students perceive this attitude, and can feel marginalised as a result. Most Cuban-trained students do, however, manage to pass within the minimum amount of time.

Opinions of senior academics as to the benefits and drawbacks of the programme differ substantially. What is clear, however, is that politics has been a major driving force in the programme. The dual burden of sudden and substantial geographical and mind mobility – both on leaving and returning to SA – has potentially profound consequences on students and this should not be ignored.

The South African experience of sending previously disadvantaged students from rural areas to be trained in Cuba is a case study in point. This is a politically motivated solution to the under-provision of medical personnel in the country.

Those students not selected on merit into one of the eight medical faculties in their home country are sent to Cuba, where they receive a mainly lecture-based education in Spanish. After their studies they return to South Africa, where they undergo clinical training in local medical schools in English before receiving their Cuban degrees, which allow them to practise in South Africa.

The system has raised resentment in the medical schools to which they did not gain admission in the first place, as the faculty see themselves as 'retraining students who failed to gain entry in the first place'. It has also proven very costly and has not gone a long way to resolve the country's lack of doctors. The government is, however, determined to increase considerably the number of Cuban-trained South African candidates but there is little optimism among academics that this mobility will provide even a short-term answer to a long-term problem.

International mobility: electives

There is considerable opinion that the opportunity to train partially in a foreign country offers benefits to students at the undergraduate level. Many institutions advocate or require such electives. Electives are not designed with the thinking that students will be taught better at institutions elsewhere; rather, their aim is to foster personal growth through new experiences. Indeed, if it were held that students who study elsewhere had an academic advantage, this could be considered unfair by those not offered the opportunity.

While arranging electives requires a substantial investment of time, effort and finances, the benefit to a student's personal growth cannot be overstated.

Whether electives represent advantages to teachers or institutions 'back home' is less sure, as the administrative work involved is not offset by reduced costs or the freeing up of places in their alma mater.

Opportunities of international electives

Students doing electives in foreign countries do feel a moral obligation to impress their hosts as they are perceived to be representing their home country. This may not be explicit, but the 'ambassadorial' role is present on a social and academic level and as such is likely to bring out the best in the visitor. Being observed as a representative of one's country evokes the Hawthorne effect, applying subtle pressure to perform at one's full potential.

It is not beyond the realms of possibility that contacts made at the undergraduate level can develop into long-term relationships leading to future visits, postgraduate exchanges or reciprocal opportunities. Foreign experience at any level is usually viewed in a positive light on a curriculum vitae.

Some students who are fee-paying are made welcome as contributors to the financial health of the hosting institution.

Challenges of international electives

To the individual

The traveller has to maintain the academic standards of her or his base institution, which may be difficult in settings of fewer resources and greater distances to a referral hospital. Diplomacy, tact and support for the receiving site could, under certain circumstances, challenge the student.

To the sending institution

The curriculum from which the student comes must accommodate 'off-site' time in its syllabus. Most curricula are over-crowded and freeing students up for a meaningful duration can mean disciplines 'finding time', which is notoriously difficult.

Administrative activities in terms of arrangements, transport costs, registration and insurance are considerable and student selection has to be judiciously handled.

To the receiving institutions

There has to be the will and capacity to receive visiting students. Unless there is some financial advantage to administrative personnel, the extra work involved in organising, teaching and assessing the visitors is not welcomed. The same may apply to tutors if not compensated, as clinical tuition is usually at a premium. The maxim of 'there must be something in it for them' applies to receiving institution, clinics or communities.

Attributes which may be enhanced by national or international mobility

Independence

Students in an unfamiliar environment have to deal with novel situations and social challenges on their own recognisances. Having to cope with and make decisions in a distant domain, sometimes in a foreign language, without familial or peer support can groom independence. Social norms, manners, hierarchical or religious customs may be subtly or vastly different and at the very least sensitivities need to be sharpened.

Curiosity

Curiosity and discovery are desirable attributes in any learner and elective visits to foreign venues foster such qualities. Apart from finding out about how 'things are done' in the medical domain, there are many comparisons for the neophyte professional to observe, not least of which are the resources available or unavailable to patients and workers.

It is of value to experience what advantages or disadvantages others have and the realisation that one's base institution is neither the best nor the worst off on an international scale of resource allocation. Students returning from electives often appreciate the teaching they receive at home more insightfully and certainly value the experiential learning opportunities at home more keenly than before. Perspective and humility are readily available by time spent 'on exchange'.

Non-prejudice

Non-prejudice is an attribute of maturity that cannot be learnt vicariously. Social norms across developed and developing countries vary enormously. It is expected that students will be confronted by considerably different norms as far as lifestyles and medical practices are concerned.

Patients from different cultures may use non-evidence-based remedies prescribed by non-medically qualified or traditional healers or have religious values or attitudes far from Western beliefs. Lifestyle habits, risk-taking behaviours and attitudes towards women, the disadvantaged or simply the 'different' all need to be accepted as part of a foreign way of life. There may be many realisations that what is 'taken for granted' in one situation may be unacceptable in another.

Exposure to different cultures in medicine and society promotes reflective practice, which is a desired graduate attribute.

Professionalism

Students arriving in foreign settings are likely to be highly aware of the level of professionalism they encounter. The manner and respect with which staff treat patients, each other and students will be keenly felt. It will be unconsciously or consciously compared with the norms of students' base experience.

Students will become aware of their own levels of professionalism and realise the universal nature of integrity, confidentiality and respect for patient autonomy, which are the basic tenets of professionalism.

The challenges of mobility

The challenges in converting non-teaching health service venues into those to be visited by students are considerable. The administrative, political and financial obstacles take great commitment to overcome and managers require 'conversion to the cause'.

This 'political will' needs to be accompanied by financial backing to provide tuition payments, transport, board and lodging and may raise issues of insurance, base residence waivers and communication costs, all of which need to be sustainable.

The choice of which students to select for distance training may present unexpected challenges. Those privileged academically and financially may not be the students who stand to gain most from visits to distant places. Those from disadvantaged backgrounds may be the most needy recipients of a travel privilege and a decision on who to send may be fraught with unintended consequences.

Take-home messages

- A broad approach to first-year intake allows for mobility of students from disadvantaged backgrounds to join the medical fraternity. This encourages 'mind mobility' for all. Interactive modules increase this benefit in terms of students' personal growth within groups.
- The pursuit of a holistic attitude in the practice of medicine needs enhancement of non-factual aspects of a student's development. The participation in training opportunities removed from the base campus is a valuable means to such growth.
- This realisation of the onus being on the student when 'off campus' is very much part of the transformative aspirations of a 21st-century medical education.
- Mobility, whether into the community or to other countries, fosters characteristics of independence, curiosity, non-prejudice and professionalism.

Bibliography

Bateman, C. (2013) 'Doctor shortages: Unpacking the "Cuban solution"', *South African Medical Journal*, 103(9): 603–5.

Bozorgmehr, K., Menzel-Severing, J., Schubert, K. and Tinnemann, P. (2010) 'Global health education: A cross-sectional study among German medical students to identify needs, deficits and potential benefits (Part 2 of 2: Knowledge gaps and potential benefits)', *BMC Medical Education*, 10(67): 1–19.

Chopra, M., Lawn, J., Sanders, D., Barron, P., Abdool Karim, S., Bradshaw, D., Jewkes, R., Abdool Karim, Q., Flisher, A., Mayosi, B., Tollman, S., Churchyard, G. and Coovadia, H. (2009) 'Achieving the health Millennium Development Goals for South Africa: Challenges and priorities', *The Lancet*, 374(9694): 1023–31.

Dhalla, I., Kwong, J., Streiner, D., Baddour, R., Waddell, A. and Johnson, I. (2002) 'Characteristics of first-year students in Canadian medical schools', *Canadian Medical Association Journal*, 166(8): 1029–35.

Hirsch, M. (2013) 'SA-Cuba medical programme criticized', *IOL News Website*. Online. Available HTTP: http://www.iol.co.za/news/south-africa/sa-cuba-medical-programme-criticised-1.1545474 (accessed 4 December 2013).

Van Schalkwyk, S., Bezuidenhout, J., Conradie, H., Kok, N., Van Heerden, B. and De Villiers, M. (2014) *Crossing boundaries: The potential for innovative medical education models to challenge traditional assessment practices*, Ottawa Conference, 26–9 April 2014, Ottawa, Canada.

PART 3

The curriculum

9
CURRICULUM PLANNING IN THE 21ST CENTURY

Ronald M. Harden

An authentic curriculum to meet the needs of the population should be designed as a collaborative activity with students and teachers playing a key role.

The changing concept of a curriculum

The concept of a medical curriculum changed dramatically over the latter part of the 20th century and the first decade of the 21st century. Fresh thinking about the education process led to the integration of previously fragmented elements and to a reappraisal of the role of the teacher as a facilitator of learning rather than simply a transmitter of information. The student came to be seen as a partner in the learning process rather than a product of it or a consumer. Within medical schools, the responsibility for the curriculum switched from departments working independently and headed by powerful professors to curriculum-planning committees representing the different stakeholders.

Curricular issues addressed related to the mission of the medical school, the learning outcomes, the curriculum content, the sequence of courses, the educational strategies, the teaching and learning methods, the assessment procedures, the educational environment, communications about the curriculum and management of the process (Harden and Laidlaw 2012). With regard to educational strategies, the SPICES model described a continuum from student-centred to teacher-centred; problem-based to information-centred; integrated to discipline-based; community-based to hospital-based; electives to uniform and systematic to opportunistic.

In this chapter we focus on four aspects of curriculum planning that reflect current educational thinking and the direction in which medical education is moving in the 21st century. These trends also recognise the importance of the international dimensions of medical education. They are:

- the authentic curriculum;
- the curriculum as a collaborative activity;
- the student and the curriculum;
- the teacher and the curriculum.

The authentic curriculum

Medical schools have been accused of working in ivory towers, out of touch with the needs of society and the community which the doctors who graduate have to serve. This is no longer acceptable politically, professionally, economically or educationally. Frenk et al. argued that, 'Professional education has not kept pace with these challenges [in healthcare delivery] largely because of fragmented, outdated, and static curricula that produce ill-equipped graduates' (2010: 1923). Relevance is today a key and much promoted principle in medical education and is reflected in the concept of an 'authentic' curriculum. Changing public and professional expectations as to what is expected of a doctor, as discussed in Chapters 2 and 3, were factors that led to the introduction of an outcome- or competency-based approach to education (see Chapter 3). In the past, curricula favoured the mastery of knowledge. The gap between the theoretical knowledge of students and their clinical competence, including their communication skills and professionalism, has been highlighted. The move to an authentic curriculum is about ensuring that on graduation students have the necessary skills to practice effectively for the patient's benefit. Learning outcomes such as communication skills, professionalism and issues such as patient safety, management of errors and teamwork are addressed. Students are trained, as described in the Mozambique case study, to be able to practise in a rapidly changing healthcare environment, to cope with unfamiliar situations, to confront the unknown and to use judgement. The emphasis on appropriate learning outcomes is highlighted in the case studies from the UK and Peru.

Case study 9.1   The University of Dundee curriculum, United Kingdom

Gary Mires and Claire MacRae

The curriculum at the University of Dundee School of Medicine is a 5-year programme with approximately 160 students in each academic year of study. The programme delivered is outcome-based, structured around the General Medical Council's (GMC's) *Tomorrow's Doctors* learning outcomes (GMC 2009) and uses an assessment-to-a-standard approach. This means that students must achieve the specified outcomes to a defined standard at each stage of the course before being allowed to progress to the next. We use a constructivist approach to curriculum planning, resulting in a 'spiral curriculum' where students are given opportunities to revisit aspects of learning, building on what they already know. As new information and skills are introduced, students are encouraged to make links between concepts, deepening their understanding (Figure 9.1).

The core curriculum emphasises the competencies necessary for a newly qualified doctor to work in the hospital or community. In Years 1–3 in the Systems in Practice (SiP) programme, students undertake a body systems-based programme where normal and abnormal structure, function and behaviour in relation to clinical medicine are studied systematically in modules (e.g. cardiovascular, respiratory and gastrointestinal systems). In Years 4 and 5, students follow the Preparation in Practice (PiP) programme. Students apply the skills and knowledge acquired in the earlier years in a variety of clinical settings in hospital and in general practice. Towards the end of this phase students serve in doctor apprenticeships and focus on preparation for early postgraduate training. Student-selected components (SSCs) provide the student with opportunities to study areas of interest in more detail while developing transferable skills such as ability to conduct literature reviews or select research methods.

We have adopted a problem-oriented approach to learning in Dundee. Around 100 core clinical problems (CCPs) are used to provide students with 'real' examples as a focus for learning. This gives

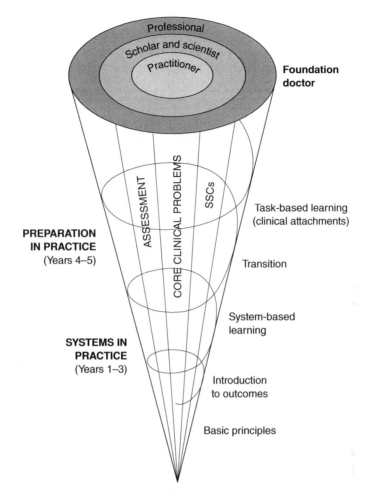

Figure 9.1 The Dundee (UK) spiral curriculum. Student-selected components (SSCs).

us the flexibility to use a wide range of educational delivery methods, including lectures, small-group teaching, traditional 'bedside' teaching encounters, elements of problem-based learning (PBL), team-based learning (TBL) and e-learning. Students are exposed to the clinical environment from Year 1, and are taught in a variety of clinical settings, including hospital wards, the community and the clinical skills centre, using models, simulators and simulated patients. Learning is integrated, with a number of longitudinal 'themes' such as medical ethics and prescribing running through the course, and this is reinforced through an Integrating Science and Specialities programme where students are encouraged to use self-directed learning and research, and to apply knowledge they have already gained in earlier parts of the course to core clinical problems to investigate solutions, think widely across systems and use basic principles when considering how to solve a problem.

Throughout the course, students use interactive online study guides designed to help them manage their own learning as they progress through the programme. The guides help students to understand what they should be learning, indicate the learning opportunities available and encourage students to assess the extent to which they have mastered the subject.

The delivery of an 'authentic' curriculum is reflected in the course content, the teaching and learning approaches, the learning opportunities provided, the student assessment and in the context for learning. The emphasis in the UK case study is on equipping the graduate with the competencies necessary to work as a doctor in a hospital or in the community. The Mozambique and Peru case studies show, even in difficult circumstances, how a community-based curriculum that pays attention to the required knowledge and skills in the local context can prepare students for practice. In Peru, students have contact with patients early in the curriculum and their attachment to health centres in the community is reported as contributing to the development of communication skills and an awareness of the local health situation, including the social dimensions of health and the need for prevention and promotion of health. As described in both the Mozambique and Peru case studies, PBL has proved to be an attractive educational strategy in part because it placed the basic medical sciences in the context of a clinical problem. This is described further in Chapter 10.

Case study 9.2 Training competent doctors for sub-Saharan Africa – experiences from an innovative curriculum in Mozambique

Janneke Frambach and Erik Driessen

Healthcare in sub-Saharan Africa faces a disproportionate share of the global disease burden as well as a radical shortage of physicians. Medical schools in the region cope with a lack of qualified faculty and poor infrastructure. Mozambique is a country in the south-east of sub-Saharan Africa that faces one of the most challenging healthcare situations in the world. The country has three doctors per 100,000 inhabitants, compared with the World Health Organization (WHO) African region average of 22 per 100,000. Mozambique's gross national income per capita is 2.5 times lower than the regional average, and prevalence of human immunodeficiency virus (HIV) is 2.5 times higher (WHO 2012).

The Faculty of Medicine of the Catholic University of Mozambique was founded in 1995, opened its doors to students in 2000 and graduates an average of 25 doctors annually. Admittance depends on academic performance after a preparatory year. The 6-year curriculum is problem- and community-based, and has been characterised as 'an instructive example of innovative African medical education' (Sub-Saharan African Medical Schools Study (SAMSS) 2009: 6). The main educational methods are small-group sessions, independent study, lectures, laboratory training, communication and clinical skills sessions with real patients in a 'university clinic' located inside the faculty building. In a community programme each student is attached to three families for 4 years, and clinical rotations in the final 2 years. Clinical training is mainly hospital-based, with a rotation in a rural area and a primary care rotation in a health centre.

Training competent doctors for a sub-Saharan African context means preparing students to confront an extremely challenging work environment. This is a difficult task for medical schools in the region, especially as they cope with shortages of adequately trained (clinical) teachers and poor resources and infrastructure. Notwithstanding these limitations, an innovative curriculum can contribute to preparing students for practice in this demanding context (Frambach et al. 2014):

- The PBL method stimulates an inquiring and independent attitude, which helps graduates deal with unfamiliar situations, e.g. as a hospital manager, in handling shortages and when encountering unfamiliar disease presentations.

> - The communication and clinical skills sessions and the community programme stimulate a holistic approach towards patients, which helps to overcome communication obstacles, to discuss traditional medicine issues and to consider the influence of socio-cultural aspects.
> - The diversity of curriculum elements stimulates a varied range of knowledge and skills in the social and cognitive domains, which helps graduates to enact the different roles expected of them in practice.
> - The school provides an overall positive learning climate, which enhances graduates' motivation to confront the challenges in practice.
>
> Clinical rotations are highly valued as a preparation for practice, but their effectiveness is compromised by a lack of adequate clinical teaching and supervision.

A clinical presentation or task-based curriculum (Harden et al. 2000), with its focus on the clinical problems and tasks facing a doctor, strongly supports the principle of an authentic curriculum. As described in the UK case study, the curriculum is built around 100 common clinical tasks facing a doctor, for example the management of a patient with abdominal pain, with the basic science and clinical skills related to the task. The use of simulators and virtual patients, augmenting but not replacing experience with real patients, provides students with practical experience not otherwise available to them and emphasises the development of the required clinical skills and at the same time the relevance of an understanding of the basic medical sciences.

The authentic curriculum is reflected also in the move in assessment from a reliance on written tests of knowledge to performance assessments such as the Objective Structured Clinical Examination (OSCE), work-based assessment and portfolio assessment, as described in Chapters 17–19.

The ethical and professional objectives that link curricula with healthcare needs are high on today's agenda. This is reflected in all aspects of curriculum planning, from the specification of learning outcomes to the integration of clinical and basic science teaching, the use of interprofessional education, the creation of appropriate learning opportunities, including experience in the community and performance-based assessment. Related to the authentic curriculum is the concept of the social accountability and responsibility of a medical school. This is one of the areas where excellence in medical education is acknowledged in the ASPIRE-to-excellence initiative (www.ASPIRE-to-excellence.org).

The curriculum as a collaborative activity

Collaboration between the key players or actors and between the different stakeholders was for the most part absent in the traditional curriculum. It can be argued that in the years ahead major advances in education will come about through collaboration among the range of stakeholders locally, nationally and internationally.

Collaboration between disciplines in the medical curriculum

Horizontal integration is now well established as a curriculum strategy. Subjects that are normally taught in the same phase of the curriculum, like anatomy, physiology and biochemistry in the early years of medicine and surgery, paediatrics and obstetrics and gynaecology in the later years, cooperate in the delivery of the education programme most commonly through system-based courses. In a cardiovascular system module, for example, students study the heart from the perspectives of the different disciplines. As illustrated in the case studies from Peru, the UK and Mozambique, this is now standard practice around the world. In vertical integration there is integration between the basic sciences and the clinical elements of the course, with students introduced to patients from the first year of the curriculum and continuing to study the basic sciences and their clinical relevance in the later years.

The rationale and benefits of integration have been described by Bandaranayake (2011) and stages on a continuum from isolation to full integration are set out in Harden's Integration Ladder (Harden 2000).

Case study 9.3 Outcome-based curriculum in a new medical school in Peru

Graciela Risco de Domínguez

Peru, located on the west coast of South America, has a population of 30 million people whose epidemiological profile is characterised by mostly preventable infectious diseases, a growing incidence of chronic conditions and some emergent health problems. One-third of the population, mostly poor and rural, is underserved or does not have access to healthcare at all. This situation is exacerbated by a critical deficit of healthcare professionals, added to their unequal distribution across the country.

Students enter medical school directly from high school. Medical studies take 7 years, including 1 year of hospital-based internship. There are 30 medical schools in Peru. The Medical School of the Peruvian University of Applied Sciences (UPC-MS), in Lima, was founded in 2007 with the vision to innovate medical education in Peru.

The design of the new curriculum took into account the main characteristics of the Peruvian medical education and major international trends in medical education informed by visits to leading foreign medical schools. The healthcare needs of the Peruvian population were analysed through indepth interviews and focus groups with the main local stakeholders and using the available statistical information. A leading consulting company in Peru (Apoyp Consultoría 2005) conducted a prospective study of the new scenarios of professional practice. Based on this information the mission of UPC-SM was established:

> To train general physicians with a broad understanding of health that includes its biological, psychological, environmental and social components; who are critical thinkers with a strong scientific formation, competent to solve the principal health problems of the individual and the community, making optimal use of available resources; oriented to service, with humane and ethical behaviour; leaders competent to work in multidisciplinary teams, motivated to change the health situation of the country through research and innovation.
>
> *(Apoyp Consultoría 2005)*

Ten learning outcomes were identified based on the Global Minimum Essential Requirements of the Institute for International Medical Education (IIME) (Schwarz and Wojtczak 2002), adapted in line with the school's mission, and the courses and the curriculum were built around them.

Horizontal integration of basic and pre-clinical sciences with clinical sciences was implemented from the first semester using initially TBL and later PBL. Vertical integration was ensured throughout four curricular threads, with each thread integrating a group of courses and curricular activities. Students' personal development was achieved through early contact with patients and health services. This helped students to acquire communication skills and ethics competences and at the same time built on the awareness about the health situation of the population. The scientific research thread ends with the completion of a thesis which is required for graduation. Clinical reasoning and clinical skills are developed using bedside training, ambulatory facilities and simulation. The Public Health and Primary Care thread, which is critical in the curriculum, begins in the first semester and continues until the eighth semester. Training is done at health centres and in the community, where students learn about prevention, promotion and social determinants of health.

Student assessment includes competence-based strategies such as OSCEs and mini-clinical evaluation exercises (Mini-CEXs). The organisational structure of the UPC-SM does not include academic departments. Curriculum thread coordinators facilitate curriculum integration.

Lessons learned from the experience included:

- the creation of a new medical school is an opportunity for innovation in medical education;
- it is possible to design a curriculum according to the modern trends in medical education, but with very particular characteristics adapted to the reality of the country;
- the implementation of an innovative curriculum requires a great deal of teacher training;
- a new curriculum requires a new organisational structure for the medical school;
- students who have just graduated from high school do well in TBL and PBL;
- a curriculum of 7 years allows the development of the general competencies by the student. It also allows the articulation of the basic sciences with professional training.

Collaboration among the different professions

High on today's agenda is a discussion about the place of interprofessional education. Many mistakes in medical practice are a result of poor teamwork and communication between doctors, nurses, midwives and other healthcare professions. If healthcare professionals have to work together effectively in clinical practice, it is argued that they should learn to do so as part of the medical curriculum. This is discussed further in Chapter 14.

Collaboration among the different stakeholders

In planning and implementing a curriculum, the need for collaboration goes beyond the different subject experts working together to deliver an integrated programme. All of the stakeholders, as illustrated in Figure 9.2, should work together in the planning and implementing of a curriculum – in specifying the learning outcomes and in planning the approaches to teaching, learning and assessment.

Collaboration among those responsible for the different phases of education

Much attention has been paid to collaboration between disciplines in the context of the undergraduate or basic medical curriculum. The situation is different across the phases of education

Curriculum planning in the 21st century

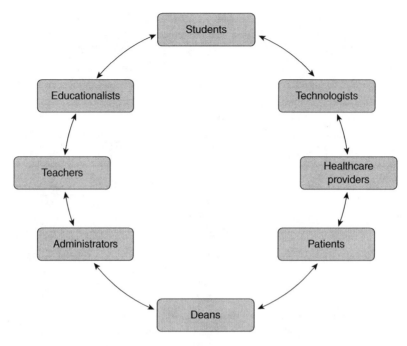

Figure 9.2 The stakeholders in curriculum development.

with the different phases – undergraduate, postgraduate and continuing education – operating in silos with little or no communication between them. Less attention has been paid by medical schools, specialty organisations and regulating bodies to collaboration across the different phases. The level of collaboration can be seen as a continuum (Table 9.1) and progress is being made from a position of isolation to a higher level of collaboration.

Local, national and international collaboration

Looking to the future, medical schools are unlikely to survive as self-sufficient entities that provide all aspects of their teaching, learning and assessment programme. Such independence will become even more difficult with increasing specialisation in medicine and with the need for students to access high-quality online learning resources and simulations. These are expensive to produce and may be beyond the budget of an individual school. At the same time there are demands to equip students with an international perspective of medicine that goes beyond their local setting and which provides them with the skills required of an international citizen. These include a sound

Table 9.1 Levels of collaboration across the different phases of education

Isolation	There is no communication between the different phases
Awareness	Each phase has a level of awareness of the training programme in other phases
Cooperation	There is a measure of collaboration with, for example, an agreement as to the learning outcomes for each phase and planned progression of students and trainees
Coordination	Some joint planning can be seen across the different phases, for example, with collaboration in the development of learning resources and learning opportunities
Integration	The boundaries between the phases become blurred or disappear

knowledge of global issues, the skills for working in an international context and the values for a global citizen.

More clearly defined learning outcomes, as described in Chapter 3, will support the unbundling of the curriculum and a sharing of learning resources, learning experiences and assessments. The experience in Peru, as highlighted in the case study, demonstrated how a curriculum can be based on international trends in medical education, but adapted to the local contexts with collaboration by local stakeholders.

The student and the curriculum

The student is a key factor in the curriculum. There has been a significant change in perceptions of the students' role and their contribution to the education process. The student is no longer seen as a product of the education system or as a consumer, but rather as a partner in the learning process.

Student-centred learning

In the traditional teacher-centred curriculum the emphasis is on the teacher and what is taught. By contrast, in a student-centred approach the emphasis is on the student and what is learned. The teacher's responsibility is to facilitate this. As described in the UK case study, students are encouraged to take responsibility for their own learning assisted by study guides and a clear statement of the expected learning outcomes.

Curriculum developments such as PBL, TBL, peer-to-peer learning, and the flipped classroom are consistent with this move toward student-centred learning. The move to student-centred learning is supported by new learning technologies, as discussed in Chapter 16.

Personalised adaptive learning

In healthcare, attention is being focused on personalised medicine, where the individual needs of each patient are addressed. In education, too, there is a move to an education programme personalised to the needs of the individual student, recognising that, just as with patients, each student is different in terms of their abilities, their previous experience, their learning styles and their aspirations. A greater understanding of how students learn and the availability of an increasingly powerful range of tools in the teacher's tool kit makes this possible. While fundamental changes to the curriculum to support adaptive learning may be some time away, there is much that the teacher can do today to move in this direction. The use of electives or SSCs is an example. Learning activities can be scheduled so that in sessions with simulators in the clinical skills laboratory, the students' time allocated is related to their mastery of the skills. What is fixed is the standard students achieve, not the time to achieve it.

Student engagement

How students engage with the delivery of the educational programme will vary from institution to institution depending on social, cultural and other issues. What is certain, however, is that the concept of the student as a stakeholder and partner in the learning process, as described in Chapter 7, is attracting increasing attention. This may manifest in different ways, as outlined in the ASPIRE-to-excellence criteria for excellence in student engagement in a medical school (www.ASPIRE-to-excellence.org). Students take on an active role on curriculum and other

Curriculum planning in the 21st century

committees and are consulted, involved and participate in the policy decisions and in the shaping of the teaching and learning experience. Students may be involved also in the delivery of the teaching programme as a peer teacher or as a developer of learning resources. Students may be engaged in the medical school's research programme and may represent the school and contribute to national and international education meetings.

The teacher and the curriculum

We have highlighted above the importance of the student. For a curriculum to be successful, the role of the teacher is also important. There is good evidence that the input of the teacher is as significant as, if not even more significant than, the design of the curriculum. Teaching in medicine is a challenging activity that requires, if the teaching is to be effective and the students' needs addressed, an understanding of medicine and the subject content as well as a mastery of a range of teaching skills. Teacher training is important, particularly as illustrated in the case study from Peru, when an innovative curriculum is introduced.

The role of the teacher has changed in recent years, reflecting different public and professional expectations of the training and the product, developments in technology, new educational approaches and increasing engagement of the student. The teacher has a number of roles in the curriculum (Figure 9.3).

Information provider

The teacher can be a direct source of information, knowledge and skills for the student directly through the delivery of lectures, small-group work and teaching in the clinical or laboratory

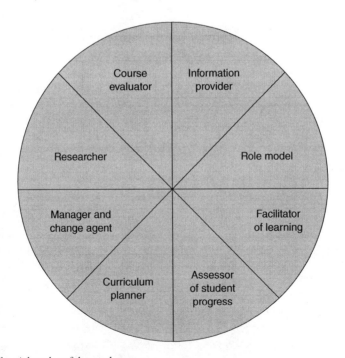

Figure 9.3 The eight roles of the teacher.

context. The teacher can also assist the student to acquire knowledge from hand-outs, textbooks and a wide range of online resources.

The teacher has a responsibility to help the student address the problem of information overload by advising on the learning outcomes and the selection of learning experiences to address the outcomes from the opportunities available. The teacher should guide the student as to how best to access, select and evaluate the rich range of possible resources. The teacher may prepare resource materials in print or electronic format and communicate with students through social networks such as blogs, Facebook or Twitter. The teacher should also identify the 'threshold concepts' essential for a student's understanding of the subject.

Role model

'We must acknowledge', suggested Tosteson (1979: 690), when Dean at Harvard Medical School, 'that the most important, indeed the only, thing we have to offer our students is ourselves. Everything else they can read in a book.' Role modelling is a powerful tool through which the medical teacher can pass on appropriate attitudes and values. Effective role models are important in medical education: they help to shape the values, attitudes, behaviour and ethics of students. They also have important influences on career choices. Role models, as William Osler advocated more than a century ago, improve students' learning by example. Students often pattern their activities on their teacher's behaviour, including their interactions with patients and their communication skills and ethical practice.

Role modelling may have a negative as well as a positive effect on the student. A dissonance is created, for example, when students having been taught the principles of ethical behaviour see a bad example in clinical practice. Many of the attributes associated with a good role model, however, can be acquired and strategies are available to help doctors to become better role models (Cruess et al. 2008).

Facilitator of learning

The role of the teacher has changed from being 'a sage on the stage' to 'a guide on the side'. Rather than the teacher's role being the transmission of information and skills to the student, the teacher now has a responsibility as a facilitator of learning: the good teacher can be defined as someone who does this most effectively. The teacher can facilitate learning in many ways. As described in the Mozambique case study, the teacher can help to create within the medical school an education environment that supports the learning of the students and encourages appropriate learning behaviour. The learning outcomes and the learning opportunities available can be made explicit and communicated to the student in such a way that learning is facilitated. Study guides can be prepared to serve as a guide or tutor for the student when the teacher is not available. In activities in the more formal curriculum, such as PBL, as described in the UK case study, the teacher has an important role to play as a facilitator.

Motivation of learning is an under-researched and often ignored aspect of medical education. The teacher should work with individual students to support, motivate and inspire them, and promote a sense of ownership of the course and their studies. Working with students on their portfolio can be a rewarding experience and can help to achieve this. Students may require particular support at times of transition, for example when they enter medical school or when they move to a clinical environment.

Assessor of student progress

Once a student is admitted to a medical school, the teacher has a responsibility to work with the student and to ensure that the student achieves the required learning outcomes. Students' progression through the curriculum should be monitored and assistance given as required. This role is reflected in the assessment-to-a-standard approach described in the UK case study. The teacher can be seen as a diagnostician, identifying any problems related to students' progress and guiding their studies to meet their individual needs, with the provision of feedback as required. Students in difficulty may require remedial teaching while those who have mastered a topic may benefit from guidance as to how they might explore the areas at a more advanced level – smoothing the pebbles and polishing the diamonds. At the same time, students should be encouraged to assess their own competence across the different domains.

Assessment of students by the teacher also has the important function of certifying when students are capable of moving on to the next part of the course and, upon completion of the course, practising as a doctor under supervision.

Curriculum planner

The development of an authentic curriculum that mirrors the mission of the medical school and relates to the needs of the community is an important task for the medical teacher. The students admitted to study medicine in the medical school and the teachers and resources available should be taken into account in the planning of the curriculum. Curriculum planning should be done in collaboration with the range of stakeholders, including teachers from the different disciplines, other healthcare professions and representatives of postgraduate programmes. Patients can also have a useful input and students should be represented on the curriculum committee. The committee should determine the expected learning outcomes and the most appropriate sequence of courses to achieve these. Decisions need to be taken about the educational strategies and the approaches to be adopted to teaching and learning. Consideration should also be given to the student assessment as an integral part of the education programme. A grid should be prepared relating the learning outcomes to the courses and assessment.

The curriculum should be built on sound education principles, including the need to encourage students to reflect and to engage in active learning. As far as possible, the curriculum should be designed to meet the different needs of the individual students.

Manager and change agent

Many management decisions at a university or medical school remain top-down with regard to strategic planning, budgeting, staff appraisals and quality assurance processes. Quality and efficiency are seen as management objectives. In general there has been a move to wider participation in management decisions and to greater flexibility, accountability and responsiveness to the needs of students. As a stakeholder, the teacher cannot afford to be disengaged from the decision-making processes within the institution. At an individual level, the teacher also has management responsibilities. These will vary with teaching responsibilities and may range from responsibility for management of a small part of the learning programme to responsibility for a module, a course or a phase of the curriculum. In terms of learning experiences, teachers are responsible for managing their own personal teaching session, which may be a lecture, a small-group activity, a clinical experience or a practical or clinical skills laboratory. Whatever the level of responsibility, the teacher will have four specific functions to perform as a manager: planning, organising, implementing and monitoring. This will require time management, delegating, communicating, team working, negotiating and conflict resolution.

We can't expect the future to be the same as the past. Significant changes are taking place in medical education in terms of curriculum planning, teaching and learning methods and assessment. Effective management is essential if we are to respond to change, whether the change arises from the internal rearrangement of functions or personnel or from external factors. Without sound management, change may result in low morale and poor end results. Potential obstacles to change must be identified and tackled. These may include a conservatism, rigidity and reluctance to change; a failure to recognise the need for change; a clear vision of the change proposed; a possible increase in staff workload and lack of resources; and a lack of an incentive to change.

The teacher as a researcher

The teacher is a professional and not just a technician delivering an education programme. With this is a responsibility to contribute to advancing the field of education, identifying what works and what doesn't work in the teaching programme and exploring ways of improving the learning experience for students. Medical education is enriched when teachers take this broader view of their role.

Teachers should be not just consumers of research, but producers of research – a move from education research *for* teachers to education research *by* teachers, from teachers as researched to the teacher as the researcher. Such practice-related or action research is an important contribution that can be made by all teachers to research in education. As a result, the teacher is empowered and the role of the teacher as a stakeholder in change is recognised. Teachers may work on their own, critically appraising and improving teaching practice, perhaps supported by staff with education research experience or as part of a larger research team with external funding.

By accepting a role as researcher, teachers can improve their own teaching practice; they can learn from their experience and a rich insight into key educational issues can be gained. The teacher as a researcher is consistent with the professionalism and scholarship of teaching and is simply an extension of what was seen as the traditional role of the teacher, not a change to the role.

The teacher as a course evaluator

As a professional, teachers have a responsibility to evaluate the courses or learning experiences for which they are responsible. The information gained is used to make decisions about the value and/or worth of an education programme. One approach to curriculum evaluation in common use is Kirkpatrick's four-level evaluation model (Kirkpatrick and Kirkpatrick 2006). Outcomes assessed are:

1   learning satisfaction or reaction to the programme;
2   learning attributed to the programme;
3   changes in the learner's behaviour by application of the knowledge to practice;
4   the impact of the programme on patient outcomes.

This model of evaluation on its own, however, does not illuminate why a programme works or doesn't work. The ten issues relating to a curriculum described by Harden and Laidlaw (2012) need to be examined if further insight is to be obtained. Other curriculum evaluation models include the logic model and the CIPP (context, input, process and product) model (Frye and Hemmer 2012).

The teacher as a professional

As professionals, teachers have a responsibility to ensure they have the necessary skills and abilities to fulfil the roles described above. Proficiency in the tasks required can be acquired through participation in staff development programmes or from following the example of more experienced teachers. Teachers have a responsibility to enquire into their own competence as a teacher and to keep themselves up to date with developments in education and how these might impact on their teaching. This can be achieved through reading medical education journals, through participation in education conferences or networking with teachers with a similar interest.

Take-home messages

- Curriculum planning should be considered in the context of the vision or mission of the medical school, the specified learning outcomes, the courses in the education programme and their sequence, the content addressed, the education strategies, the teaching and learning methods, the assessment approaches, the educational environment, communication about the curriculum to staff and students and the education management.
- Increasing attention is being paid to the need for an authentic curriculum where the focus is on equipping graduates with the competence to work as a member of a team and to practise medicine as a doctor.
- Curriculum planning and delivery should be a collaborative activity involving all of the stakeholders. It should include interdisciplinary and interprofessional education, collaboration between those responsible for the different phases of undergraduate, postgraduate and continuing education, and collaboration with other schools locally, nationally and internationally.
- A feature of a curriculum should be student engagement in curriculum planning and in delivery of the teaching programme. Students can also be engaged in the school's research programme and in representing the school nationally and internationally at medical education conferences.
- The success of a curriculum will depend on the teachers. Roles for the teacher include information provider, role model, facilitator of learning, assessor of students' progress, curriculum planner, education manager, researcher and course evaluator.

Bibliography

Apoyo Consultoría (2005). *Estudio del mercado de formación de médicos y su futura demanda laboral*, Lima: Apoyo Consultoría.

ASPIRE (2014). Online. Available HTTP: http:www.aspire-to-excellence.org (accessed 8 September 2014).

Bandaranayake, R. (2011) *The integrated medical curriculum*, London: Radcliffe Publishing.

Cruess, S.R., Cruess, R.L. and Steinert, Y. (2008) 'Role modelling – making the most of a powerful teaching strategy', *British Medical Journal*, 336(7646): 718–21.

Frambach, J., Manuel, B., Fumo, A., Van der Vleuten, C. and Driessen, E. (2014) 'Students' and junior doctors' preparedness for the reality of practice in sub-Saharan Africa', *Medical Teacher*, 37: 64–73.

Frenk, J., Chen, L., Bhutta, Z.Z., Cohen, J., Crisp, N., Evans, T., Fineberg, H., Garcia, P., Ke, Y., Kelley, P., Kistansamy, B., Meleis, A., Naylor, D., Pablos-Mendez, A., Reddy, S., Scrimshaw, S., Sepulveda, J., Serwadda, D. and Zurayk, H. (2010) 'Health professionals for a new century: Transforming education to strengthen health systems in an interdependent world', *The Lancet*, 376(9756): 1923–58.

Frye, A.W. and Hemmer, P.A. (2012) 'Program evaluation models and related theories. AMEE guide 67', *Medical Teacher*, 34(5): e288–99.

General Medical Council (2009) *Tomorrow's doctors: Outcomes and standards for undergraduate medical education*, London: GMC. Online. Available HTTP: www.gmc-uk.org/New_Doctor09_FINAL.pdf_27493417.pdf_39279971.pdf (accessed 10 June 2014).

Harden, R.M. (2000) 'The integration ladder: A tool for curriculum planning and evaluation', *Medical Education*, 34(7): 551–7.

Harden, R.M. and Laidlaw, J.M. (2012) *Essential skills for a medical teacher: An introduction to teaching and learning in medicine*, Edinburgh: Churchill Livingstone/Elsevier Publishing.

Harden, R.M., Crosby, J., Davis, M.H., Howie, P.E. and Struthers, A.D. (2000) 'Task-based learning: The answer to integration and problem-based learning in the clinical years', *Medical Education,* 34(5): 391–7.

Kirkpatrick, D. and Kirkpatrick, J. (2006) *Evaluating training programs: The four levels* (3rd edn), San Francisco, CA: Berrett-Koehler.

Schwarz, M.R. and Wojtczak, A. (2002) 'Global minimum essential requirements: A road towards competence-oriented medical education', *Medical Teacher*, 23(2): 125–9.

Sub-Saharan African Medical Schools Study (SAMSS) (2009) *Site visit report: Faculty of Medicine, Catholic University of Mozambique*, Washington, DC: SAMSS.

Tosteson, D.C. (1979) 'Learning in medicine', *New England Journal of Medicine*, 301(13): 690–4.

World Health Organization (2012) *Mozambique: Health profile*. Online. Available HTTP: http://www.who.int/gho/countries/moz.pdf (accessed 8 September 2014).

10
AUTHENTIC LEARNING IN HEALTH PROFESSIONS EDUCATION

Problem-based learning, team-based learning, task-based learning, case-based learning and the blend

Hossam Hamdy

Medical schools around the world have moved towards more interactive learning situations using problems scenarios and cases.

'Authentic' has been defined as 'genuine, real and worthy of trust' by www.freeonlinedictionary.com and 'learning' has been described as measurable and relatively permanent change in behaviour through experience, instruction or study by www.businessdictionary.com.

A deeper definition of 'authentic learning' is 'when the learning is integrally related to the understanding and complex solutions of real life complex problems' (Lombardi and Oblinger 2007). Lave and Wenger (1991) argue that all learning, in any discipline or profession, needs to be 'enculturated' into the discipline, and the earlier the better. Educational researchers have described the key features of authentic learning experiences in ten design elements (Von Glasersfeld 1989), which can be adapted to any discipline. These could be further clustered under four main key features:

1. real-world relevance – activities matching professional practice as near as possible, e.g. high-fidelity simulation;
2. challenging problems – around and within which learning takes place. These activities require investigation and inquiry by students over a period of time and synthesis from multiple resources;
3. collaborative activities – among learners and reflection about their learning;
4. interdisciplinary perspectives – integrated curricula and assessment.

Students in the early phases of authentic learning environments and activities therein may be disoriented or even frustrated with this new experience. This may have more to do with their prior learning experiences and development rather than preference for more or less passive learning approaches. However, this changes when problems, tasks and activities are relevant

Table 10.1 Comparing key features of four authentic learning methods

Key features	Task-based learning	Cased-based learning	Problem-based learning	Team-based learning
Underpinning learning theories	• Experiential learning • Adult learning theory • Constructivism	• Cognitivism • Constructivism	• Social constructivism • Cognitivism • Guided discovery learning	• Social constructivism • Guided discovery learning
Curriculum	• Integrated • Course-based • Mixed	• Integrated • Course-based • Mixed	Integrated	• Integrated • Course-based
Faculty role	Several experts	Several experts	Several facilitators, non-expert	Expert One faculty
Student – self-directed learning	+++	++	++++	+++
Class size	Large	Large	Small: approx. 8–10	Large, can be more than 100
Physical resources: 'classroom'	Standard – large classrooms or wards	Standard – large classrooms / lecture halls	Multiple – small classrooms	Standard – large class / lecture hall which can allow small-group formation

to what really counts in real life (Herrington et al. 2003). Authentic learning privileges the 'messiness' of real-life decision making, where there are no completely right or wrong answers and all depends on the context and what is fit for purpose. This requires considerable reflective judgement that goes well beyond the memorisation of content (Dede et al. 2005). In this chapter, examples of authentic learning practices used in health professional education (HPE) are described.

If we apply these definitions to the context of HPE, authentic learning should be relevant, closely linked to the future profession of the learner and lead to relatively permanent change in the learner's behaviour by demonstrating competence considered essential for the job. To achieve these outcomes, educational strategies should be different from the traditional teacher-centred didactic teaching. Adult students prefer to learn by doing rather than listening (Knowles 1980; Taylor and Hamdy 2013). During the last three decades, HPE has focused more on outcome competencies, 'what the graduate is able to do' rather than 'how much s/he knows'. This goal influenced the move towards designing and implementing outcome-based, competency-based curricula (Harden et al. 1999). This trend necessitates the implementation of authentic learning and relevant teaching strategies, student assessment and programme evaluation systems and methods. More and more institutions have moved towards interactive learning situations using small groups, student-centred learning, integrated curricula, the early introduction of clinical sciences and skills and the creation of more realistic and authentic settings for learning. Authentic learning cuts across disciplines and brings students into meaningful contact with the real world, future work environment and patients.

This chapter focuses on the key features, theories and principles underpinning authentic learning; the application of strategies in different contexts and phases of the curriculum; and implementation problems that can lead to failure in achieving its objectives. It is not intended to provide a comprehensive review of the different types of authentic learning. Rather, four common strategies supportive of student-centred learning will be presented, discussed and compared:

1 problem-based learning (PBL);
2 team-based learning (TBL);
3 task-based learning (TkBL); and
4 case-based learning (CBL).

In addition, case studies are presented with messages applicable in multiple contexts. The key elements of each of these teaching approaches are summarised in Table 10.1.

Educational theories underpinning authentic learning

The four learning strategies highlighted above derive from different contemporary learning theories.

Behavioural theory

Behavioural theories emphasise the stimulus that can be a problem/case scenario, a task or an encounter with a real patient. The reaction 'behaviour' of the learner to the stimulus is influenced by the context and the history of those involved. Feedback and reinforcement are important to support and inculcate the behaviour and for it to become a 'habit' (Schmidt 1993).

Cognitive theory

Cognitive theory looks at authentic learning activities that promote critical thinking, reasoning processes and particular mechanisms of processing, storing and retrieving new information (Dolmans et al. 2002).

Constructivist theory

Constructivist theory is a philosophical view on how we come to understand or know (Von Glasersfeld 1989; Rorty 1991). As a theory and philosophical perspective of modern education, it is characterised by:

- Understandings developed from interactions with the environment. What is learned is not separate from how it is learned and the context in which it is learned.
- The goal of the learner is central in considering what is learned.
- The learner builds and constructs understanding based on prior experiences and knowledge.
- The social environment is critical to the development of knowledge and understanding (Von Glasersfeld 1989). Collaborative learning, as in PBL and TBL, fits with constructivism. They test students' understanding about a problem, compare it with others', expand it and facilitate its storage in deep memory and its retrieval. This proposition is also similar to the cognitive perspective.
- Reflection on and in action, together with the role of the teacher in providing support, is thought to provide a scaffold on which the student can build learning.

Experiential learning theories

Experiential learning theories (Kolb 1984) and social constructivism (Schon 1983) are closely related to PBL, TBL and TkBL. Experiential learning relates to learning professional tasks in the work environment. Students at an early or advanced phase of their learning link experience with learning of knowledge, skills and attitude, emphasising relevance. Knowledge, if not applied, is quickly forgotten. The teacher's role in social constructivism is one of facilitating learning rather than providing information. The teacher values and challenges the learner's thinking. The concept of the learning scaffold and the zone of proximal development (Vygotsky 1978) represent the role of the teacher and the teacher's interaction with the student, attempting to extend the student's development into the gap between the learner and teacher.

Social theories of learning

Social theories of learning (Bandura 1977) emphasise the importance of learning from each other and creating a community of learners. Ideas are discussed, elaborated and challenged by teams and group of learners. Social media and electronic communication networks are examples of this principle. The social perspective supports students' and teachers' reflection on content, process and the learning experience itself, all of which need training for students to develop this skill, do it well and record it (reflective portfolio). Teachers require the ability to guide students, evaluate the reflective portfolio and give and receive timely constructive feedback.

Problem-based learning

PBL is an approach that emphasises students' active and self-directed learning individually and in small groups. It was introduced into medical education in the late 1960s at McMaster University, Canada (Barrows 1986) and rapidly spread all over the world to become a symbol of innovation. It was a response to the perceived lack of relevance in the early years of medical education and was a break from the existing focus of teacher-centred, passive student role that emphasised how much students knew and could recall rather than the relationships among things. It is characterised by small groups of students (six to ten) who worked around a problem to seek to understand its different facets. The main outcome is learning from the problem, not solving the problem. The tutor's role is to facilitate group learning activities rather than to be a primary source of information. Typically, the curriculum design of PBL is the integrated, organ system in which students study a new problem each week. Problems have different learning objectives related to basic medical sciences, clinical sciences and behavioural sciences. Two to three tutorial sessions of small-group learning typically take place each week.

The roles of students and the tutor in PBL have been well described (Schmidt 1993; Barrows 1996; Dolmans et al. 2002). What happens in the first tutorial session of a new problem and the second tutorial session (the reporting phase) have also been well described (Schmidt 1993). On the other hand, what students and the programme provide in between and beyond the sessions is vague. Other structured educational activities arranged by the programme vary and may include lectures, resource sessions, review sessions, laboratory work, clinical skills and more. This blend of educational strategies and instructional methods characterises PBL as implemented in the first decade of the 21st century.

Over the last four decades, hundreds of studies have described, analysed and evaluated PBL (Maudsley 1999). The way PBL is implemented varies widely from 'window dressing' to an orthodox implementation, as originally described in the 1960s, i.e. no lectures. The fuzzy world of PBL (Hamdy 2008) requires attention and flexibility in relation to the context of implementation while at the same time being vigilant in maintaining key principles, values, objectives and rationale.

It is common to see PBL programmes become inattentive to some of the underlying assumptions that make it work best. This is one of the most common and important problems encountered by PBL programmes internationally. The case study of the Faculty of Medicine, Suez Canal University, Egypt, illustrates how one institution adjusted its PBL programme to maintain its viability.

Case study 10.1 Implementation of computer-assisted PBL sessions to medical students at Faculty of Medicine, Suez Canal University, Egypt

Somaya Hosny and Yasser El-Wazir

The Faculty of Medicine Suez Canal University (FOM-SCU) adopted PBL as one of its main learning strategies from its inception in 1978. We started to replace the paper-based educational problems with interactive digital problems in 2009 in order to motivate students and increase engagement in the learning process. The newly designed problems were enriched by multimedia to improve the learning environment and to increase the opportunity for more diverse elaboration of learning, connecting their knowledge and analytical thinking skills. Students see images and video clips and hear sounds of the relevant clinical manifestations of the patient problem during discussions. The underlying assumption was that this would improve the diversity of their learning experiences and enhance their understanding of the case while at the same time providing better learning.

Student satisfaction was assessed at the end of the first year of implementation. Questions addressed various aspects of the learning process, such as brainstorming, knowledge acquisition and the impact on their assessment. A total of 175 of 330 students responded to the questionnaire. Analysis showed that students believed that e-problems helped them to understand better (79 per cent), participate more in discussions (70 per cent), render PBL sessions more interesting (79 per cent), focus their discussion (63 per cent) and improve their achievement in problem solving (49 per cent) and written exams (39 per cent). Analysis of the open-ended comments showed that students asked for more multimedia and less text (36 per cent) and more training for tutors on how to facilitate e-problem discussions (12 per cent). The analysis of tutor responses showed that e-problems helped students to understand better (83 per cent), participate more in discussions (83 per cent) and render PBL sessions more interesting (83 per cent) and focused (50 per cent).

The second phase of the project began in 2011 by adding digital problems to the clerkship phase. Here the aim was to improve clinical reasoning skills. This was done by presenting students with a video tape of a simulated patient encounter interrupted by pause intervals to trigger reflection. A similar assessment of this phase of the project showed that 84 per cent of the students agreed that e-format was better than the conventional paper format and 80 per cent believed that it improved their clinical reasoning skills.

PBL, in most medical colleges, is implemented mainly in the pre-clerkship phase of the curriculum and disappears in the clerkship phase. To avoid this disconnection, the written scenario, 'The Problem', is replaced by a real patient problem while maintaining the small-group learning structure.

Initially, as students learn to use PBL, there is a high degree of uncertainty about the depth and breadth of study required and expected. As the tutorial sessions unfold, students can compare and contrast what they have studied and learned and the extent to which it is similar and different to what other students have done. A broad overview of the 'block/unit' objectives and a tutor guide can help both students and tutors ameliorate this problem of uncertainty of depth and breadth of learning.

Another problem is a tendency of students to regress to discipline-focus thinking. For example, it is not uncommon for students, during the first tutorial session of a new problem, to split the problem into discipline-related objectives and forget about the problem scenario and how new information relates to the findings and presentation of the problem.

Students are advised that they are responsible for all the objectives generated from the problem (Dolmans et al. 2005). In PBL, the development of a concept map is another mechanism which has been effective in ameliorating this problem (Kassab and Hussain 2010), as it can illustrate the relationships between the different concepts and disciplines.

Assessment and learning are inseparable. In PBL, if the assessment is not in alignment with the learning objectives derived from the problems and the process as a whole related to PBL, the learning strategy may fail. The case study from the Arabian Gulf University in Bahrain is a good illustration of this. They addressed this problem through adjusting the assessment to promote integration.

Case study 10.2 Integrated assessment in problem-based learning promotes integrated learning

Raja C. Bandaranayake

PBL has become increasingly popular in medical education over the past four decades. There are strong educational reasons for this. It is worthwhile stepping back and considering the extent to which the many different forms of PBL practised in schools do, in fact, take advantage of the educational benefits of this strategy to promote authentic learning.

The College of Medicine and Health Sciences in the Arabian Gulf University in Bahrain has practised PBL in its undergraduate medical curriculum since its inception in 1982. Almost two decades later it became evident that a practice that tended to detract from the authentic characteristics of PBL was occurring in many student groups during the pre-clerkship phase of the curriculum. For example, during the first meeting for a given problem, discussion of the sequence of triggers, which should have formed the basis by which learning needs were identified, quickly focused on the disciplines which impinged on the problem. Each discipline was considered separately by the group and students allocated responsibility amongst themselves to learn according to discipline. Returning after a period of self-study for the second meeting, students shared their learning by discussing each discipline in turn. Individual students were often unaware of related concepts from other disciplines. Integrated learning, one of the main advantages of PBL, was becoming disintegrated. Instead, the problem was seen as a summation of concepts from different disciplines, rather than a whole formed by the relationships among the concepts.

A closer examination of this undesirable practice showed that it was, in part, related to the nature of student assessment. Examinations took place at the end of each organ system, and sometimes after combinations of organ systems, as well as at the end of the pre-clerkship phase. These examinations purported to be 'integrated'. However, they consisted of a collection of test items constructed by individual departments/disciplines. Students know how to survive and play the education game. They resorted to a learning strategy that addressed their immediate concerns, i.e. negotiating the impending examination successfully. Each examination consisted of a multiple-choice question (MCQ) paper, a short-answer question (SAQ) paper and an Objective Structured Practical Examination (OSPE). Students preferred to learn discipline-wise rather than to use the problems to integrate their learning among different disciplines. They did what the teachers asked them to do in the examinations.

A decision was made to make the SAQ paper integrated. Themes were identified within each organ system module and assigned to each assessment committee member for that module. A skeleton of an SAQ was drafted by a member of an interdisciplinary subcommittee consisting of representatives from disciplines related to that theme. Each subcommittee member added 'flesh' to the related part of the question. At a subsequent meeting, links between the parts were sought and deliberate attempts made to test the interdisciplinary links within the theme. The question was then submitted to the assessment committee for further discussion and clarification before being accepted into a bank of questions from which the SAQ part of the examination was set.

While a study has not been undertaken since this system was adopted in the school, students self-study differently, in a more integrated manner.

It must be recognised by schools wanting to introduce PBL that it is a strategy to achieve desirable learning habits and relevant outcomes among students, rather than an end in itself. In this sense, it is similar to cadaver dissection in anatomy, and clinical skills training, both a means to an outcome rather than the outcome itself. The same applies to all the other methods of authentic learning outlined in this chapter. The practice of a method by itself should not be the determinant of authenticity. Rather it should be the effect the method has on student learning in preparation for practice in the real world of medicine.

Unsubstantiated claims have been made that PBL is more expensive than subject-based learning or other learning strategies in which large numbers of students are taught in a class with one faculty. These claims are contradicted by studies that have demonstrated that, up to a class size of 100 students, PBL is not more expensive (Mennin and Martinez-Burrola 1986; Hamdy and Agamy 2011). PBL does, however, require a different set of skills, commitment and preparation.

Class size and infrastructure make a difference when implementing and sustaining PBL programmes. Sudden increases in class size, often as an attempt to meet increased demands from the healthcare system, can disrupt the underlying assumptions and practices of the tutorial, as seen in the following case study from the Faculty of Medicine and Health Sciences, Universiti Malaysia Sarawak, Malaysia.

Case study 10.3 Authentic learning via problem-based learning – reflections from a Malaysian medical school

William K. Lim

The medical school at the Universiti Malaysia Sarawak (UNIMAS) became the second in Malaysia to employ a PBL curriculum upon its inception in 1995 (Malik and Malik 2002a). The continuing challenge in UNIMAS is to implement PBL in ways that enable students to benefit maximally from its educational philosophy. In the initial years of the school's inception all teachers were trained as tutors. They sat in all the lectures and guided their respective PBL groups. The assessments they designed tested the entire taught curriculum. However, as the school was directed to increase its student intake continually, teachers were continuously recruited. Most came from schools with lecture-based curricula, where it was assumed students learned mainly by transfer of information via lectures (Margetson 1997).

After the fifth year, when the school had the full complement of Phase One and Phase Two students, teaching in Phase One and PBL tutorials were handled almost exclusively by pre-clinical teachers while specialist clinicians taught mainly in Phase Two. Phase One lecturers no longer attended each other's lectures and only knew the PBL teaching content in the few blocks in which they tutored. Hence their assessment questions mainly tested the content of their own lectures. Over-recruitment of teachers in a particular discipline resulted in the creation of new teacher-centred lectures in that discipline. Consequently, time for self-directed learning was progressively reduced (Malik and Malik 2002b) and information from lectures frequently duplicated PBL content. Without the services of a medical education specialist, tutor training sessions were irregular and PBL case review became infrequent. Tutor training focused mostly on the steps of PBL, without its underpinning pedagogical principles. When student numbers outgrew tutors, PBL group size increased up to 13 students per group.

(continued)

> *(continued)*
> To improve this situation, a PBL coordinator was appointed, tutoring of one trigger was accorded the same workload value as giving a lecture, tutor training was conducted regularly and incorporated the PBL philosophy, PBL rooms were uniformly equipped, student training in PBL increased, the PBL group sizes reduced and the PBL scenarios were reviewed.
>
> The successful implementation of PBL requires suitable infrastructure for tutorials, regular training of faculty and students and constant review. At the UNIMAS medical school the challenge is now to harmonise the lecture and PBL content so that authentic learning prompted by real-world problems is underpinned by appropriate and complementary teaching with balanced assessment.

The take-home message is that PBL, like any educational work, requires continuous attention and multiple small adjustments on a regular basis. Failing to do this leads to much more difficult and expensive problems that are avoidable.

Team-based learning

TBL is a strategy for teaching and learning first described by Larry Michaelsen for business education (Michaelsen et al. 2002) and later introduced to HPE (Seidel and Richards 2001; Hunt et al. 2003; Parmelee and Hudes 2012). Embedded in this approach is the ability to be a critical thinker and work effectively in a team. TBL is a 'guided discovery learning' model. Social constructivist theory (Savery and Duffy 1995) constitutes the main theoretical framework of TBL. Three phases are typically described for TBL:

1. Phase One – 'Pre-class study' in which students prepare for class by going through the objectives and pre-class assignments assigned in advance by the teacher.
2. Phase Two – This starts with an Individual Readiness Assurance Test (IRAT). Students answer individually a number of questions, usually MCQs. Next, the same test is discussed in small groups, the Group Readiness Assurance Test (GRAT). The elaboration and collaboration to find the best answer and problem solution create an interactive learning environment. Faculty members direct the session, provide feedback and wrap up at the end.
3. Phase Three – This is the application phase, where groups work on another problem that encourages them to apply their newly acquired knowledge to solve another similar problem. This can take place during the same session, if time allows, or in a separate session.

TBL has the advantage of cost-effectiveness, as large numbers of students can be in one classroom, and it fits well with a subject- or course-based curriculum. The teacher is a subject matter expert whose role changes from purely that of an information giver to one that includes planning and facilitating learning. Students are active as learners before, during and after the class session. TBL can also be combined with other teaching methods, lecture-based and even PBL (Abdelkhalek et al. 2010; Anwar et al. 2012).

The 'flipped classroom' (McLaughlin et al. 2014) is a buzzword which is spreading at all levels of education – primary, secondary and higher. It is an active learning strategy coupled with advancements in instructional technology like video-taping lectures, use of social media and others. Learning is student-centred, before coming to the class, in the classroom and beyond. The flipped classroom has many features of TBL in that learning takes place before coming to the classroom and the in-class activities are explanations and applications of the pre-class-acquired knowledge.

The initial testing of students' preparedness is similar to the IRAT of TBL. It increases the student's commitment to study and prepare before coming to the class. The in-class small-group activities and discussion in a flipped classroom are close to the GRAT. In the two approaches, the role of the teacher changes from provider of information to facilitator of learning.

Case study 10.4   The effect of team-based learning on students' learning in a basic science course at the Universidad Peruana de Ciencias Aplicadas Medical School

Denisse Champin

The School of Medicine of the Universidad Peruana de Ciencias Aplicadas (UPC-MS) was founded 7 years ago in Lima, Peru and based its curriculum planning on Harden's spiral curriculum model, using PBL as the integrating axis (Harden et al. 1997). Prior to implementing a PBL methodology, it was decided to use TBL as a transition from working in large groups to small groups.

A curriculum change in 2010 provided an opportunity to study the benefits of implementing TBL with students studying biology. TBL sessions were offered in the curriculum in the second semester. They were developed in three sessions of 4 hours per week, with a facilitator-to-student ratio of 2:30 per classroom. The structure of TBL consisted of:

- first session, reading or viewing a video about a biology topic, then concluding the session with a reading test;
- second session, individual and group assessment (multiple-choice tests that are discussed at the end of the training session);
- third session, case solution (clinical cases are presented about some topics developed in the biology course).

Case study resources included biology class material, reference texts and the internet. The results were better performance on tests in the group exposed to TBL. Teacher training in TBL was an important factor, which should always be considered.

Task-based learning

TkBL is an approach in which learning is built around a specified task. Learning results from the process of understanding the concepts and mechanisms underlying those tasks (Harden 1996). It is an example of experiential learning (Kolb 1984). The student learns about the different facets related to the task, basic sciences, pathology, pharmacology, decision making, communication skills and ethics. The approach also has been described as 'service-based learning' (Grant and Marsden 1992). The same task can be presented at different phases of the curriculum and in different learning and practice environments, for example skill labs, hospitals and general clinics, and it can also be presented at different dimensions of complexity.

TkBL offers a practical approach to integration in the curriculum as students learn by building activities around a number of tasks. They seek to understand the concepts related to the task and at the same time develop skills and proficiency in doing the task. Learning outcomes are products of the contributions of the individual learner, the task and the context of the 'situation'. Tasks occupy a central place in a three-way relationship between teachers, learners and learning outcomes. The tasks can represent the outcome competences of a programme. One example is the Dundee curriculum (Harden et al. 1997). Tasks can be integrated with different types of curricula, as described in the case from University of Sharjah, United Arab Emirates, where they combine PBL, TBL and TkBL. The following case study describes how TkBL is implemented in the pre-clerkship phase of an integrated PBL curriculum.

Case study 10.5 Teaching and learning basic medical sciences in the clinical environment using a task-based learning approach at the University of Sharjah, United Arab Emirates

Hossam Hamdy

Basic medical sciences constitute a major component of the pre-clerkship phase regardless of whether the curriculum is discipline-based or integrated. The pre-clerkship phase of medical education is characterised by most of the teaching taking place in classrooms – lectures, PBL tutorials and clinical skills labs using simulators and simulated patients. In many colleges, there are lab sessions related to disciplines, e.g. anatomy, physiology, biochemistry.

The College of Medicine, University of Sharjah, United Arab Emirates created a strong link with teaching hospitals, allowing students in the pre-clerkship phase of the integrated, PBL, organ system curriculum to work around tasks that demonstrate the clinical application of the basic medical sciences in action. They are related mainly to clinical investigation, monitoring and/or management of patients in the hospital. A number of tasks are identified in relation to each organ system, for example, in the cardiovascular system, electrocardiography, echocardiography, measuring central venous pressure, lipid profiles, cardiac enzymes; in the respiratory system, respiratory function tests, ventilatory support, blood gas analysis and chest physiotherapy; and in the gastrointestinal system, upper and lower endoscopy, microbiology of *Helicobactor pylori*, stool culture, rectal pressure studies and oesophageal manometry. The radiological anatomy of each system is taught in the radiology department, including conventional x-rays, computed tomography, magnetic resonance imaging and invasive radiology.

There is a list of objectives for each task that students work towards during a visit to the hospital. Clinical teachers receive training in how to explain the tests and relate them to underlying basic medical sciences. Each student reflects after each session about the experience framed by six questions:

1   What have I observed?
2   What did I do?
3   What did I learn?
4   What am I uncertain about?
5   What do I need to do to address the uncertainty, the gaps I see and understand?
6   How will I evaluate progress?

This programme is in its second year of implementation. Attention to the logistics of implementation in the hospital is crucial. Important issues to be considered to promote success include: limiting the number of students in each session (approximately ten); preparatory training for clinical teachers; and coordination and communication between the programme director and the clinicians.

Case-based learning

CBL is characterised by small groups of learners working around a written problem using creative problem-solving strategies with some advance preparation. Students use previous experiences (cases) to suggest approaches to solving the problems and to help interpret findings in the new situation. CBL requires combining reasoning with learning. The tutor, who is a facilitator and subject matter expert, actively shares responsibility for reaching key learning points (Srinivasan et al. 2007). A 'tutor guide' provides questions and a flexible framework for discussion. Students prepare in advance and, in contrast to PBL, the objectives of the problem are declared at the end of the session and feedback from the tutor is given to the students. Of particular interest in this method is when and how the tutor sees, understands and acts to influence learning in the role of a facilitator, and when and how she or he and the group choose the tutor's role as one of sharing expertise in various forms, commonly as a lecture. The relationship between these roles is dynamic and depends on what is happening in the group at the time. Learning to see, understand and influence learning in this approach requires sensitivity to oneself, the group, to individuals, to the goals of the case, and sometimes all of these together.

Learning strategies such as CBL can be implemented in different formats and contexts:

- descriptive, narrative cases, parts of which may be given successively (progressive disclosure);
- mini-cases;
- directed case study – discussion of cases that may be long or short and are followed immediately with highly directed questions;
- 'bullet cases' – two or three sentences with a single teaching point, akin to examination questions.

CBL can approximate PBL and it can become like a lecture (Dufuis and Persky 2008) depending on conditions including class size, teachers' training, capability and experience, students' preparation, and the form and structure of the assessment system. It can be used with other learning strategies in a subject-based, coordinated or integrated curriculum.

It has been proposed that CBL may be better used to prepare younger learners in becoming better self-learners (Dufuis and Persky 2008). Learners using CBL are active and focused on application and problem solving. The following case from Sweden describes how CBL was introduced in the clerkship phase of a discipline-based curriculum.

Case study 10.6 Improving students' decision-making skills on the surgical rotation

Jonas Nordquist

Karolinska Institute is a bio-medical university located in Stockholm, Sweden. Its medical programme is 5.5 years with an undergraduate intake of 250 students.

The curriculum has an integrated character divided into seven thematic areas. Students are exposed to patient contact during the first semester through primary care centres. Clinical rotations

(continued)

(continued)

starts in the third year and are conducted at four different hospitals in Stockholm. The rotation in surgery is placed in the fifth year and consists of 16 weeks, including general surgery, anaesthesia, orthopaedic surgery and radiology.

The programme management of the surgical rotation at the Karolinska University Hospital Solna introduced CBL in 2008 with the intention of further activating students during their learning process and fostering integration of different medical subspecialties. CBL is a well-documented educational method originating from the Harvard Business School (Barnes et al. 1987). It fosters effective learning in groups (Thistlethwaite et al. 2012) and has the advantage that it can accommodate large groups with one facilitator. The method focuses particularly on analytical and decision-making skills. CBL has been adapted for medical students and was chosen by the University Hospital because of its potential to bridge the gap between traditional theoretical teaching and clinical experience (Barnes et al. 1987; Nordquist et al. 2012).

Fifteen cases were developed during 2009. Faculty development in facilitating case seminars took place during two semesters, with teachers being observed and receiving feedback from an educational consultant. Students were introduced to the new method during the introduction to the semester.

It was a challenge to produce 15 new cases in a rather short period of time. Medical doctors are not used to writing authentic cases in a narrative open-ended format from the perspective of one protagonist. Also, many faculty members were new to facilitating learning in a group of approximately 40 students, rather than giving a lecture. In addition, most students had never actively participated in case-based seminars during which they had to make their voice heard and to defend their decisions and positions publicly in a group of peers. Most importantly, students were not used to reasoning about possible solutions to a case.

Formative assessment focused on the level of implementation after two semesters. The managers of the programme were content with the assessment results and improvement of reflective skills among the students and how challenges were addressed (Nordquist et al. 2012).

It is crucial to dedicate adequate time for developing cases and for faculty development in facilitating skills. It is also very important to prepare students and to help them be aware of the programme expectations and what students should expect from the new teaching/learning method. It is clear that both faculty and students hold different expectations about CBL compared to the managers and educationalists planning the course. CBL works in harmony with other educational methods like subject-based learning and one does not need to change an entire curriculum as a result of its introduction.

In education a 'one size fits all' approach cannot be applied. Although a learning strategy of PBL, TBL, TkBL and/or CBL could be employed as the main learning method, in reality different methods are combined depending on the context, learning environment and the outcomes of learning.

Take-home messages

- Social constructivism is a common theoretical perspective of authentic learning strategies.
- Successful translation of an authentic learning method from a 'curriculum on paper' to actions ensures that student learning is the main challenge.

- Proper implementation of authentic learning needs knowledgeable and experienced leadership in medical education, faculty development, sensitivity to the context and institutional culture.
- The cost of introducing an authentic instructional method is an important element to be considered to ensure its sustainability.
- Monitoring what is happening and taking corrective actions needs to be built into all approaches. It is easy to keep the label of PBL or TBL while what is happening is a distorted version of one or the other.
- Assessment of students is a key part of success that must be in alignment with the strategies for learning, assessing both process and content.
- Authentic learning methods for health professionals will continue to evolve based on personal and contextual experiences. The current trend is to use a blend of learning methods guided by experience and general programme outcomes.
- All educational work requires continuous attention and multiple small adjustments on a regular basis. Failing to do this leads to much more difficult and expensive problems which are avoidable.

Bibliography

Abdelkhalek, N., Hussein, A. and Hamdy, H. (2010) 'Using team based learning to prepare medical students for future problem-based learning', *Medical Teacher*, 32(2): 123–9.

Anwar, K., Shaikh, A.A., Dash, N.R. and Khurshid, S. (2012) 'Comparing the efficacy of team based learning strategies in a problem based learning curriculum', *ACTA Pathologica, Microbiologia et Immunologica Scandinavica*, 120(9): 718–23.

Bandura, A. (1977) *Social learning theory*, New York: General Learning Press.

Barnes, L., Christensen, C. and Hansen, A. (1987) *Teaching and the case method*, Cambridge, MA: Harvard University Press.

Barrows, H.S. (1986) 'A taxonomy of problem-based learning methods', *Medical Education*, 20(6): 481–6.

Barrows, H.S. (1996) *What your tutor may never tell you: A medical student's guide to problem-based learning (PBL)*, Springfield, IL: Southern Illinois University School of Medicine.

Dede, C., Korte S., Neson, R., Valdez, G. and Ward, D.J (2005) *Transforming learning for the 21st century: An economic imperative*. Naperville, IL: Learning Point Associates. Online. Available HTTP: http://net.educause.edu/section_params/conf/eliws061/Dede_Additional_Resource.pdf 9 (accessed 24 April 2007).

Dolmans, D.H., Gijselaers, W.H., Moust, J.H., De Grave, W.S., Wolfhagen, J.H. and Van der Vleuten, C.P. (2002) 'Trends in research on the tutor in problem-based learning: Conclusions and implications for educational practice and research', *Medical Teacher*, 24(2): 173–80.

Dolmans, D.H.J.M., De Grave, W., Wolfhagen, I.H.A.P. and Van der Vleuten, C.P.M. (2005) 'Problem-based learning: Future challenges for educational practice and research', *Medical Education*, 39(7): 732–41.

Dufuis, R.E. and Persky, A.M. (2008) 'Initial experience in using case-based learning in a clinical pharmacokinetics course', *American Journal of Pharmaceutical Education*, 72(2): 29.

Grant, J. and Marsden, P. (1992) *Training senior house officers by service-based learning*, London: Joint Centre for Education in Medicine.

Hamdy, H. (2008) 'The fuzzy world of problem based learning', *Medical Teacher*, 30(8): 739–41.

Hamdy, H. and Agamy, E. (2011) 'Is running a problem-based learning curriculum more expensive than a traditional subject-based curriculum?', *Medical Teacher*, 33(9): e509–14.

Harden, R.M. (1996) 'Task based learning: An educational strategy for undergraduate, postgraduate and continuing medical education, Part 1 (1996) AMEE medical education guide no. 7', *Medical Teacher*, 18(1): 7–13.

Harden, R.M., Davis, M.H. and Crosby, J.R. (1997) 'The new Dundee medical curriculum: A whole that is greater than the sum of the parts', *Medical Education*, 31(4): 264–71.

Harden, R.M., Crosby, J.R. and Davis, M.H. (1999) 'AMEE guide no. 14: Outcome-based education: Part 1 – an introduction to outcome-based education', *Medical Teacher*, 21(1): 7–14.

Harden, R.M., Davis, M.H. and Crosby, J.R. (2000) 'Task based learning: The answer to integration and problem based learning in the clinical years', *Medical Education*, 34(5): 391–7.

Herrington, J., Oliver, R. and Reeves, T.C. (2003) 'Patterns of engagement in authentic online learning environments', *Australian Journal of Education Technology*, 19(1): 9–71. Online. Available HTTP: http://www.ascilite.org.au/ajet/ajet19/herrington.html (accessed 20 June 2014).

Hunt, D.P., Haidet, P., Coverdale, J.H. and Richards, B.F. (2003) 'The effect of using team learning in an evidence-based medicine course for medical students', *Teaching and Learning in Medicine*, 15(2): 131–9.

Kassab, S. and Hussain, S. (2010) 'Concept mapping assessment in a problem-based medical curriculum', *Medical Teacher*, 32(11): 926–31.

Knowles, M.S. (1980) *The modern practice of adult education: From pedagogy to andragogy* (2nd edn). New York, NY: The Adult Education Company.

Kolb, D.A. (1984) *Experiential learning: Experience as the source of learning and development*, Englewood Cliffs, NJ: Prentice-Hall.

Lave, J. and Wenger, E. (1991) *Situated learning: Legitimate peripheral participation*, Cambridge, MA: Cambridge University Press.

Lombardi, M. and Oblinger, D. (2007) 'Authentic learning for the 21st century: An overview', *EDUCAUSE*. Online. Available HTTP: http://net.educause.edu/ir/library/pdf/eli3009.pdf (accessed 20 June 2014).

Malik, A.S. and Malik, R.H. (2002a) 'The undergraduate curriculum of Faculty of Medicine and Health Sciences, Universiti Malaysia Sarawak in terms of Harden's 10 questions', *Medical Teacher*, 24(6): 616–21.

Malik, A.S. and Malik, R.H. (2002b) 'Implementation of problem-based learning curriculum in the Faculty of Medicine and Health Sciences, Universiti Malaysia Sarawak', *Journal of Medical Education*, 6(1): 79–86.

Margetson, D. (1997) 'Why is problem-based learning a challenge?' In D. Boud and G.E. Feletti (eds) *The challenge of problem-based learning*, London: Kogan Page.

Maudsley, G. (1999) 'Do we all mean the same thing by problem based learning? A review of the concepts and formulation of the ground rules', *Academic Medicine*, 74(2): 178–85.

McLaughlin, J.E., Roth, M.T., Glatt, D.M., Gharkholonarehe, N., Davidson, C.A., Griffin, L.M., Esserman, D.A. and Mumper, R.J. (2014) 'The flipped classroom: A course redesign to foster learning and engagement in a health professions school', *Academic Medicine*, 89(2): 236–43.

Mennin, S.P. and Martinez-Burrola, N. (1986) 'The cost of problem-based vs traditional medical education', *Medical Education*, 20(3): 187–94.

Michaelsen, L.K., Kinght, A.B. and Fink, L.D. (2002) *Team based learning: A transformative use of small groups in college teaching*, Sterling, VI: Stylus Publishing.

Murphy, J. (2003) 'Task-based learning: The interaction between tasks and learners', *English Language Teaching Journal*, 57(4): 353–60.

Nordquist, J., Sundberg, K., Johansson, L., Sandelin, K. and Nordenstrom, J. (2012) 'Case-based learning in surgery: Lessons learned', *World Journal of Surgery*, 36(5): 945–55.

Parmelee, D. and Hudes, P. (2012) 'Team-based learning: A relevant strategy in health professionals' education', *Medical Teacher*, 34(5): 411–13.

Roberts, C., Lawson, M., Newble, D., Self, A. and Chan, P. (2005) 'The introduction of large class problem-based learning into an undergraduate medical curriculum: An evaluation', *Medical Teacher*, 27(6): 527–33.

Rorty, R. (1991) *Objectivity, relativism and truth*, Cambridge, MA: Cambridge University Press.

Savery, J.R. and Duffy, T.M. (1995) 'Problem based learning: An instructional model and its constructivist framework', *Educational Technology*, 35: 31–8.

Schmidt, H.G. (1993) 'Foundations of problem-based learning: Some explanatory notes', *Medical Education*, 27(5): 422–32.

Schon, D.A. (1983) *Educating the reflective practitioner*, San Francisco, CA: Jossey-Bass.

Seidel, C.L. and Richards, B.F. (2001) 'Application of team learning in a medical physiology course', *Academic Medicine*, 76(5): 533–4.

Srinivasan, M., Wilkes, M., Stevenson, F., Nguyen, T. and Slavin, S. (2007) 'Comparing problem-based learning with case-based learning: Effects of a major curriculum shift at two institutions', *Academic Medicine*, 82(1): 74–82.

Taylor, D. and Hamdy, H. (2013) 'Adult learning theories: Implications for learning and teaching in medical education: AMEE guide no. 83', *Medical Teacher*, 35(11): e1561–72.
Thistlethwaite, J., Davies, D., Ekeocha, S., Kidd, J., MacDougall, C., Matthews, P., Purkis, J. and Clay, D. (2012) 'The effectiveness of case-based learning in health professional education: A BEME systematic review: BEME guide no. 23', *Medical Teacher*, 34(6): e421–44.
Von Glasersfeld, E. (1989) 'Cognition, construction of knowledge and teaching', *Synthese*, 80(1): 121–40.
Vygotsky, L.S. (1978) *Mind in society. The development of higher psychological processes,* Cambridge, MA: Harvard University Press.

11
INTRODUCING EARLY CLINICAL EXPERIENCE IN THE CURRICULUM

Ruy Souza and Antonio Sansevero

The advantages of early exposure in the curriculum to clinics and communities are now well documented.

Early clinical exposure (ECE) is one of the most significant paradigm shifts in modern medical education. The hegemonic model of medical education in the 20th century, derived from the Flexner Report (Flexner 1910), reflected the enchantment of the positivist movement with the development of science at the end of the 19th century (Doll 1993). Flexner proposed a division of the medical curriculum into two branches, beginning with 2 years of a laboratory branch, where the student would receive the foundation of the biomedical sciences, followed by 2 years of training at a hospital branch (Flexner 1910). During the second half of the 20th century, medical education was confronted with new challenges. The rapid growth of biomedical knowledge brought about a progressive separation between the basic and clinical sciences. The pre-clerkship curriculum, based almost exclusively on the transmission of knowledge with little emphasis on the professional aspects of medicine, was slowly dehumanising the formation of physicians.

In the 1950s Case Western Reserve University, USA, introduced a series of reforms to integrate the foundation sciences with clinical practice (Funkestein 1971). The World Federation for Medical Education (WFME), co-sponsored by the World Health Organization, promulgated the 1988 Edinburgh Declaration, setting a climate for change, promoting the integration of science and clinical practice and requiring medical competence to go beyond knowledge recall (Walton 1999). Evidence emerged in the 1990s that most US medical schools did not offer adequate clinical skills training (Nelson and Traub 1993) and in 1993 the UK General Medical Council (GMC) published *Tomorrow's Doctors,* defending early exposure to clinical skills (GMC 1993). Almost 100 after publishing the Flexner Report, the Carnegie Foundation issued a new call for reform in all higher education (Sullivan and Rosin 2008) and subsequently in medical schools, advocating a learning process connected to patient care 'at all levels' (Cooke et al. 2010).

An integrated curriculum has been adopted by several schools as a way to overcome the gap between basic and clinical science. It presents enriched learning experiences and logistical challenges for all concerned. What worked well in both of the following case studies was that an ECE programme was tried, followed by an evaluation. Reflection with feedback resulted in new adjustments being tried that improved the experience for all. In experimenting with ECE what we try, how we try it, and the meaning we make from it are key points in the case studies of the Bond University in Australia and the Gulf Medical University in the United Arab Emirates. In the case of Bond University, the use of active methodologies, such as problem-based learning (PBL), proved to be an effective strategy. However, despite all the advantages of the method, it is still an artificial (*in vitro*) education performed inside classrooms, and it lacks the authenticity necessary for students to understand indepth the practical nuances involved in the complexities of healthcare. As a second step, Bond University defined a series of clinical practices to align with the content of basic sciences to promote ECE.

Case study 11.1   The challenges of integrating early clinical experience into the curriculum – Bond University, Australia

Richard Hays

Bond University, a new medical school in Australia, chose a curriculum model that was highly integrated, both 'horizontally' and 'vertically'. The former reflects integration across disciplines within each year (e.g. anatomy, physiology, genetics) and the latter integration of 'pre-clinical' sciences and clinical practice across years. The conceptual framework was a graduated, 'overlapping-wedge' design that required approximately 10 per cent of Year One to be clinical experience demonstrating the clinical relevance of the foundation sciences. PBL was the chosen integration pedagogy, with relevant clinical scenarios/cases used from the commencement of Year One. These clinical scenarios were relatively simple early in Year One, with complexity increasing by the end of Year Two as the curriculum 'spiralled' twice through material that was presented according to lifecycle stages and then broad disease/illness categories.

The more detailed plan involved aligning the clinical practice proportion, wherever possible, to the content and sequence of the PBL clinical scenarios, which in turn were aligned to the foundation science content. For example, cardiovascular structure and function could be a primary source of learning objectives for a PBL case that involved some form of cardiac emergency, e.g. somebody collapsing in a public place and requiring cardiopulmonary resuscitation. Relevant clinical experiences might include simple cardiovascular and examination skills (pulse rate and blood pressure), attending basic first aid and cardiopulmonary resuscitation training, and observing an ambulance or paramedic service shift. Students would then 'debrief' and integrate within the PBL process what was learned in all of the activities that week. It was realised that mainstream healthcare services (hospitals and primary care practices) might be of limited value for very junior medical students, as their knowledge of healthcare was limited, and so a wider range of broader, community-based, health and social care sector experiences was considered. The result was a list of useful and interesting activities that involved visits to various agencies where nominated supervisors would provide contact with people either in, or at the doorstep of, healthcare. In overview, the planned curriculum appeared to be innovative, exciting for students and potentially supportive of integrated learning.

As with many great ideas, the devil was in the detail of implementation. While the system worked, in that students attended PBL tutorials, several on-campus learning activities (lectures, workshops, skills sessions) and off-campus clinical experiences, the logistical complexity was high. It proved difficult to arrange for all students to have the clinical experience concurrently with the

(continued)

(continued)

relevant science. Such a model required the whole cohort to have the same clinical placement during a single week, which was rarely possible. It did however prove possible for some experiences to take place for all students during a 4-week block, while other experiences were dispersed over the whole semester. Additional challenges came from the training of the local supervisors, many of whom were new to medical education, and to managing the expectations and confidence of students. More work than had been anticipated proved necessary to make explicit the links to the curriculum and the specific roles at each location of both supervisors and students. Examples of extreme misunderstandings included junior students being asked to perform intimate examinations at a women's health clinic (where the goal was talking with women about general health issues) and inviting junior students to observe challenging forensic autopsies (when the goal was understanding cancer and death) (Yardley et al. 2013). Further, students perceived that the clinical experiences were not assessed explicitly and some therefore regarded the visits as irrelevant to their goals.

Aligning ECE with an integrated curriculum proved more challenging than expected. A formative evaluation of the initial implementation proved helpful to address issues, resulting in modification to the curriculum that is now well regarded by students, staff and the accreditation agency. One issue that has emerged, however, is that where training capacity is being fully utilised, using mainstream health facilities to provide clinical experiences to junior students may not be the most efficient use of scarce clinical resources. As a result, medical educators should be very thoughtful and deliberate in deciding where to allocate more junior students, and prioritise mainstream acute healthcare facilities for more senior students (Colquhoun et al. 2009).

In the second case study ECE was introduced to the curriculum via a communication skills course based in practices in the university hospital. Many schools adopt communication skills as a gateway to clinical practice for learners early in their education. An important advantage is that communication skills can be fully and safely practised at primary and secondary healthcare facilities where there is an abundance of people and cases, and where patients frequently have a more active role in medical education than in tertiary hospitals.

Case study 11.2 Integrating early clinical experience in the curriculum – experience from a teaching hospital in United Arab Emirates

Manda Venkatramana and Pankaj Lamba

In 2008 Gulf Medical University (GMU) changed from a traditional discipline-based curriculum to an organ system-based integrated curriculum. A communication skills course was utilised as a means of integrating ECE into the curriculum.

The communication skills course lasts for 3 weeks during Phase I of the integrated MBBS curriculum. Initially it had been taught by didactics, interactive lectures and role play. The revised curriculum sought to provide students with an opportunity to learn communication skills in an authentic, clinical context, thus the 'early patient contact' (EPC) was introduced as an additional teaching / learning strategy.

Two batches of first-year GMU medical students were offered elective posting of early patient experience at Gulf Medical College Hospital at Ajman, United Arab Emirates as part of the communication skills course during the first month of medical school. The EPC was undertaken for 10 hours per week outside routine study hours within the clinical faculties of the Departments of Medicine, Surgery, Obstetrics, Paediatrics, Ophthalmology and Ear, Nose and Throat. Each student was expected to shadow the designated clinical faculty in the ambulatory setting of the hospital for 2 hours per day for a 5-day period. No more than two students were assigned to a clinical faculty member.

The learning objectives for the EPC were provided both to the students and to the faculty supervisors and concerned focusing on the communication skills aspect of the doctor–patient contact, including observing history taking, verbal and non-verbal cues, interpersonal skills and the development of 'right attitudes' by shadowing their role model. The students were instructed to follow all rules and regulations of the Gulf Medical College hospital, adhere strictly to the dress code and wear an identity badge and lab coat at all times while in the hospital. Assessment of communication skills was conducted using a written examination by the Van Dalen paper-and-pen test (Van Dalen et al. 2002) and a video-based Objective Structured Clinical Examination (OSCE) at the end of the communication skills course. Student and faculty feedback were obtained at the end of the EPC posting.

Some social issues and logistical problems were encountered during this experience, including a shortage of clinical training sites; the lack of motivation amongst clinical faculty to accept students at this stage of their education; limiting the number of students per clinician to two at a time; the need for parental permission, especially for female students, to stay back outside routine hours; evening postings and providing transportation to students outside routine hours. The first batch of students was posted with the same clinician for the entire duration of their rotation. This did not find favour with some students. A meeting with the faculty and students was convened to resolve difficult issues. Making it a formal part of the curriculum would overcome some of the logistic issues and the need for parental permission, motivate more clinicians to accept students at an early stage, while rotating the students with different clinical faculty addressed other issues encountered.

The assessment results showed that the EPC programme helped students to improve their communication skills, as indicated by scores obtained on communication skills tests, especially in the OSCE. Students with EPC experience obtained higher scores than those without this experience. The analysis of the feedback showed that faculty and students had positive perceptions about the programme, particularly in relation to student motivation, professionalism, documentation and communication skills (Ventakramana and Lamba 2010 ; Ventakramana et al. 2011, 2012; Lamba and Ventakramana 2012).

ECE needs to be a regular part of the curriculum, starting from the first day of medical school. It enhances communication skills of students and influences the development of positive attitudes.

Bridging the great divide

There exists a great divide in medical education between what is taught and the dynamic context of the medical profession. The educational practice of teaching facts dissociated from patient realities can result in a 50 per cent loss in memory (Custers 2008). There is a popular fable about an old professor of surgery who said in his retirement speech,

> In my first years I used to teach peptic ulcer as a surgical disease, then I had to change and teach it as a clinical disease. Now that I am retiring, it has become an infectious disease. I really do not know where it will stop . . .

We cannot predict what will be important to teach students in the future. It makes sense to focus on the more practical, relevant and essential aspects of the medical profession. As Osler said, 'We can only instil principles, put the student in the right path, give him method, teach him how to study, and early to discern essentials and non-essentials' (Nussbaum 2008: xiii).

Going 'back to the future', the medical teacher now has the task of promoting early discernment of essential and non-essential aspects of medicine, for example, perception of community health necessities, basic clinical and communication skills and interprofessional learning in the workplace, just to name a few. The agenda in medical education is challenged to go beyond isolated content to embrace a competency framework as the basis for undergraduate medical programmes (Harris et al. 2010). The complexity of these themes cannot be explored fully inside the walls of the schools, not even in the most realistic skills laboratory. Effective ECE requires the school to expand and make more permeable its traditional boundaries, its 'walls and halls', to privilege the authenticity of the workplace. Once again, medical education is facing a transformation. Traditionally, the hospital was thought to be the ideal place for training. Not any more. The cost of a tertiary care hospital has become prohibitive. Patients are more acutely ill, they spend less time in the wards, their care is more highly specialised and the teaching and learning opportunities are more limited than ever. The essential lessons from community health and epidemiology are that most threats to human health are better managed outside of the tertiary hospitals.

Responding to contemporary demands and challenges requires that medical schools build networks with the health services to provide students multiple authentic learning opportunities at different levels of complexity. We can see an example of one response to this challenge in Swansea University, in the UK, and how they have approached creating learning opportunities in authentic clinical settings.

Case study 11.3   Early clinical exposure in graduate-entry medicine at Swansea University – Learning Opportunities in the Clinical Setting (LOCS)

Paul Kneath Jones and Judy McKimm

Swansea College of Medicine is the second smallest medical school in the UK, admitting 70 students per year. The graduate-entry medicine (GEM) programme is a 4-year course, open to graduates from any background, and its curriculum philosophy is summarised below as the six Ss:

1. *situated* in the clinical setting, where students learn to be doctors by doing what a doctor does, where a doctor does it;
2. *student*-driven – maximising opportunities for students to work things out for themselves;
3. *spiral* – topics are revisited, reinforcing learning throughout the curriculum;
4. *simulates* clinical practice – centred on patient presentations and clinical cases;
5. *small* – a small cohort with teaching utilising small-group learning as one of the main modalities;
6. *serving* the needs of patients and the public, 'thinking globally, acting locally'.

Many accelerated programmes restrict students' early clinical contact. The GEM curriculum redresses this trend by embedding clinical experience from the first weeks in four ways during the first 2 years:

1. Students have 20 community-based learning days, working in pairs with a general practitioner.
2. Teaching clinical skills with simulation teaching based on a clinical 'case' contextualises learning in the clinical setting.
3. Students spend 5 weeks totally immersed in clinical practice three times during the first 2 years in innovative, 'modern clinical apprenticeships'.
4. All students choose a minimum of 20 LOCS (at least ten per year) to complement and extend learning in other parts of the course.

LOCS are half-day, student-selected, self-managed, experiential clinical encounters, during which students are supervised directly by a clinician. Students select LOCS from a bank of approximately 1,000 that include activities such as working with a paramedic on an ambulance, working alongside a prison doctor, attending a postmortem, accompanying a consultant on a postintake ward round and attending a surgical outpatient clinic. Students learn directly from the supervising clinicians on the job with appropriate safeguards for patient and student safety.

Published findings on the LOCS reveal positive feedback from both students and clinicians (Noor et al. 2011), including: identifying early opportunities to integrate basic science concepts into clinical practice; developing hands-on clinical skills from an early stage of the programme; and tailoring these clinical encounters to their own interests and needs.

Some of the limitations of the LOCS are that opportunities to engage directly in clinical activity are sometimes restricted and limited to observation; maintaining the organisation of so many encounters is sometimes difficult, e.g. students not being expected in a clinical area by clinicians; and the need for greater curriculum alignment with the LOCS.

Improvements have been made and further evaluation of the LOCS through student and teacher feedback is ongoing. Changes include: signposting for greater curriculum alignment; highlighting the relevance of the LOCS to the course; and linking the personal development of the student with a tailored programme to meet individual student needs. This is leading to the identification of specific LOCS which should enhance learning and professional development.

LOCS are one of the innovative ways in which ECE is achieved in the GEM programme in Swansea. The LOCS scheme facilitates the incorporation of student-selected experiential learning into an undergraduate medical education programme which, with careful planning and curriculum alignment, has been tailored to meet students' learning needs.

The three previous case study experiences demonstrate the importance of formative assessment, where effective feedback is the key element of a well-designed educational programme (Wood 2010). Learning opportunities in clinical settings have special implications for the junior medical student. With fewer opportunities in tertiary hospitals, the healthcare services in the communities, especially at the level of primary care, frequently offer the ideal context for learning the medical profession in consonance with the local reality.

Meeting the community health needs

The community can be the ideal 'context for student learning' (Harden 2005), and most schools that adopt ECE do it at a primary care level (Basak et al. 2009). ECE is not about teaching some mechanical procedures to the novice, as is commonly the case with many medical teachers. It is about giving medical students a comprehensive view of the health system and the realities of the medical profession from the beginning of their formation and socialisation into the profession. Advantages of promoting ECE at primary and secondary settings include:

- opportunities to experience the authentic context of the community where students are learning medicine;
- opportunities to understand the therapeutic itinerary of a patient, that is, the path that a person takes until the final healthcare, and which is influenced by economic, social and cultural aspects, reflecting the different concepts of health between individuals;
- multiple situations in which to learn the care of the most prevalent diseases, with a focus on prevention and promotion of health;
- rich and diverse scenarios in which to develop communication skills in an environment where the patient has more autonomy and can participate more fully in the learning experience of the student;
- deeper understanding of the health system and model of health assistance;
- more opportunities to work at an interprofessional level.

When planning an ECE programme in the community, there are four fundamental challenges:

- First, align the programme to the healthcare model of the region where the school is located; for example, the insertion of students into family health teams.
- Second, develop specific and assessable learning objectives with increasing complexity over time, and publicise them among students and health workers.
- Third, promote faculty development towards a comprehensive programme of assessment, with an emphasis on formative assessment as part of an overall programme offering continuous feedback.
- And fourth, train the health team to be an active part of the programme with a significant role in teaching and assessing the students.

The programme at the Suez Canal University in Ismailia, Egypt, provides a good example of community-based education in the early phases of the curriculum, associated with new learning technologies.

Case study 11.4 Integrating early clinical experience in the curriculum of the pre-clinical years at the Faculty of Medicine, Suez Canal University, Egypt

Somaya Hosny and Mirella Youssef Tawfik

At Suez Canal University, the early integration of clinical experience throughout the pre-clerkship phase provides students with earlier patient interactions in order to develop sufficient basic clinical skills training, and the experience and attitudes necessary to become competent, caring physicians. ECE is provided through community-based education activities and clinical skills lab training, with computer-assisted training sessions being introduced for medical students in 2006.

Training in the clinical skills laboratory takes place during Years One through Three (pre-clinical phase) with the aim of standardising the training and evaluation of basic clinical skills, helping students to recognise the clinical relevance of the basic sciences and appreciate how the social, psychological and ethical dimensions of medical practice are interrelated. Students are trained using their peers or mannequins, instructed by trained junior faculty members and guided by regularly updated and standardised checklists.

Recently, increasing class sizes have threatened the level of students' performance in clinical skills. Reported problems include students' inability to watch skills' demonstration properly, insufficient practice time for individual students and more difficulty arranging time for feedback from tutors. To overcome these difficulties, a new instructional method using computer-assisted training (CAT) sessions was introduced. The aim was to create an educational setting that facilitates the maximum use of available scheduled time for training, to increase the mastery of skills. The CAT provides standardised audio-visual and computer-generated multimedia programmes of different skills. These programmes are interactive, self-explanatory, enable proper skill demonstration and ensure enough time for practising skills for all students.

CAT was implemented between 2005 and 2007 in three phases: preparation, implementation and evaluation. The first phase (preparation) involved updating checklists, preparing training settings and materials (models, supplies and equipment) and developing movies. Captured movies were revised and edited to match the updated checklists. Movies were also prepared in a format and installed as links together with a web interface for different links. A server with a local network connected to 16 stations (representing training rooms) was established. Training rooms and materials were prepared to suit the new training method.

The finalised multimedia programmes were implemented with second-year students in 2006. Tutors showed the movie, ensured proper audio-visual demonstration for all students, supervised practice for every student with the revised checklists, gave feedback, replayed sections of the movie which appeared difficult or unclear for students, instructed and supervised re-practice. Students were asked to navigate through the links for the required scientific information. Movies were available outside of the schedule times.

Evaluation consisted of a quality check to determine the extent to which each computerised skill was done using two questionnaires, one for the faculty and one for the students. Results showed both to be satisfied with the product and considered its quality good to excellent. Most faculty agreed on its suitability for self-directed learning. Most students considered the product suitable after few modifications. The percentage of student failures after implementation of the project was significantly lower compared to that of the previous 3 years.

Modifications were done according to suggestions from students and tutors and implemented with students in Years One and Three. In addition, materials were made available for revision by students in the clerkship phase of their education. The method continues to be useful and has been adopted by other faculties of medicine inside and outside Egypt.

The early integration of computer-assisted learning materials improved self-learning and was associated with lower failure rates among students and helped students to be better prepared for the clerkship phase.

Authenticity is key

What we have seen in the case studies so far is that effective integration of students with the health team through authentic tasks is essential. Both the students and the health team need to have a clear idea of the learning goals and the goals should be consistent with the working goals of the health unit. Students should have an active role with health workers and be involved in different tasks (Kachur 2003), thus directing the pedagogy towards an intrinsic component of ECE apprenticeship.

Apprenticeship as an approach to learning is being re-examined in medical education (Dornan 2005; Morris and Blaney 2010). To have a meaningful role as part of the vast domain of medical education, it needs to be approached as a programme designed for learning in the workplace. Authentic patient care and appropriate supervision are essentials aspects of ECE. Faculty development programmes of medical schools will need to be expanded to include health workers from the facilities where students are placed, with special focus on the ability to provide feedback. Student-run clinics (SRCs) during the pre-clerkship years can provide authentic learning scenarios for students, as described in the next case study.

Case study 11.5 Student-run clinics provide authentic patient care roles and activities for early learners, University of California, San Francisco, USA

H. Carrie Chen

The pre-clerkship and classroom-based curriculum in the first 2 years of a 4-year medical programme at the University of California, San Francisco (UCSF) School of Medicine, USA, includes a longitudinal clinical skills course. Students practise interviewing and physical exam skills with peers as well as with real and standardised patients. In addition, they participate in half-day preceptorship experiences in authentic clinical settings approximately every 3 weeks over the 2 years. Despite emphasising preceptorships as a laboratory for hands-on practice of clinical skills with actual patient encounters, many students remain in the observational role with little active participation in the clinical practices of their preceptorship settings. Preceptors are challenged to find appropriate roles and activities for these very early learners, and both preceptors and students may feel the students are not yet capable of contributing to patient care. Students frequently contrast their observational experiences in preceptorships with their more active clinical roles and activities in their elective volunteer clinical experiences.

Approximately 70 per cent of first- and second-year students at UCSF elect to participate in one of four SRCs at the institution, and 20 per cent of second-year students assume leadership roles in these clinics. SRCs are relatively unique to, and increasingly common in, the USA. These clinics are often initiated by students, provide free or low-cost care for underserved (e.g. poor, uninsured, homeless, marginalised) populations, and routinely rely on pre-clerkship student volunteers to provide direct patient care services under the supervision of licensed volunteer physicians.

A published study showed that students in the UCSF SRCs actively engage in authentic patient care activities (Chen et al. 2014) such as patient triage, histories and physical examinations, patient education, minor procedures (phlebotomy and vaccinations), prescription writing, documentation and even billing. Students in leadership roles organise and run the clinics. They manage patient flow, supervise procedures, ensure patient follow-up and take responsibility for community outreach, clinic supplies, budgeting, procurement of funding and quality improvement activities. The SRC preceptors mainly serve as resources to support student work and ensure quality of care by verifying findings, supervising clinical decision making and finalising management plans. In contrast to the preceptorship experiences in our required or formal curriculum, students in our SRCs take on key roles performing authentic activities that contribute meaningfully to patient care, clinic function and professionalisation as part of the learning. They assume roles and activities generally reserved for more advanced learners such as clerkship students.

The SRCs are able to achieve this depth of early learner engagement and clinical participation by constraining the breadth of activities and providing concentrated learner support. Due to focused missions and limited resources, the clinics have a very narrowly defined scope of practice. For example, one clinic focuses entirely on a single disease entity, hepatitis B. Patients present with a small and well-anticipated range of problems, and the clinics only offer a reduced number of available procedures and interventions. Each SRC provides learning experiences to students focusing on the specific areas of knowledge and skills necessary to participate and contribute to that particular clinic. Students learn the clinic's patient population, common presenting problems, basic clinical skills and selected procedural skills (e.g. hepatitis B vaccination). The SRCs also provide students with support in the form of history questionnaires, handbooks containing disease-specific information sheets, illness protocols and operations manuals.

When given adequate focused support, pre-clerkship students are capable of meaningful participation in and contribution to clinical practice. One approach to successful integration of ECEs may be to provide focused experiences in legitimate patient care roles and supervised activities in highly structured/supported environments. UCSF has incorporated SRCs and subspecialty clinics as preceptorship sites in the required pre-clerkship curriculum. Pre-clerkship students are now also provided with practical learning in health coaching skills to support their participation in clinic-specific patient education activities.

The UCSF SRCs demonstrate that, in authentic settings, the preceptor can be responsible for formative assessment of students and represent the main resource from which learners find support. The role of the medical teacher in the workplace has to be more deeply explored in faculty development programmes.

The art of learning a craft

Learning a craft through direct authentic experience in any health profession is reserved for the workplace rather than the classroom. The present chapter illustrates some principles that can be useful for the planning and introduction of an ECE programme. Some necessary steps for an effective ECE programme are suggested.

Coaching: plan a faculty development programme to facilitate coaching

Coaching requires a special eye from the teacher to deliver real-time and specific feedback for special tasks (Collins 2006). It is necessarily linked to an action by the student and implies a formative feedback approach inclusive of knowledge, skills and attitudes together with experience from the coach. A faculty development programme directed to coaching needs to contemplate an educational role for all the health workers involved in the programme rather than only medical teachers.

Developmental: plan authentic learning objectives of increasing dimensionality (low – simple to high – complex)

Students and teachers/preceptors should know what is expected from them in every phase of their training and be well informed of the careful planning of the learning objectives. Learning activities should be reflective and recursive and thus progressively more complex (Doll 1993).

Reflection with action (praxis): plan a formative assessment programme

Offering students opportunities to reflect and to compare their actions to those of an expert, and afterwards to have a chance to modify their performance and do it again, is an effective way to promote learning. This is best achieved through a comprehensive assessment programme with emphasis on the formative assessment.

Exploration: plan an ECE programme with multiple scenarios

Offering tasks in both similar and different contexts helps stimulate learners to reinforce what they can already do and strengthen their ability to adapt and extend their understanding to different scenarios as they become more experienced and sophisticated health team collaborators. This is achieved by offering multiple scenarios of increasing dimensionality in primary, secondary and tertiary levels.

Conclusions

In the 21st century, the learner is becoming progressively less dependent on the teacher to gain factual information and knowledge that can be accessed by simulation and electronic media. There is a growing demand for authentic work-based scenarios where students are able to experience integrated basic and clinical science beginning at the early stages of medical school. The role of the teacher as a support for the apprentice in the process of learning the medical profession is re-emerging. It becomes imperative, therefore, to promote faculty development programmes for a new generation of medical teachers. We can once again embrace the wisdom of Osler (1925: 407), who said, 'I taught medical students in the wards, as I regard this as by far the most useful and important work I have been called upon to do'.

Take-home messages

- Learning objectives need to be linked with and, as much as possible, embedded in authentic tasks.
- Students learn better when actively involved; therefore, when possible, avoid planning a passive role for students limited to observation of the workplace.
- An ECE programme has to be planned collectively and involve the medical school, health units, patients and students. Leaving the health team outside the planning is one of the major reasons programmes fail.
- Plan activities in multiple scenarios and with increasing complexity over time. This requires planners to understand the health network of their region at multiple levels.
- Align and embed the school programme within the regional health assistance model.
- Assure that health workers are an integral part of the team and are involved in the faculty development plan.
- Formative assessment is essential to apprenticeship learning and requires real-time feedback and opportunities to compare, review and replay performance.
- Formative developmental evaluation of new and ongoing ECE programmes is necessary to keep them aligned to the needs of learners, preceptors and health units – fit for purpose.

Bibliography

Basak, O., Yaphe, J., Spiegel, W., Wilm, S., Carelli, F. and Metsemakers, J.F. (2009) 'Early clinical exposure in medical curricula across Europe: an overview', *European Journal of Medical Practice*, 15(1): 4–10.

Chen, H.C., Sheu, L., O'Sullivan, P., ten Cate, O. and Teherani, A. (2014) 'Legitimate workplace roles and activities for early learners', *Medical Education*, 48(2): 136–45.

Collins, A. (2006) 'Cognitive apprenticeship,' in R.K. Sawyer (ed.) *The Cambridge handbook of the learning sciences*, New York, NY: Cambridge University Press.

Colquhoun, C., Hafeez, M.R., Heath, K. and Hays, R.B. (2009) 'Aligning clinical resources to curriculum needs: the utility of a group of teaching hospitals', *Medical Teacher*, 31(12): 1081–5.

Cooke, M., Irby, D.M. and O'Brien, B.C (2010) *Educating physicians: A call for reform of medical school and residency*, San Francisco: Jossey Bass/Wiley.

Custers, E. (2008) 'Long-term retention of basic science knowledge: A review study', in M. Cooke (ed.) *Educating physicians: A call for reform of medical school and residency*, San Francisco: Jossey Bass/Wiley.

Doll, W. (1993) *A post-modern perspective on curriculum*, New York, NY: Teachers College Press.

Dornan, T. (2005) 'Osler, Flexner, apprenticeship and the 'new medical education',' *Journal of the Royal Society of Medicine*, 98(3): 91–5.

Flexner, A. (1910) *Medical education in the United States and Canada. A report to the Carnegie Foundation for the Advancement of Teaching*, Boston: Updyke.

Funkestein, D.H. (1971) 'Medical students, medical schools and society during three eras', in R.H. Coombs (ed.) *Psychosocial aspects of medical training*, Springfield, IL: Charles C. Thomas.

General Medical Council (1993) *Tomorrow's doctors: Recommendations on undergraduate medical education*, London: General Medical Council.

Harden, R. (2005) 'Curriculum planning and development', in J. Dent and R. Harden (eds) *A practical guide for medical teachers*, London: Elsevier.

Harris, P., Snell, L., Talbot, M. and Harden, R.M. (2010) 'Competency-based medical education: implications for undergraduate programs', *Medical Teacher*, 32(8): 646–50.

Hosny, S., Mishriky, A.M. and Youssef, M. (2008) 'Introducing computer-assisted training sessions in the clinical skills lab at the Faculty of Medicine, Suez Canal University', *Medical Teacher*, 30(2): e35–40.

Kachur, E. (2003) 'Observation during early clinical exposure – an effective instructional tool or a bore?', *Medical Education*, 37(2): 88–9.

Lamba, P. and Ventakramana, M. (2012) 'Student's and teacher's perceptions of Early Patient Contact program at the Gulf Medical University', poster presented at Association of Medical Education in Europe conference August 2012, Lyon, France.

Morris, C. and Blaney, D. (2010) 'Work-based learning', in T. Swanwick (ed.) *Understanding medical education. Evidence, theory and practice*, London: Wiley-Blackwell.

Nelson, M.S. and Traub, S. (1993) 'Clinical skills training of U.S. medical students', *Academic Medicine*, 68(12): 926–8.

Noor, S., Batra, S. and Byrne A. (2011) 'Learning opportunities in the clinical setting (LOCS) for medical students: a novel approach', *Medical Teacher*, 33(4): e193–8.

Nussbaum, M.S. (2008) 'Preface to the first edition', in W. Stehr (ed.) *The Mont Reid surgical handbook*, Philadelphia, PA: Saunders/Elsevier.

Osler, W. (1925) *AEQUANIMITAS, with other addresses to medical students, nurses and practitioners of medicine*, Philadelphia, PA: P. Blakiston's Son & Company.

Sullivan, W. and Rosin, M.S. (2008) *A new agenda for higher education: Shaping a life of the mind for practice*, San Francisco, CA: Jossey-Bass.

Van Dalen, J., Kerkhofs, E., Verwijnen, G.M., van Knippenberg-van den Berg B.W., van den Hout, H.A., Scherpbier, A.J. and van der Vleuten, C.P. (2002) 'Predicting communication skills with a paper-and-pencil test', *Medical Education*, 36(2): 148–53.

Ventakramana, M. and Lamba, P. (2010) 'Perceptions of first year medical students regarding experience of early patient contact program during the communication skills course at Medical University in UAE'. Oral presentation at International Conference in Medical Education (ICME 2010), 4–7 December 2010, Abu Dhabi.

Ventakramana, M., Lamba, P. and Ajay, S. (2011) 'Perceptions of first year medical students about importance of professionalism during early patient contact program at Medical University in UAE', poster presented at Association of Medical Education in Europe conference, August 2011, Vienna, Austria.

Ventakramana, M., Lamba, P. and Ajay, S. (2012) 'Performance of students in communication skills after EPC program in UAE', poster presented at Association of Medical Education in Europe conference, August 2012, Lyon, France.

Walton, H. (1999) 'The Edinburgh declaration: Ten years afterwards', *Journal of the International Association of Medical Science*, 9: 3–7.

Wood, D.F. (2010) 'Formative assessment', in T. Swanwick (ed.) *Understanding medical education: Evidence, theory and practice*, New Jersey, NJ: Wiley-Blackwell.

Yardley, S., Brosnan, C., Richardson, J. and Hays, R. (2013) 'Authentic early experience in medical education: A socio-cultural analysis identifying important variables in learning interactions within workplaces', *Advances in Health Sciences Education*, 18(5): 873–91.

12
BENEFITS AND CHALLENGES ASSOCIATED WITH INTRODUCING, MANAGING, INTEGRATING AND SUSTAINING COMMUNITY-BASED MEDICAL EDUCATION

Regina Helena Petroni Mennin

> *Some schools have successfully integrated the academic-based and community-based activities necessary for a comprehensive education of tomorrow's doctors.*

Community-based medical education (CBME) offers unique, foundational learning opportunities in the praxis of local healthcare as an integral part of regional and national healthcare systems. It works well to provide a broad spectrum of authentic, accessible learning experiences that embody the social determinants of health.

As a broad concept, CBME has been well discussed in the literature (Boaden and Bligh 1999; Magzoub and Schmidt 2000; Thistlethwaite et al. 2013). Considering that an important role of a medical school is to prepare students to work with and improve the health of populations, the school must be capable of providing learning activities for students related to primary care for people and families in the local community (Starfield et al. 2005) as well as opportunities to continue to study toward specialisation, thus making available the full spectrum of healthcare resources, services and learning opportunities. The introduction, management, integration and sustainability of CBME have been challenging for medical schools, communities, preceptors, students, teachers, citizens and health workers. The questions and issues addressed in this chapter are about 'what works', what it means for all concerned and what can be done to continue the development of CBME and improve community health.

Education placed in the community requires the revision of teaching and learning methods, especially in relation to learning from practice, reflection, feedback, assessment and curriculum evaluation (Mann et al. 2009). Education placed in the community works best when it involves the participation of all stakeholders, including students, teachers, health professionals, community members and representatives of other sectors, all actively engaged in bringing a higher dimension to learning than that available in the classroom. The authenticity of early and sustained CBME is challenging for hospital, clinics and university-based teachers. Sustainable success is possible if community and university-based learning are linked in an interdependent way. Otherwise, students are conflicted and have to play games with mixed loyalties, survival and power at the expense of their learning.

The use of different settings for teaching and learning is not new. Some of the elements that favour the implementation of medical education in community settings are based on health policies adopted by local, regional and national institutions, and these vary between countries. The relationship between the delivery of healthcare services and education is complex in all countries (Boaden and Bligh 1999). Societal need for healthcare remains the driving force behind the need for physicians (Takahashi et al. 2011). The choice of government, the role of ministries of health and education, the freedom of medical schools to choose the curriculum and the relationship between private and public educational systems all play a role in the education of health professionals. Other important problems to address in many countries concern severe staff shortages and/or maldistribution of health personnel, often aggravated by the disintegration of health systems that can have damaging effects on the production, recruitment and retention of health professionals (Lehmann et al. 2008).

If that weren't enough, healthcare continues to change from a focus on the episodic care of individuals in hospitals to the promotion of healthy families in the community. Medical schools need to be part of this change (Jones et al. 2001). How can a school choose to prepare future healthcare professionals, adopt a broader view of social reality, deal with the problems of society and address contemporary issues related to students wanting to specialise too early in their educational trajectory? Early specialisation reduces a student's freedom of opportunity to learn.

What works for all concerned with CBME is when medical schools establish professional relationships between general practitioners and students, when the school provides clear learning objectives and guidelines, and when there is adequate and sufficient infrastructure and university support. Flinders University Medical School in Adelaide, South Australia is recognised for its innovations in CBME. Student competencies are established by an interdisciplinary team that embraces the complexities of medical education without the hegemony of reductionism and fragmentation, and it works well.

Case study 12.1   Flinders University Parallel Rural Community Curriculum

Jennene Greenhill

The Flinders University Parallel Rural Community Curriculum (PRCC) provides a novel approach to studying medicine. The PRCC enables students to learn in a complex adaptive system via an innovative model called symbiotic clinical education (Prideaux et al. 2007). The underlying philosophy is one of mutually beneficial partnerships between health services, universities, individual students, clinicians, governments and communities.

The PRCC was established in 1997 in the Riverland South Australia, for a group of eight students, and was the first longitudinal integrated clerkship programme in Australia. The programme has now grown, with up to 36 students spending the entire third year of their MD programme in rural communities. In some regions, they can stay until they complete their internship. Groups of eight to ten students are based in four distinctive rural regions: the Riverland, Greater Green Triangle, Hills Mallee Fleurieu and the Barossa Valley.

Students live in small rural communities while they learn by being immersed in general practices and health services. The university employs rural general practitioners (GPs) as clinical educators and provides them with faculty development. Their role is to organise and deliver the education programme, undertake assessments and liaise with other clinicians and academics who teach. Clinical educators have time to develop long-term relationships with their students and help them to move out of their comfort zone towards 'the edge of learning'. This continuity of learning helps them to deal with the uncertainty and unpredictability of clinical practice (Hirsh et al. 2007). Clinicians orchestrate learning opportunities and guide students as they develop clinical reasoning. They encourage their students to practise skills, explore different roles, reflect on the wider implications and provide quality and safety for patients. Students transform over time and shape their new professional identity as doctors.

The university also provides infrastructure at each general practice by building multipurpose consulting rooms that can be used for visiting specialists, Indigenous health clinics and student consulting. Students see patients every day under supervision and 'in parallel' with the GPs (Walters et al. 2011). Students are integrally part of the multidisciplinary team in their practice. All rural general practices enjoy being fully engaged in the students' learning experiences and many have recruited graduates who are now also involved in teaching. Therefore, the future sustainability of the PRCC programme and rural medical workforce is assured.

Each of the four regions has a dedicated administration team that organises high-quality accommodation within each community and schedules weekly study days. Study days consist of problem-based learning tutorials, visiting specialists' lectures and clinical simulation sessions. The administrators all live locally and assist the students to care for their own well-being and that of their family. They also have a network of community groups and individuals who ensure students are socially connected and thoroughly enjoy the rural lifestyle. A decade of research and evaluation demonstrates positive programme outcomes, excellent academic achievement, rural retention and community engagement.

The PRCC brings human and social capital to underserved rural areas; there is employment for local rural people and it has also brought young professionals, clinicians and academics to live in rural towns. There have been added socio-economic benefits to rural communities: a university presence in a small rural town makes a significant impact. The PRCC has won several national awards and the clinical simulation team has won awards for excellence in teaching from the Australian Learning and Teaching Council, presented at a glittering ceremony at the Sydney Opera House. The university has also built physical infrastructure with several new buildings constructed at hospitals. There are several PhD students and research has been undertaken on health priorities, including mental health, Indigenous health, stroke epidemiology, cardiac rehabilitation and rural health workforce issues.

Benefits of CBME

The above case study from Flinders illustrates several benefits of CBME at the level of the local community, society, teachers and learners. Students develop skills and performance capabilities through real problems that influence the attitudes of future professionals (Mennin and Petroni-Mennin 2006). At the same time, students can develop skills in health education and health promotion, work in multidisciplinary teams and increase social commitments and responsibilities. They can learn how to work with diversity and can go beyond the health sector to understand the interactive roles that economics, education, sanitation and housing have in people's health.

CBME depends on the focus of the curriculum developed in the medical school, i.e. the extent to which public health and preventive medicine are a central or a peripheral part of the curriculum. The International Conference on Primary Healthcare Declaration of Alma-Ata (World Health Organization (WHO) 1978) underlined the importance of primary healthcare. It was recognised as the principal means for attainment of health for all, and as the first level of national healthcare systems. However, many governments are still struggling to launch and sustain primary healthcare at an adequate level (Hall and Taylor 2003). Attention to improve the health of the population is a necessary measure that goes beyond timely intervention at a hospital. The World Federation for Medical Education Edinburgh declaration strongly recommended student learning in authentic scenarios (World Federation for Medical Education 1988).

Other competencies students can achieve in CBME include a practical feel for both a rural and urban community as a geographic area. This can be done by mapping frequency and distribution of health problems, establishing epidemiological studies to address and solve local health problems, prioritising areas with the worst problems, knowing the social programmes and including the participation of the community in decision-making processes at the primary care level. The following case study from Indonesia demonstrates the ways in which a community-oriented medical curriculum seeks to combine the development of theoretical knowledge, and its application through teaching and research to identify and tackle local health problems.

Case study 12.2 Community-oriented education, Faculty of Medicine, University of Airlangga, Indonesia

Nancy Margarita Rehatta and Adrianta Surjadhana

Our medical school was established in 1913 as Nederlands Indische Artsen School in East Java, Indonesia. During the era of Japanese occupation it became known as Ika Daigaku, before becoming the state-run Faculty of Medicine, University of Airlangga (FMUA) in 1954. The curriculum is conducted over 11 semesters, in two stages: the academic phase (seven semesters), after which the graduate obtains a *Sarjana Kedokteran* (equal to Bachelor of Medicine); and professional phase (four semesters), after which the graduate becomes a medical doctor. The medical doctor then undertakes a 1-year internship managed by the Ministry of Health.

Medical schools need to be socially accountable, in directing their education, research and service activities towards addressing the priority health concerns of the community, region and/or nation they have mandated to serve (Boelen and Heck 1995). In line with this, the vision of FMUA is to ensure that research and education programmes aim to improve the health of the community. Research is conducted to identify the community health needs, and the results translated into a set of competencies that should be achieved by all Indonesian medical school graduates with primary health as the basic concern (Indonesian Medical Council 2012).

Teaching community medicine began at FMUA in 1971, when the WHO conducted a seminar on community medicine for medical teachers with participants from Association of South East Asian Nations (ASEAN) countries. In 1979 the WHO South East Asia Regional Office (SEARO) had a meeting at FMUA regarding the reorientation of medical education, and community-oriented medical education (COME) was accepted as a part of medical education content. It took another 17 years before community medicine became formally included in the curriculum.

The FMUA has a hybrid curriculum, with basic science lectures within integrated blocks to provide detailed understanding on certain topics. The educational programme is not solely based on community objectives or delivered in a community setting; rather, the community-oriented curriculum is achieved by embedding the community needs in the basic science and clinical programmes, and having a holistic perspective in managing healthcare. Interactive lectures provide a theoretical understanding of basic sciences, while the integrated blocks provide a more applied understanding of topics such as human interaction, holistic health and concepts such as wellness and illness. Table 12.1 provides an overview of the content of the academic phase, while Table 12.2 presents the community medicine programmes of the professional phase, which are all about working and researching in the community.

Our learning strategy includes special initiatives, such as:

- community service learning, which starts early in the semester to encourage the development of empathy and 'soft' skills;
- a joint palliative home care team;
- a 1-day programme for children with special needs/disabilities arranged in collaboration with external social organisations.

Assessment is based on the students writing short essays on their experiences and must be submitted directly after the programme. We have been surprised at the major impact even such short experiences can have on students' attitudes, particularly their awareness of the need to give a helping hand to people with disabilities. The availability of high-quality healthcare that is culturally sensitive is an important issue in a country like Indonesia with numerous ethnic groups.

Table 12.1 Academic phase

Semester	Topic	Learning strategy
1	Integrated module: Human interaction	Interactive lecture, problem-based learning session
1	Integrated module: Holistic approach – host, agent and environment	Interactive lecture, problem-based learning session
2	Public health and preventive medicine 1	Interactive lecture
2	Integrated module: wellness illness concept	Interactive lecture, problem-based learning session
4	Public health and preventive medicine 2	Interactive lecture
4	Integrated module: Tropical medicine	Interactive lecture, problem-based learning session, community survey and counselling, laboratory work
6	Social internship programme: Learn with community (university-based)	Interprofessional working in the community
7	Public health and preventive medicine 3	Interactive lecture

Table 12.2 Professional phase

Topic	Learning strategy
Public health and preventive medicine	Research inspired by (local) community needs
Community medicine	Work in the community with the community

(continued)

(continued)

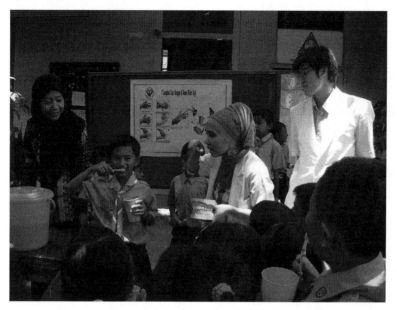

Figure 12.1 Guidance and counselling on the right way of brushing teeth. (Courtesy of Adrianta Surjadhana.)

After being introduced to social medicine in the academic phase, the students spend 1 month in the district health centre during the professional stage. This is a part of a community medicine programme that is intended to offer practical experience of working in the natural environment of various culture groups, including underserved and marginalised groups (Figure 12.1). These programmes are managed by FMUA in partnership with the community, healthcare providers and local government.

Learning from experience, professional behaviour, leadership and effective communication are all competencies needed in serving the community. Of vital importance is supporting the teacher and encouraging the teacher's responsibility as a role model of professional performance. This has been hard to achieve, and we are still looking for a better approach.

In conducting research as a part of their educational programme, the students are free to choose the topic, but are asked to ensure that the research question is inspired by community needs and could be implemented to address community health problems. In the last 5 years several research projects have provided valuable insights for addressing community health issues and changing the existing health system.

Through the implementation of a community-oriented curriculum, we have sought to improve the social accountability of our educational programme to the community we serve. The community needs high-quality healthcare, and for this we need to produce high-quality students with appropriate knowledge and levels of professionalism. Teachers are important role models, and their standards will influence the quality of performance.

The experience of placing students in the community with an emphasis on primary care gives students the opportunity to approximate the different environments of human caring and technology.

Personal responsibility for health at the local level increases the understanding of the diverse factors involved in the social determination of health and disease and the impact of class differences on people's health. The programme established in the Nelson Mandela School of Medicine, South Africa, illustrates the importance of CBME in improving population health.

Case study 12.3 The Selectives Programme for undergraduate medical students, Nelson R. Mandela School of Medicine, University of KwaZulu-Natal, KwaZulu-Natal, South Africa

Stephen Knight and Jacqueline van Wyk

Using the community-oriented primary care (COPC) approach and a social accountability framework, the Selectives Programme aims to develop medical students who are responsive to the needs of local communities and who will become socially accountable agents of change in the ailing South African healthcare system.

The Nelson R. Mandela School of Medicine, at the epicentre of the human immunodeficiency virus (HIV), acquired immunodeficiency syndrome (AIDS) and tuberculosis epidemics in KwaZulu-Natal, serves a predominantly rural population of about 10.6 million people. The COPC model was developed by Sidney and Emily Kark in the rural Pholela district in the 1940s and became an integral part of the Durban Medical School in the 1950s. Moving from the traditional disease-focused approach, COPC responded to the social determinants of health based on community needs, especially where primary healthcare interventions could be measured using epidemiological principles involving multidisciplinary teams. It also acknowledged the proactive role of primary healthcare providers as stakeholders in integrated prevention, health promotion and curative services. The social medicine philosophy that emphasises equal and good healthcare for all contradicted the apartheid government's plans that neglected to address indigenous health. The initial curriculum at the school had a strong eurocentric, biomedical and tertiary hospital-based focus.

The medical curriculum was reviewed following the democratic elections of 1994, with the recognition that healthcare was failing the poor and majority rural population. It was realigned with the Millennium Development Goals, and the Selectives Programme based on COPC was introduced.

Three Selectives modules are now undertaken in the second, third and fourth academic years. Clear learning outcomes are prescribed for these modules, unlike with an elective, where students decide how to spend their time. Academics from family medicine, public health medicine and rural health are collectively responsible for the design, coordination, delivery and assessment of students on the programme. Students choose their own Selectives site, usually near their home town, and are encouraged to work in groups of two to four. During each 4-week block, the self-selected groups identify a local primary care practitioner as a facilitator with whom to liaise for placement.

Portfolios are presented as evidence of learning. These individual assignments in the form of records and reflections are submitted electronically and include descriptions of observed primary healthcare consultations, a practice profile based on the basic patient data collected and a description and assessment of primary healthcare resources in the Selectives site. Students identify a patient with a chronic condition (or a newborn baby) and conduct home visits over the 3 years, describing the individual, family and environmental situation in which the patient lives to gain a greater understanding longitudinally of the psycho-social factors that have an impact on patients' well-being.

(continued)

(continued)

As a group they formulate a community diagnosis based on disease patterns they have identified. Each student then conducts a brief referenced literature review on an identified community health problem, emphasising a psycho-social perspective of the problem.

The group returns to the same community in their third year, having prepared a protocol for a community-based research survey following instruction in research methods and obtaining ethical approval from the Institutional Ethics Review Board. The fieldwork is conducted on 100 participants from the Selectives site. When back in the community, they follow up on the patients from their previous year and record their participation in primary healthcare patient examinations, building on what they learned during earlier Selectives, and these reports are submitted electronically for assessment. The group presents a scientific research poster at a research day, where they are assessed by their peers and a panel of assessors as evidence of learning.

The research findings and community diagnosis are then used to develop a community-based health promotion activity plan in their fourth year. Students have to evaluate the intervention and present their findings to peers and assessors from a population perspective, detailing the health promotion activity and its evaluation, reflections of the longitudinal patient follow-up and an evaluation of the prescription and primary healthcare facility usage.

The value of the programme lies in the local engagement of students with real situations in the community, which serves to improve their knowledge of health systems and clinical skills through experience with both rural and clinical environments. The community engagement extends the learning platform, and students form long-term relationships with their peers and community members while they gain a deeper understanding of the healthcare system and its responsiveness to community health needs. Students also develop self-reliance, teamwork and research skills through real projects that show them how research can be made relevant to impoverished communities.

Challenges for implementing CBME that works

Classification and taxonomy of CBME and COPC have helped to clarify terminology and description of the field, promoting greater understanding of community medical education (Magzoub and Schmidt 2000). The field has grown and extended to include learning about the integral relationship of political and economic aspects of society that have an important role in policy decisions about population health at the level of the community (Thistlethwaite et al. 2013). The development of a greater appreciation of the importance of the relationship between early and sustained community experience, social responsibility and medical education is a welcome development, although still in its infancy (Boelen and Woollard 2009).

A significant challenge, now gaining some traction, relates to who goes to medical school. Most students who access medical schools come from well-to-do families, bringing a bias to the future role of the physician in society (Almeida-Filho 2011). Strong competition for entry to medical courses that carry high social prestige often involves expensive preparatory courses that effectively make medicine a monopoly of the affluent classes and further reinforces individualistic values and practices and for-profit approaches to healthcare (Almeida-Filho 2011). The historical development of universities in countries previously colonised by Western powers has a bias toward individualism and self-interest more than collective health and community health experiences (Bleakley 2006). Students and professionals prefer to do what they know best, which favours big-city life over life in rural communities. Some factors that influence medical students' decision to choose a career in primary care have been shown to be related to the students' social class, the extent of their exposure to a rural area, having a rural background, the influence of role models and working conditions (Puertas et al. 2013).

Wealth and money have other, sometimes more subtle, influences on CBME and COPC. There is a romantic, naïve point of view that developing countries are immune to pressure from for-profit managed care and the push to privatise local and regional health systems, when often the opposite happens (Waitzkin et al. 2001). Health systems and health professionals in economically developing regions are pressured by technology and pharmaceutical industries, and practitioners are lured by the promise of large profits that often accompany the practice of specialties compared with primary care (Iriart et al. 2011). This monetary culture influences what students see and with whom they learn. For example, the private sector promotes an individualistic ideology in which public service is sometimes considered as merely underpaid employment that, although stable compared with private entrepreneurship for-profit health enterprises, is less financially rewarding (Almeida-Filho 2011).

The presence of affirmative action in medical schools is relatively new and requires further study. It was only in 2012 that affirmative action become law in Brazil for federal schools and colleges, and advanced the debate about the democratisation of universities and a more equitable public policy mechanism to address the comparatively low numbers of economically disadvantaged young people entering higher education in Brazil (Brasil 2012).

Another challenge at a national level is that economically developed countries promote and export their medical educational models internationally to underdeveloped countries that seek to attain similar 'high standards of practice'. There is a risk of neo-colonisation of minds and hearts toward a replication of individualistic educational models which may be less fit for purpose in developing economies given local resources and realities (Bleakley 2006, 2010; Bleakley et al. 2008, 2011).

It is not easy to attract teachers and health professionals to work at the community level, especially when the urban and rural areas are poor, under-resourced and, at times, violent (Lehmann et al. 2008). There is a continuous struggle to convince the medical school, students, parents and teachers to assume social responsibility for health work in these areas. The social class of medical students and health professionals plays a significant role in decisions to work or not to work in particular communities and in particular geographic locations (Hall 2005). Moving educational experiences into authentic scenarios such as the community health centres creates a challenge to provide qualified preceptors for students. There was, and still is, a need for more physicians able to work in the area of health profession education. Preceptors are by and large without sufficient pedagogical guidance and financial support to prepare them for primary healthcare and CBME responsibilities. Academic incentives and recognition for teaching and training physicians vary from low to non-existent. Primary healthcare still carries a negative stigma and social devaluation in relation to specialty practices in medicine.

Another challenge not yet fully appreciated across the medical education field is the density of the medical curriculum that leaves little time and space for other, more general studies necessary to promote broad humanistic views of caring and curing among health professionals (Todres et al. 2009). A related challenge concerns the differences in learning experiences of students working with preceptors where access to healthcare is a right of all citizens and those working in systems where access is based on ability to pay. In both cases it is important to recognise that CBME is not poor medicine for poor people in communities being exploited by universities and students practising on underserved populations (Mennin and Petroni-Mennin 2006). It is important to understand that in many countries it is common to use poor people to practise medicine, which would not be acceptable or possible with more affluent people.

Cultural competencies

CBME offers experiences related to culture, ethics and professionalism that cannot be achieved in the classroom (Kodjo 2009). Cross-cultural understanding in healthcare is essential to overcome barriers between patients and healthcare providers to ensure effective healthcare delivery and medical compliance. This dimension of the health profession is learned best in authentic experiences like those described in the next two stories about 'going home', meaning going back to the community.

Case study 12.4 '... and my patient died happy and cured', an experience in Brazil

Ruy Souza

My Yanomami patient had his first seizure in the middle of a festival in his village in northern Brazil, near the border with Venezuela. He was immediately separated from his family. The tribe knew the risks that certain neurological diseases could bring to the community. A few years ago an outbreak of meningococcal meningitis had devastating effects on the village. Moreover, as a member of an extremely ancient nomadic Indian society that survives by hunting and gathering natural resources in the rainforest, the situation could bring serious risks to families.

The case evolved into a status epilepticus, and my patient had to be transferred to a tertiary hospital, where the diagnosis was quick: glioblastoma multiforme, a highly aggressive tumour that occupied much of the right cerebral hemisphere, totally beyond therapeutic possibilities. After a palliative treatment, the patient experienced significant improvement. His movements partially returned and he could now communicate with the healthcare team with the help of a translator. However, in the second week of hospitalisation, the patient was isolated in what appeared to be a severe depression; a psychiatric evaluation diagnosed psychotic depression. He refused to eat and talk with members of the staff. He even refused to return to his community. It was necessary to initiate parenteral nutrition.

After 3 weeks, with the help of an anthropologist, it was suggested that we try a consultation with an Indian medicine man. Arriving at the hospital, the healer wanted to talk to me before seeing the patient. He was concerned whether the disease was transmissible and the possible risks to other members of the village. After being assured about the safety of the situation for the others members of the tribe, he performed a religious ritual at the bedside, and declared the patient cured. The result was dramatic. My patient began to interact with everyone, quickly recovered his nutritional status and then asked to return to his tribe. When asked why he did not express his wish to return to his tribe earlier, he told me that it was because now he was feeling healed. With the help of an indigenous agency, he returned to his tribe. After a few months, I found the medicine man and asked how my former patient was. He told me that the patient returned and was able to reintegrate into his community, and after 4 months he died. When I said I was sorry, the healer said, 'You shouldn't be, because he died happy and cured!'

A similar, yet different, case illustrates the interwoven relationship between hospital and community at an urban setting when a preceptor's responsibility goes beyond the hospital.

> **Case study 12.5   Beyond the hospital, Brazil, South America**
>
> *Regina Helena Petroni Mennin*
>
> I had just begun to work in the university hospital as a health educator in 1984 when I was asked to speak with Mr Manuel, who had been hospitalised with cirrhosis of the liver and abdominal ascites due to alcohol abuse. He owned a bar in the *favela* (slum) beside the hospital where he sold and consumed alcoholic beverages. It was the first time the university hospital had hired a health educator, so it was not clear what my role was. I was asked to convince him to go home, so he could be discharged from the hospital, as they needed the bed.
>
> Mr Manuel explained that many medical students had come to palpate his belly until it hurt and that they talked and talked about things with words he could not understand. He did not want to go home with a big belly because he had come to the hospital to treat it. He wanted the physician to remove more liquid from his belly. He was ashamed to go back home with the same big belly. After so many days in the hospital, he thought he should be cured by now. He showed me the dietary plan he had received from the dietician and asked me, 'Who will cook like this for me?'
>
> There was an impasse. The hospital needed the bed and wanted to discharge him, knowing that they could not cure his problem and he would probably be back in few days. Mr Manuel did not understand his prognosis and no one had made it clear for him. What Mr Manuel did know was that he would not be able to take care of himself and there was nothing the hospital could do about that. There was no one who could help him and he did not want to go home with a big, swollen belly.
>
> At that time, there was no way to interweave hospital care and home care for Mr Manuel. Students were taught to treat diseases, not sick people, and follow-up home care was not considered part of hospital care. It made a big impression on me that physicians and students couldn't communicate effectively with Mr Manuel. They didn't ask him about his life's circumstances and couldn't understand his context. Who cared? Who was caring? Who treated him? It is not always possible to cure, yet it is always possible to care.
>
> Brazil changed their healthcare model from one based principally on emergency care predominantly in large hospitals to a primary care model in which the family in their own environment became the focus for delivery (Saúde 1998). These changes were necessary to address the preponderance of specialised hospital patient care that had become fragmented to the detriment of the patient. The new model included actions for health promotion, prevention, recovery and rehabilitation of diseases and common injuries, and included medical students at different levels.
>
> Today, if Mr Manuel were to be seen in that same hospital, he would be discharged with home healthcare services, including medical and nursing care. The new model is implemented in a way that is developing and staying responsive to local population healthcare needs. Still, there remain many challenges to improve continuity of healthcare.

CBME: what works?

CBME provides students with authentic learning experiences that promote actions necessary for health promotion, prevention, recovery and rehabilitation from common diseases and injuries. At the same time, students learn the imperative of integrating the relevant physiological, sociological and psychological impact of patient problems in the face of healthcare disparities. The opportunity to learn in scenarios in which the vast majority of the population is cared for by health services, and to experience medicine in a more integrated and inclusive manner, has made learning experiences more meaningful (Muller et al. 2010).

Early community education experience orients medical curricula towards the social context of practice, eases students' transition to the clinical environment, enhances their motivation to learn, contributes to increased confidence in approaching patients and makes them more aware of themselves and others (Dornan and Bundy 2004). Early and sustained CBME experiences work. Students' theoretical knowledge is enhanced, becomes stronger, deeper and more contextualised and CBME strengthens the role of professionals working with students in their approach to learning (Dornan and Bundy 2004; Muller et al. 2010).

Key factors, benefits and challenges for students learning with CBME

- CBME provides authentic connections among students, patients and families.
- CBME provides continuity for students in authentic community settings for longer periods of time and during different phases of their education.
- CBME enhances engagement of students and preceptors.
- CBME provides early experiences of working in multidisciplinary teams and being part of a health network.
- CBME demands clear learning outcomes.
- It benefits from timely assessment and feedback.

Key factors, benefits and challenges for teachers, community and the medical school when CBME is present

- Promotes curriculum change.
- Raises questions about the processes of student selection and admission to medical school.
- Establishes and recognises the functional relationship between the university and health services.
- Requires different faculty development for teachers and preceptors.
- Promotes a career pathway for preceptors as clinical educators.
- Requires the university and community to establish an infrastructure to receive students.
- Requires a plan to have an impact on the community, developing local solutions for local needs and developing health promotion practices.
- Engages community providers and key partners collaboratively to conceive and sustain the CBME programme.
- Establishes a CBME team inside the medical school as well a health professional team in the community.

CBME relates to the place, practice, subjects involved and the nature and substance of learning activities that constitute the complex inter-relationships among teaching and learning, practising and experiencing. It includes technologies as well as the moral and ethical precepts of individual and collective behaviours. It is related to students' comprehension and practice grounded in the nature of the problems they will face in the future as professionals. It brings authenticity to the identification of the social, economic, biological and environmental factors in the process of health–disease and provides cultural competence facing uncertainty.

Take-home messages

- The value of CBME lies in the local engagement of students with authentic situations in the community, the goals of which include improving the local and regional health system and enhancing the relevance of student knowledge and clinical skills through the collaborative involvement of the medical school and community.
- Implementing sustainable CBME, like healthcare itself, is a continuous challenge.
- CBME engages students and universities in the full spectrum of the social determinants of health.
- Making CBME work depends on the broadness of the conception of the programme, the capacity of medical and health professionals to work effectively within the health system for healthcare delivery and the degree of clarity of the activity expected from health personnel and medical students.

Bibliography

Almeida-Filho, N. (2011) 'Higher education and healthcare in Brazil', *The Lancet*, 377(9781): 1898–1900.

Bleakley, A. (2006) 'Broadening conceptions of learning in medical education: the message from team working', *Medical Education*, 40(2): 150–7.

Bleakley, A. (2010) 'Social comparison, peer learning and democracy in medical education', *Medical Teacher*, 32(32): 878–9.

Bleakley, A., Brice, J. and Bligh, J. (2008) 'Thinking the post-colonial in medical education', *Medical Education*, 42(3): 266–70.

Bleakley, A., Bligh, J. and Browne, J. (2011) *Medical education for the future: Identity, power and location*, Dordrecht: Springer.

Boaden, N. and Bligh, J. (1999) *Community-based medical education: Toward a shared agenda for learning*, London: Arnold.

Boelen, C. and Heck, J.E. (1995) *Defining and measuring the social accountability of medical school*, Geneva: WHO. Online. Available HTTP: http://whqlibdoc.who.int/hq/1995/WHO_HRH_95.7.pdf (accessed 1 July 2014).

Boelen, C. and Woollard, B. (2009) 'Social accountability and accreditation: A new frontier for educational institutions', *Medical Education*, 43(9): 887–94.

Brasil (2012) Lei nº 12.711, de 29 de agosto de 2012 dispõe sobre a reserva de 50% das matrículas por curso e turno nas 59 universidades federais e 38 institutos federais de educação, ciência e tecnologia a alunos oriundos integralmente do ensino médio público, em cursos regulares ou da educação de jovens e adultos. Lei nº 12.711. C. Nacional. Brasília, DF, *Diário Oficial da União*. Lei nº 12.711: 1–2.

Community Medicine Unit Faculty of Medicine (2012) *Community medicine profile*, Surabaya: Faculty of Medicine Airlangga University.

Dornan, T. and Bundy, C. (2004) 'What can experience add to early medical education? Consensus survey', *British Medical Journal*, 329(329): 834–7.

Hall, P. (2005) 'Interprofessional teamwork: professional cultures as barriers', *Journal of Interprofessional Care*, 19(Supp 1): 188–96.

Hall, J.J. and Taylor, R. (2003) 'Health for all beyond 2000: The demise of the Alma-Ata Declaration and primary health care in developing countries', *The Medical Journal of Australia*, 178(1): 17–20.

Hirsh, D., Ogur, B., Thibault, G. and Cox, M. (2007) 'New models of clinical clerkships: 'continuity' as an organizing principle for clinical education reform', *New England Journal of Medicine*, 356(8): 858–66.

Indonesian Medical Council (2012) *Standard competence for Indonesian doctor*, Jakarta: Indonesian Medical Council.

Iriart, C., Franco, T. and Merhy, E.E. (2011) 'The creation of the health consumer: challenges on health sector regulation after managed care era', *Global Health*, 7(2): 1–12.

Jones, R., Higgs, R., de Angelis, C. and Prideaux, D. (2001) 'Changing face of medical curricula', *The Lancet*, 357(9257): 699–703.

Kodjo, C. (2009) 'Cultural competence in clinician communication', *Pediatrics in Review*, 30(2): 57–64.

Lehmann, U., Dieleman, M., and Martineau, T. (2008) 'Staffing remote rural areas in middle- and low-income countries: a literature review of attraction and retention', *BMC Health Services Research*, 8: 19.

Magzoub, M.E.M.A. and Schmidt, H.G. (2000) 'A taxonomy of community-based medical education', *Academic Medicine*, 75(7): 699–707.

Mann, K., Gordon, J. and MacLeod, A. (2009) 'Reflection and reflective practice in health professions education: a systematic review', *Advances in Health Sciences Education*, 14(4): 595–621.

Mennin, S. and Petroni-Mennin, R. (2006) 'Community-based medical education', *The Clinical Teacher*, 3(2): 90–6.

Muller, D., Meah, Y., Griffith, J., Palermo, A.G., Kaufman, A., Smith, K.L. and Lieberman, S. (2010) 'The role of social and community service in medical education: The next 100 years', *Academic Medicine*, 85(2): 302–9.

Prideaux, D., Worley, P. and Bligh, J. (2007) 'Symbiosis: A new model for clinical education', *The Clinical Teacher*, 4: 209–12.

Puertas, E.B., Arósquipa, C. and Gutiérrez, D. (2013) 'Factors that influence a career choice in primary care among medical students from high-, middle-, and low-income countries: a systematic review', *Revista Panamericana de Salud Pública*, 34(5): 351–8.

Saúde, M.D. (1998) *Saúde da família: uma estratégia para a reorientação do modelo assistencial*, Ministério da Saúde Brasília. Online. Available HTTP: http://bvsms.saude.gov.br/bvs/publicacoes/cd09_16.pdf (accessed 26 June 2014).

Starfield, B., Shi, L. and Macinko, J. (2005) 'Contribution of primary care to health systems and health', *Milbank Quarterly*, 83(3): 457–502.

Takahashi, S.G., Bates, J., Verma, S., Meterissian, S., Rungta, K. and Spadafora S. (2011) *Environmental scan synthesis report, Future of medical education in Canada postgraduate (FMEC PG) project environmental scan consultant group*. Online. Available HTTP: https://www.afmc.ca/pdf/fmec/Synthesis-Report.pdf (accessed 26 June 2014).

Thistlethwaite, J.E., Bartle, E., Chong, A.A., Dick, M.L., King, D., Mahoney, S., Papinczak, T. and Tucker, G. (2013) 'A review of longitudinal community and hospital placement in medical education: BEME guide no. 26', *Medical Teacher*, 38(8): e1340–64.

Todres, L., Galvin, K.T. and Holloway, I. (2009) 'The humanization of healthcare: a value framework for qualitative research', *Medical Teacher*, 4(2): 68–77.

Waitzkin, H., Iriart, C. and Lamadrid, S. (2001) 'Social medicine in Latin America: Productivity and dangers facing the major national groups', *The Lancet*, 358(9278): 315–23.

Walters, L., Prideaux, D., Worley, P. and Greenhill, J. (2011) 'Demonstrating the value of longitudinal integrated placements for general practice preceptors', *Medical Education*, 45(5): 455–63.

World Federation for Medical Education (1988) 'The Edinburgh declaration', *The Lancet*, 8068: 464.

World Health Organization (1978) *Primary health care. Report of the International Conference on Primary Health Care, Alma-Ata, USSR, 6–12 September 1978*, Geneva: WHO. Online. Available HTTP: http://whqlibdoc.who.int/publications/9241800011.pdf (accessed 01 July 2014).

13
INTEGRATION OF THE SCIENCES BASIC TO MEDICINE AND THE WHOLE OF THE CURRICULUM

Stewart Mennin

> *A number of programmes have successfully brought together the sciences basic to medicine and clinical practice.*

Integration is a keystone in the arc of medical education that warrants a much deeper understanding of its interdependence with the purpose and function of the curriculum. As Beane (1997) notes in the following quotation, claims are often made of integrated curriculum.

> Of course, all curriculum designs claim to create connections of some kind or another – with the past, with the community, across subjects, and so on. But here is a curriculum design that seeks connections in all directions, and because of that special kind of unity, is given the name curriculum integration.
>
> *(Beane 1997: 2)*

What works for the integration of the sciences basic to medicine[1] and the whole curriculum has been, is now, and will continue to be challenging as new information, ideas, experiences and approaches to learning emerge. Integration in the present context refers to the interactions, exchanges and interrelationships that unify different subjects and objects forming a whole. The perception of the 'whole' is relative to the scale at which observations and measurements occur. The whole that comes from curriculum integration exists, and is co-embedded at multiple levels of an even larger and greater whole. This chapter argues that an awareness of different levels of integration, the *whole* (e.g. the curriculum), the *part* (e.g. individual learners, patients and teachers) and the *greater whole* (the university, the health system and the well-being of society), is fundamental for the emergence of an ecology of medical education that fulfils its social contract with society. Integration of the sciences basic to medicine and the whole involves complex interrelationships that necessarily function within and across constraints that serve to organise, liberate and optimise a self-organising, learning curriculum. Integration occurs within, and as a consequence of, conditions and constraints that are a variable consequence of the circumstances. It is the author's contention that it is the qualities of sensitivity and adaptive responsiveness to variations in local conditions that produce a coherent sustainable adaptive whole, i.e. fit for function.

The present chapter begins with a view of integration expressed in terms of the recent history of medical education. The focus then turns to the ability of integration of the sciences basic to medicine to exist at many levels of curriculum and the organisation. Finally, a perspective view of an adaptive integrated curriculum is considered that can be relevant to the needs of society while conditions and problems continue to evolve and change (Doll 1993; Beane 1997; Fogarty and Pete 2009; Mennin 2010a; Bleakley et al. 2011; Patterson et al. 2013).

Integration: where are we and how did we get here?

The story of the integration of the sciences basic to medicine with the whole of the medical curriculum is one of episodic evolution of new concepts, pedagogies, methods and technologies at every level (Papa and Harasym 1999). Over 100 years ago Flexner sought to bring together and integrate research in the basic sciences with hospital-based care to reconstitute the whole of medical education with the basic sciences taught separately as a necessary prerequisite to clinical studies (Flexner 1910). Over 40 years later, Case Western Reserve University, USA, loosened the constraints on single-subject-specific curricula by integrating (co-mingling) the basic science disciplines within patterns of organ systems (Patterson 1956). McMaster University, Canada, went even further in the mid-1960s, significantly reducing the constraints on curriculum integration using 'authentic' clinical cases in small-group, problem-based learning (PBL) tutorials promoting integration and relevance among and across the basic and clinical sciences (Neufeld and Barrows 1974). The primary driving force for learning in their PBL approach was the 'need to know', derived from students' systematic inquiry and questions created by them at the frontier of their understanding in the context of a particular problem (Barrows and Tamblyn 1980; Schmidt 1993). PBL popularised and made accessible the integration of self-directed 'independent' study, collective elaboration and the reflective application of what was being learned to 'more realistic' problems; initially in the sciences basic to medicine and later in the greater whole of health professions education and beyond. It also promoted greater collective accountability for what and how sense making occurred in small-group learning and cleared the way for the emergence of increased reflection, feedback and formative assessment in medical education. Small-group, problem-oriented learning promoted more equity in the curriculum for areas such as professionalism, ethics and communication, among others. Maastricht University, the Netherlands, since the early 1980s, has had a major integrative role nationally and internationally, promoting the development of research in medical education and the dissemination of PBL (van der Vleuten et al. 2004; Mennin 2010b). The University of New Mexico (USA) School of Medicine's parallel curriculum track, the Primary Care Curriculum (1979–94), further decreased constraints on the teaching and learning of the sciences basic to medicine by integrating community-oriented learning and PBL together, focusing on early and sustained clinical skills as the nidus around which the sciences basic to medicine, community-oriented learning, clinical experiences and PBL were oriented (Kaufman 1985; Kaufman et al. 1989). A focus on the whole, the part and the greater whole was further strengthened by the publication of two reports by the Association of American Medical Colleges (AAMC) General Professional Education of the Physician (GPEP) (AAMC 1984) and *Assessing Change in Medical Education – The Road to Implementation* (ACME-Tri) (Anderson and Swanson 1993), and the adoption of the General Medical Council's (GMC's) *Tomorrow's Doctors* (GMC 2003, 2009) and 'the Scottish doctor' (Simpson et al. 2002).

Significantly, a loosening of constraints around the concept and purpose of assessment brought a greater emphasis on formative assessment as integrative and co-embedded with learning (Schuwirth and van der Vleuten 2006; Hodges 2013). The rise of portfolio assessment as part of learning further integrated and legitimised narrative and qualitative perspectives in the lexicon of curriculum and research in medical education (Friedman Ben-David et al. 2001). Progress testing deepened the temporal dimensions of assessment and integration in medical education (Wrigley et al. 2012).

Many other significant integrative advances in medical education included the classification of knowledge into hierarchies and sequences from least to most complex, with workplace authenticity being defined as the greater whole (Bloom et al. 1956; Miller 1990). The advent of simulated and standardised patients (Stillman et al. 1986; Barrows et al. 1987) and the explosion of technologies for low- and high-tech simulation fostered the integration of clinical skills, clinical care, assessment and the sciences basic to medicine in ways not previously possible (Motola et al. 2013).

The relatively recent emphasis on outcomes and competency-based curricula is influencing medical education by integrating the emphasis on the process of learning with clearly defined and measurable learning outcomes (Harden et al. 1999; Morcke et al. 2013). The rise of interest in ethics, professionalism and communication, among other complex capabilities, required integration with the whole of the curriculum, including the basic sciences (Epstein and Hundert 2002; Stepien and Baerstein 2006; O'Sullivan et al. 2012). Sustained clinical and community experiences were recognised as authentic opportunities for the integration of the sciences basic to medicine across a wide spectrum of healthcare and workplace scenarios. Assessment and learning in the workplace extended our experiences and ideas of how the whole of integrated learning looked (Norcini and Burch 2007).

Longitudinal integrated clerkships decreased the constraints on clinical education, breaking new ground in what had previously been clerkship-dominated specialties, taught separately and sequentially. Entrustable professional activities (EPA) established the capacity for mutual interrelated responsibility and accountability (integration) in the clinical setting with high degrees of freedom for the learner and preceptor, further decreasing the constraints on the concept of curriculum and medical education (Worley et al. 2000; ten Cate 2005).

What's next for integration in medical education? It's not possible to predict. It does seem clear that 'what works,' and what will continue to work in the future, requires an increased awareness, recognition, acceptance and understanding of the role of constraints on the dynamics of the interrelationships among educational activities, programmes, curricula and practices. Current trends in medical education towards earlier authentic learning experiences change the fundamental nature of learning as the problems and issues selected as learning activities become more immediately meaningful for learners both in the here and now and in their future careers.

In summary, the evolution of contemporary medical education has been marked by a progressive decrease of constraints (conversely, a progressive increase in the degrees of freedom) around how the sciences basic to medicine fit with the whole of the curriculum, and a progressive revision of how the whole of medical education has been perceived, understood and influenced during the last 50 years. The organisation of curriculum activities based on real-life problems that involve the learners in the here and now, rather than learning something that will be useful at some time in the future, is a fundamental change that has enhanced meaningful and coherent integration necessary for capacity building (Beane 1997).

The landscape of curriculum integration

How to make sense of changes in curriculum integration in the face of varying degrees of freedom and constraints? The adaptive action landscape diagram (Figure 13.1) is one way to visualise relationships and interactions in a complex environment (Kauffman 1993). It has been widely adopted in the field of leadership, organisational development and adaptive action (Stacy 1996; Zimmerman et al. 2001; Eoyang and Holladay 2013) and more recently in education (Patterson et al. 2013) and curriculum integration.

Integration of the sciences

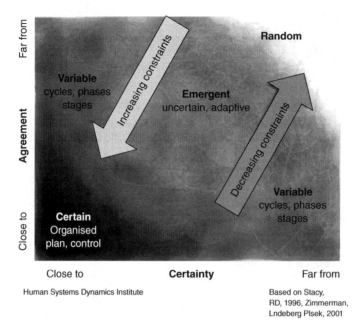

Figure 13.1 Adaptive action landscape diagram. A composite from several authors, illustrating the conditions for integration along a continuum of certainty and agreement (Stacy 1996; Zimmerman et al. 2001; Eoyang and Holladay 2013; Patterson et al. 2013).

The horizontal (*x*) axis in Figure 13.1 is the degree of certainty in any system (e.g. curriculum) along a continuum from close to certainty on the left to far from certainty on the right. The closer to certainty, the more predictable, stable and controllable are the patterns of connections, interactions and teaching, assessing and integration in the curriculum. The further from certainty, the greater the unpredictability and the weaker and more short-lived are the patterns of connections and integration in the curriculum. For example, vaccine production and use, pacemakers and insulin pumps have to be very stable, accurate, reproducible and predictable. High-stakes assessments are highly constrained and need to be accurate, reliable and controlled.

By contrast, far from certainty is privileged when what has worked in the past isn't working now; when expertise is not useful and when you're stuck and not sure what to do. Under these conditions, creativity, innovation and educated trial and error with reflection and feedback are fit for function. Integrated curricula with low constraints (far from certainty) accumulate tension and are sensitive and responsive to small changes in the environment that affect learning, integration and the curriculum. Examples are found in entrustable activities for residents (ten Cate 2005), longitudinal clerkships (Worley et al. 2000) and community-based medical education (Mennin and Petroni-Mennin 2006).

The vertical (*y*) axis in Figure 13.1 represents agreement in a curriculum (system) along a continuum from close to agreement to far from agreement. When teachers and students are close to agreement, things are predictable; there is a strong similarity in ways that teachers and students respond to challenges and stimulation. Clearly defined specific objectives and outcomes indicate to both students and teachers exactly what to expect. Close to agreement, disagreements are minimised. When a system is far from agreement, everyone does their own thing; there is little to no coordination and agreement among teachers and students; satisfaction with and productivity of the learning environment are low. Here one finds a large gap between what is taught, assessed and actually done in practice (Hafferty 1998).

The sciences basic to medicine: day-to-day integration within a phase of a curriculum

A coherent curriculum is one in which the patterns of practice and understanding present across the whole of any given education programme are similar, without losing the richness of difference at the same time (Eoyang and Holladay 2013). Four case studies from medical schools in Malaysia, Argentina, Saudi Arabia and the USA respectively illustrate how integration of the sciences basic to medicine are shaped by constraints at different levels of the whole. The case studies also illustrate and reinforce the organising effect of constraints on the interrelationships of different elements, parts and subjects, and how they combine and coordinate to form a more complete, harmonious and emergent whole (Beane 1997; Harden 2000; Fogarty and Pete 2009; Mennin 2010a; Eoyang and Holladay 2013).

The organisational framework for the discussion of the case studies is based on and adapted from the work of Beane (1997), Fogarty (1991), Fogarty and Pete (2009) and Harden (2000). Fogarty's classic work proposed three dimensions of curriculum integration: (1) within a single discipline; (2) across disciplines; and (3) within and across learners; and ten models of integration within the three dimensions (Fogarty and Pete 2009) (Table 13.1). The reader is referred to these authors for a more indepth explanation of the models.

The first case study focuses on integration within a single discipline, anatomy.

Table 13.1 Summary of three domains (within a single discipline, across several disciplines and inside the mind of the learner) and ten models of curriculum integration

	Fragmented 	Topics isolated within a single discipline, separate and distinct. Teachers unaware of other subjects and disciplines. Discipline-based and mastery testing. Integration by prioritising, ranking topics. Gastrointestinal physiology, neurophysiology, muscle physiology
Within single discipline (certainty)	Connected	Topics, ideas and details connected within a single discipline over time. Teachers relate subjects within a discipline. Muscle physiology in the gut, in the respiratory system, in the vascular system. Integration by relating topics within a discipline
	Nested	Different skills within a single discipline. Muscle physiology, sports physiology, muscle strength measurement. Teachers cluster and combine related topics and skills within a single discipline. A wider, more systemic view within a discipline
Across several disciplines (variable)	Sequenced	Separate subjects arranged by teachers to form a related and synchronised sequence. Requires teachers to plan collaboratively. Pharmacology and physiology coordinate and sequence their teaching about muscle
	Shared 	A module or unit of study combining two separate disciplines into a single topic. Emphasis is on common skills, elements and concepts. Cross-disciplinary planning by teachers. For example, a module on the neuropharmacology of muscle

(continued)

Table 13.1 (continued)

	Webbed	Based on central broad themes combining several disciplines. Collaborative planning. Assessment focuses more on relationships among topics. For example, the multiple dimension of movement (subcellular, cellular, tissues, organs, people, groups, cultures)
	Threaded 	Synthesis of several themes. No single discipline or subject is emphasised. Emphasis is on broader thinking and ideas. Students in small-group learning studying an issue across multiple subjects. For example, a worker's injury in a factory. How do they reflect on their learning?
	Integrated	Interdisciplinary and cross-disciplinary models and themes overlap creating patterns of thought and understanding that emerge from combined topics not present when viewed as in single-disciplinary learning. Integration emerges from shared commonalities among subjects, topics and disciplines. Emphasis on interconnections and authentic relationships among topics and interests
Inside the mind of the learner (emergent)	Immersed	Integration comes from a sustained immersion of attention and reflective through the learner's life experience. It is more like a labour of love. The interest is authentic and generated without the need for outside stimulation
	Networked 	Networked and dynamical interaction with others in related areas of interest and study. Networks are self-selected as needed and continue to grow over time. The immersion expands as the network evolves and develops

Source: Adapted from Fogarty and Pete (2009). See Harden (2000) for specific examples applied to medical education.

Case study 13.1 Integration of simulation-based clinical correlation pedagogy within an anatomy curriculum, Kuala Lumpur, Malaysia

Nicole Shilkofski and Carmen Coombs

Perdana University Graduate School of Medicine (PUGSOM) in Kuala Lumpur is the first graduate-entry medical school in Malaysia, developed in collaboration with Johns Hopkins University School of Medicine (JHUSOM) to introduce the American-style 4-year medical curriculum in Southeast Asia. Simulation-based clinical correlation pedagogy was integrated into the Introduction to Human Anatomy course for Year 1 medical students at PUGSOM, which, unlike at JHUSOM, is non-cadaveric in its pedagogy as a result of resource and cultural constraints. Cadavers for purposes of dissection are not widely available in Malaysia, necessitating a novel pedagogy to teach surgical and radiological approaches to anatomy.

A simulation-based curriculum was designed to teach the clinical relevance of anatomical principles and surface anatomy correlates utilising high-fidelity mannequin simulators, partial task trainers and standardised/simulated patients (SPs). Modules were designed around the major anatomical regions studied concurrently in the course, with specific measurable learning objectives related to clinically relevant anatomy. Students rotated each week between simulation stations in small groups, overseen by a faculty preceptor. For example, students encountered a high-fidelity mannequin simulating tension pneumothorax. They discussed the simulator's clinical findings of decreased breath sounds, hypoxia and tachypnoea, requested diagnostic studies and made a provisional diagnosis. Faculty reviewed radiological images and discussed treatment options in light of the relevant anatomical concepts, emphasising surface anatomical landmarks for the procedure of needle decompression. Students practised the procedure on the mannequin under faculty supervision and guidance. Additional stations included clinical anatomy procedures for the thorax, abdomen, extremities and head and neck regions. Engagement, self-assessed pragmatic learning and knowledge retention were evaluated favourably by students. Knowledge of clinically related anatomical concepts was assessed as significantly better after participation in the curriculum.

This type of applied simulation is feasible and effective for integration into pre-clinical sciences such as anatomy, particularly in settings where access to cadaveric specimens for dissection may be limited.

This case study presents integration using aspects of the 'nested' and 'shared' curriculum models in collaborative planning with clinical skills and anatomy as required (Table 13.1), in which multiple skills such as needle decompression of a tension pneumothorax are used to enhance the relevance of the anatomy of the thorax (Fogarty and Pete 2009). Integration of knowledge is the primary focus, with some 'social integration' in working with peers and teachers around case diagnosis and treatment (Beane 1997).

Constraints that organise the integration include the lack of cadavers, a single discipline sequenced early in a new 4-year curriculum, organisation by disciplines and specific anatomical regions, defined problems and diagnoses, radiological correlates and surgical procedures. Advantages of this approach to integration include enhancing the relevance of specific anatomical regions, hands-on simulation, practical procedures and clinical radiological and surgical skills stimulating interest in the subject.

It is worth noting that the integration is geared towards future practice rather than application now, to real problems of consequence that could be within the skill level of first-year students. For example, it might be possible to decrease further the constraints on learning anatomy by extending learning activities to include basic screening history interviews with simulated and real patients whose problems require sense making with knowledge of anatomical correlates related to the story of the present illness and its history. Most history questions have anatomical and other sciences basic to medicine underlying their purpose. For example, 'How often, if at all, do you wake up at night to go to the bathroom (heart, pulmonary, kidneys, urogenital diaphragm, drug-induced, etc.)? What is the anatomical structure of the heart and lung sounds you are hearing in this person? How do they relate to the person's chief complaint? What is the structural explanation for wheezing in this person? Is your pain localised (patient points to area with one finger) or diffuse (patient moves the whole hand over a region)?' In this way, typical history questions can be interpreted anatomically as well as with most of the sciences basic to medicine. The basic screening history and physical examination provide all the anatomical correlations students need in the here and now as they learn and practise basic clinical skills early in their education. It is also possible to be multidisciplinary, to add other disciplines sequenced within the basic screening clinical skills approach. It could even lead to a sequenced and shared integration (Table 13.1) with planning between the anatomy and clinical skills teachers.

The next case study combines several basic science disciplines with clinical correlations in a slightly different way.

> **Case study 13.2   Clinical odontologists teaching basic sciences for health, integrating basic/clinic, different methodologies and disciplines in Argentina at the National University of Rio Negro Dental School – why it works**
>
> *Elena I. Barragán*
>
> A multidisciplinary course comprised of anatomy, histology, embryology, physiology, biochemistry and biophysics involved 60 students in the second year of a 6-year course at the Dental School in the National University in Patagonia, Argentina. The purpose was to use clinical correlations to engage clinical practitioners and enhance teaching.
>
> The teachers of the basic sciences are practising dental health professionals. They apply examples and metaphors from their everyday practice to their teaching. The integration is between the disciplines involved in the course and the practical applied experience of the teachers. Teachers also emphasise and highlight relevant content from the appropriate texts related to professional practice. Students identify with practising odontologists. They see themselves in the future with the help of a teacher who can translate clinical situations for students and use clinical examples to explain the importance of concepts to both the present course and to their future practice. This motivates students to integrate the complex arena of the basic sciences with the management of clinical situations. In return, the reward of engaging students in significant learning is an important motivation for teachers learning new methodologies and seeking to enhance their capability as teachers. Pedagogy is integrated by mixing teacher- and student-centred methods. In addition, internet platforms, email, PowerPoint and communication contribute to the course.
>
> One problem encountered is that professionals and teachers have become specialised and, consequently, someone who teaches anatomy may have difficulty teaching embryology or physiology. Similarly, dentists who practise orthodontics may not be familiar with mandible junction problems. The challenge is to build teams that know how to work together, support each other and give the ability to someone else to take the lead when their expertise is required. Knowing when and how to shift roles to be supportive of someone else's abilities is very important for effective teamwork (Arrow and Henry 2010). Without this ability among the teachers, students find it difficult to learn from and within teams and struggle to develop their own collaborative and collective integrated vision of effective teamwork.
>
> What works with students is centring education where it is fit for purpose, sometimes on students, sometimes on teachers and at other times on texts, internet materials, community-based experiences, field-based practice and family practice. A dynamic approach blends teaching methodologies that are responsive to the variable mix of the disciplines. Teachers use real situations to integrate content and practice and students find this effective for their learning and professional growth.

The integration described crosses disciplines and could combine aspects of Fogarty's 'sequenced' and 'shared' models of curriculum (Table 13.1). 'Sequenced' refers to topics and ideas arranged serially to coincide with one another, i.e. practising dentists bringing practical experiences and metaphors to particular disciplines and content. 'Shared' refers to planning in two disciplines organised around shared concepts or ideas (Fogarty and Pete 2009). The integration described in the dental school could also have aspects of the 'webbed' model that presents a central theme linked to different subject areas (Table 13.1). It is not clear to what extent teachers are using their practical experience and metaphors to organise the course content or whether the subject content is the organisational centre around which practice themes and metaphors are selected; probably some of both, depending on individual teachers, the conditions and their comfort with the subject. 'Knowledge integration' and 'social integration' (Beane 1997) are expressed by practising dentists serving as role models for early socialisation of students into the profession. In addition, there is some 'integration' in curriculum design as knowledge is developed and used to address both basic sciences and practical applications. The motivation for and relevance of learning the basic sciences are enhanced by clinically relevant examples, stories and metaphors. As with the case study from Malaysia, the application of what is being learned is deferred to the students' future, a constraint on the continuity of learning and coherence across the curriculum.

The example from Saudi Arabia seeks to integrate learning across the entire curriculum rather than within a particular subset of disciplines.

Case study 13.3 Basic science integration into the whole curriculum at the Faculty of Medicine, King Abdulaziz University, Saudi Arabia

Abdulmonem Al-Hayani

The medical curriculum at Abdulaziz University begins with and follows an outcome-based approach linked to the attributes students must have at graduation. Two phases are described:

- Phase I (first 2 years) includes core courses in the basic medical sciences and system-based modules, such as musculoskeletal, immune-blood-lymph. Basic sciences are integrated horizontally at different levels of Harden's ladder of integration (Harden 2000). In addition, some clinically relevant topics are included in different modules, promoting vertical integration among basic and clinical sciences.
- Phase II includes core clerkships and subspecialties, special clinical, biomedical and ethics electives. Special study modules promote self-directed, indepth learning in various fields as students explore their career preferences and/or remedy deficiencies in a subject or specialty. Extended elective modules provide students with opportunities to acquire research abilities, to enhance skills in collection, evaluation, synthesis and presentation of evidence and to participate in community services.

Different teaching approaches and strategies include lectures, tutorials, self-directed learning, student-prepared presentations, practical learning and PBL. PBL emphasises the elaboration of learning goals and discussion in small groups across disciplines. Formative and summative assessment methods include: written examinations, multiple-choice questions, matching, short and long essay, Objective Structured Practical Examination (OSPE) and Objective Structured Clinical Examination (OSCE). Central management of the curriculum is overseen by Phase I and II committees and a main curriculum committee that oversees the whole curriculum.

Integration occurs within a curriculum organisation constrained in two phases in a '2 + 2' Flexnerian organisation with clinical correlates in core courses and systems-based modules in the first 2 years (Phase I). Phase II resembles Fogarty's 'shared' and 'threaded' curriculum integration model (Table 13.1), with teaching organised around connected sections, such as core clerkship topics, where the final outcome competencies are defined within and across all sections. Electives can be understood to function as both a 'webbed' and a 'themed' curriculum model, allowing deeper development of a particular area of interest (Fogarty and Pete 2009). Electives that are extended over a long period of time allow for more 'immersion' (Table 13.1), with aspects of the third of Fogarty's categories: integration within and across learners. The curriculum described has an overall 'threaded' and 'webbed' theme (Table 13.1) with a progressive decrease in constraints on student learning over the 4 years. Integration works to the extent that it is present across the curriculum (coherence) rather than within particular subsections.

A further case study of relevance to this chapter ('The Primary Care Curriculum at the University of New Mexico School of Medicine' by S. Scott Obenshain) can be found in Chapter 15. This New Mexico case study illustrates aspects of 'webbed', 'threaded' and 'integrated' models (Table 13.1) in which clinical skills and community are the organising focus around which the rest of the curriculum is organised, including the sciences basic to medicine. There were also some aspects of the 'immersed' and 'networked' model (Table 13.1) in that the primary care curriculum remained responsive to real-time health issues and to the growing needs of the community. Networking also promoted responsiveness to students as they participated in decision making about the programmes itself (Beane 1997).

Assessment and integration of the sciences basic to medicine

The assertion that assessment of learners and learning are co-embedded, interrelated and interdependent (Schuwirth and van der Vleuten 2004, 2006; Dijkstra et al. 2010; Schuwirth et al. 2011; Hodges 2013) specifies that the level of complexity of the assessment must match the level of complexity of the teaching conditions of the whole for which the assessment is valid. Another way to say this is that the assessment is 'fit for function'. What might this look like in the sciences basic to medicine?

Imagine you are at the end of your first year of a 4-year, or the end of the second year in a 6-year, medical curriculum. You are in an anatomy laboratory practical examination with a series of timed stations, one of which has a bisected human heart with an arrow pointing to a part of it (in this example the arrow points to a hole in the interventricular septum). The question reads, 'Describe the chief complaint that brought this person to seek assistance from their health provider. Explain how it is interrelated with the structure indicated by the arrow.' Students have to recognise the interventricular septum and know its structure, embryology and function. They would need to understand the dynamics of pressure in the heart chambers during the cardiac cycle and how this hole in the interventricular septum is a difference that makes a difference. Many of the sciences basic to medicine are integrated with the whole of this 'simple short question' and it is relevant to early clinical experiences in the curriculum.

Another example of an assessment question for integrating sciences basic to medicine at a higher dimension of interrelationships comes from a pilot assessment written collaboratively by the author and the late Miriam Friedman Ben-David in 1991 for what was to become an integrated Student Progress Assessment of the Primary Care Curriculum at the University of New Mexico School of Medicine. The question was developed for students at the end of their second year of their study in that programme. The question begins with a brief problem that Mrs Pereira brings to her physician, followed by some history about her problem, some physical examination data, and laboratory data and images (Box 13.1).

Box 13.1 Sample question illustrating an approach to assessing the integration of the sciences basic to medicine and clinical skills

History

Regina Pereira is a 48-year-old woman who visited her family physician, Dr Wernicke, complaining of increasing fatigue and shortness of breath on minimal exertion (such as carrying the groceries from the car). She has noted progressive worsening of her symptoms over the previous few months. She had no history of heart or lung problems. Her husband has noticed that she is pale.

Review of symptoms is notable for many months of menstrual irregularity with quite heavy menstrual flow. She has not had this problem previous to this year and has no history of other bleeding problems or easy bruising.

Past medical history is negative for rheumatic fever, hypertension and diabetes. She has had three pregnancies that were uncomplicated.

Social history: non-smoker, works in the home, married 15 years.

A) Physical examination

- Mrs Pereira is a pleasant but somewhat apprehensive woman who appears pale.
- Temperature 37.2°C; blood pressure 120/55 mmHg; pulse 110 beats/minute; respiration 16 breaths/minute.
- Sclera anicteric. Neck: No jugular venous distension.
- Heart. Prominent point of maximal impulse, S1, S2, no S4 or S3, a systolic murmur was heard.
- Lungs. Normal to percussion. No rales or rhonchi noted.
- Abdomen. Normal bowel sounds, no hepatosplenomegaly. Stool Hemoccult negative.
- Extremities. No cyanosis or oedema.
- Neurological exam: Normal.

B) Laboratory data

White blood cells 5.5×10^9 litre	(Normal 4.8×10^9 litre)
Differential: 74% neutrophil; 21% lymphocyte; 4% monocyte; 1% eosinophil	
Red blood cells 3.0×10^{12}/litre	(Normal $4.7–6.1 \times 10^{12}$/litre)
Haemoglobin 7.0 g/dl	(Normal female 12.0–16.0 g/dl)
Haematocrit 23.0%	(Normal female 37–47%)
Platelet count 450×10^9/litre	(Normal $150–400 \times 10^9$/litre)
Mean cell volume 76.6 fl	(Normal 81–99 fl)
Mean cell haemoglobin concentration 30.4 g/dl	(Normal 31.5–36.6 g/dl)
Reticulocyte count (uncorrected) 2.8%	(Normal 0.5–1.5%)
Total bilirubin 1.1 mg/dl	(Normal 0.2–1.2 mg/dl)
Direct bilirubin 0.2 mg/dl	(Normal 0.–3 mg/dl)
Lactate dehydrogenase 361 IU/ml	(Normal 300–600 IU/ml)

(continued)

(continued)

Task 1: Using the figures below, choose a letter of the blood smear which illustrates the red blood cell morphology that is most consistent with this patient's situation (1 point) and then explain your choice (2 points).

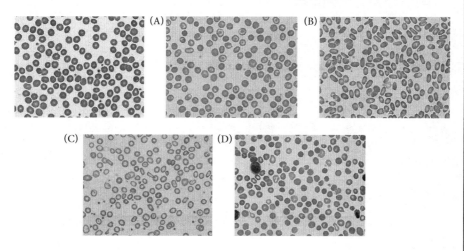

Source: Images provided by Carla S. Wilson MD PhD, Department of Pathology, University of New Mexico School of Medicine.

Task 2: Calculate the corrected reticulocyte count (1 point) and then explain its significance in this patient (2 points).

Task 3: Explain what the bilirubin value tells you about this patient's problem (2 points).

Task 4: Below are several tracings synchronised in time; ECG lead II, aortic pressure and four heart sounds: A, B, C and D. Using this illustration (below), choose the one tracing, A, B, C or D, that most accurately represents the heart sounds for this patient (1 point) and explain your choice (2 points).

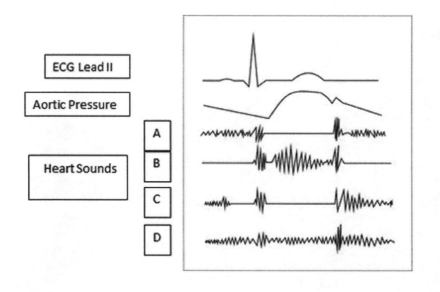

Mrs Pereira's story cannot be understood without making some sense of the relationships among the sciences basic to medicine. The question is still somewhat discipline-oriented and can fit with 'webbed' and 'integrated' models of curriculum (Table 13.1). The question is derived from a need to understand a real problem in the here and now rather than at some time in the future. Furthermore, it is not possible to receive a passing mark on this question by only correctly identifying structures, as explanation is worth twice as much as identification. This gives a strong message to students and teachers about the relevance of integration to understanding health problems and the need for understanding that informs actions.

The integration of the sciences basic to medicine is an interactive process of interrelating, combining, forming, emerging and working together to form a whole. The perception and understanding of an 'integrated whole' of the curriculum are relative to the scale at which it is observed and measured. Thus, curriculum integration can be viewed at multiple levels: the whole (a module or unit, the curriculum), the part (a single event, discipline or subject, a person), and the greater whole (the university, the hospital, the health system and society). The expression of what works with respect to the integration of the sciences basic to medicine, and its integration across the continuum of possibilities, can be understood as a function of the limits and constraints (degrees of freedom) affecting the interactions and exchanges among people, ideas, things and environments. Learning situations close to certainty and agreement are organised and integrated as single disciplines with linear, additive, reliable and replicable characteristics. A little further away from certainty and agreement, learning situations exhibit more variations and possibilities organised and integrated in predictable phases, steps and cycles – a main theme in contemporary medical education. Still further from certainty and agreement, when there are too many factors involved in the learning situation to control in a predictable way, the conditions become complex and unpredictable and are far from equilibrium.

Tension builds up in the system and its release functions to reorganise the structure of the situation (self-organisation) spontaneously such that a new structure emerges that is more appropriate, i.e. a better fit for function. This is a fundamental mechanism and explains why complex adaptive systems are learning systems (Davis et al. 2008). Examples are seen in the nervous and immune systems, socio-cultural interactions with health systems, collective problem solving through group and teamwork, authentic educational settings, complex health professional–patient relationships, and the process of learning to become a practising health professional.

It is in this context that the integration of the sciences basic to medicine into the whole of the curriculum can be understood and explained. The adaptive action landscape diagram (Figure 13.1) combined with Fogarty's dimensions and models of curriculum integration (Tables 13.1 and 13.2) (Fogarty 1991; Fogarty and Pete 2009), as seen through the lens of the case studies from Malaysia, Argentina, Saudi Arabia and the USA, can be used to visualise the dynamics of the relationships between learning situations far from certainty and agreement (emergent) and those closer to certainty and agreement (certain and variable) (Figure 13.2).

It also suggests a meaningful strategy for change through modification of the conditions (constraints) in the workplace to which people respond rather than directly persuading and pressuring people to change (Heifetz 1994; Heifetz et al. 2009; Eoyang and Holladay 2013).

The significance of the proposed synthesis of levels of curriculum organisation and the continuum of integration of learning situations as a function of agreement and certainty is that both linear and non-linear conditions can be embraced without the necessity of resorting to reductionism and fragmentation when confronted with complex high-dimensional learning, teaching, assessment and research situations. To go further in medical education, to achieve a responsive, integrated curriculum across the full spectrum of learning and practice situations,

Integration of the sciences

Table 13.2 The relationship between landscape categories and Fogarty's three stages and ten curriculum models

Landscape diagram *(Figure 13.2)*	***Fogarty's ten curriculum models*** *(Fogarty and Peat 2009)*
Certain Highly constrained curriculum integration patterns and activities. Predictable, reliable, reproducible	**Within a single discipline** Fragmented, connected, nested
Variable Moderately constrained curriculum integration patterns and activities expressed as recognisable variations in phases, cycles, stages and steps. Variations on the theme are common	**Across disciplines** Sequenced, shared, webbed, threaded, integrated
Emergent (uncertain) Very low constraints on curriculum integration; patterns are complex and unpredictable. Innovation and creativity in response to changing conditions	**Within and across learners** Immersed, networked

requires seeing, understanding and influencing both linear (additive) and non-linear (multiplicative) learning situations (West 2010).

Non-linear, complex adaptive situations are essential to creativity and innovation and are especially useful when what has worked before is no longer working. What is needed is integration of the full range of learning conditions in the curriculum from day one to the last day and beyond, so students learn and become more comfortable with the different conditions that favour certainty, variability and emergent complex adaptive situations. The

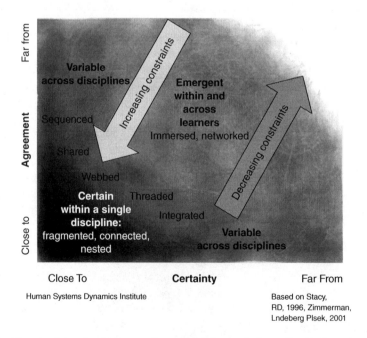

Figure 13.2 The adaptive action landscape diagram with Fogarty's three dimensions and ten curriculum models (Fogarty and Pete 2009), woven together with the continuum of certainty and agreement.

presence of integration of certain, variable and emergent learning situations from day one of the curriculum until graduation and beyond contributes to a comfort and capacity building among students of their ability to deal with the sticky reality of uncertainty much earlier, and therefore have more experience learning about and with it during their professional education. This proposed approach to integration keeps learners, teachers and the curriculum continuously curious about, and sensitive and responsive to, variability, creativity and innovation while assuring the quality of knowledge, skills and attitudes for what needs to be learned, understood and embedded through authentic experiences as a way to move forward in the dynamic context of 21st-century health professions education.

Take-home messages

- Integration in the curriculum is the combination and coordination of separate and diverse elements into a more complete and harmonious whole.
- The recent history of medical education is one of progressive decreases in the level of constraints on integration in the curriculum.
- There are different degrees of integration of the sciences basic to medicine depending on the constraints and conditions that can be visualised in an adaptive action landscape diagram of close to certainty and agreement (certainty), further from certainty and agreement (variable) and far from certainty and agreement, depending on the number of factors involved.
- Three stages of integration (within a single discipline, across disciplines, across learners) and ten curriculum models are described.
- Integration of the sciences basic to medicine applies equally to assessment of learners, and the level of complexity of the integration questions must match the level of complexity of the teaching conditions for the assessment to be valid.
- A curriculum model is proposed in which curriculum constraints can be illustrated within a landscape diagram with axes of certainty and agreement, upon which Fogarty's three forms and ten methods of integration are superimposed.

Note

1 The concept of the sciences basic to medicine is preferred as it provides a more expansive, inclusive and relevant framework (i.e. the physical, biological, social, political sciences and more) than the concept of the basic sciences (i.e. traditionally limited to anatomy, physiology, biochemistry, microbiology, pharmacology and pathology).

Bibliography

Anderson, M.B. and Swanson, A.G. (1993) 'Educating medical students – the ACME-TRI report with supplements', *Academic Medicine*, 68(6, Suppl.): S1–46.

Arrow, H. and Henry, K.B. (2010) 'Using complexity to promote group learning in healthcare', *Journal of Evaluation in Clinical Practice*, 16(4): 861–6.

Association of American Medical Colleges (1984) 'Physicians for the twenty-first century: Report of the project panel on the general professional education of the physicians and college preparation for medicine', *Journal of Medical Education*, 59(11, Part 2): 1–208.

Barrows, H.S. and Tamblyn, R.M. (1980) *Problem-based learning: An approach to medical education*, New York, NY: Springer Publishing.

Barrows, H.S., Williams, R.G. and Moy, R.H. (1987) 'A comprehensive performance-based assessment of fourth-year students' clinical skills', *Journal of Medical Education*, 62(10): 805–9.

Beane, J. (1997) *Curriculum integration: Designing the core of democratic education*, New York, NY: Teachers College Press.

Bleakley, A., Bligh, J. and Browne, J. (2011) *Medical education for the future: Identity, power and location*, Dordrecht: Springer.

Bloom, B.S. (ed), Engelhart, M.D., Furst, E.J., Hill, W.H. and Krathwohl, D.R. (1956) *Taxonomy of educational objectives: The classification of education goals. Handbook I: Cognitive domain*, New York, NY: David McKay.

Davis, B., Sumara, D. and Luce-Kapler, R. (2008) *Engaging minds: Changing teaching in complex times*, New York, NY: Routledge.

Dijkstra, J., van der Vleuten, C.P.M. and Shuwirth, L.W.T. (2010) 'A new framework for designing programmes of assessment', *Advances in Health Sciences Education*, 15(3): 379–93.

Doll Jr, W.E. (1993) *A post-modern perspective on curriculum*, New York, NY: Teachers College Press.

Eoyang, G.H. and Holladay, R. (2013) *Adaptive action: Leveraging uncertainty in your organisation*, Stanford, CA: Stanford University Press.

Epstein, R.M. and Hundert, E.M. (2002) 'Defining and assessing professional competence', *Journal of the American Medical Association*, 287(2): 226–35.

Flexner, A. (1910) *Medical education in the United States and Canada: A report to the Carnegie Foundation for the Advancement of Teaching*, bulletin no. 4, New York, NY: The Carnegie Foundation for the Advancement of Teaching.

Fogarty, R. (1991) '10 ways to integrate curriculum', *Educational Leadership*, 49(2): 61–5.

Fogarty, R. and Pete, B.M. (2009) *How to integrate the curricula* (3rd edn), Thousand Oaks, CA: Corwin.

Friedman Ben-David, M., Davis, M.H., Harden, R.M., Howie, P.W., Ker, J. and Pippard, M.J. (2001) 'AMEE medical education guide no. 24: Portfolios as a method of student assessment', *Medical Teacher*, 23(6): 535–51.

General Medical Council (2003) *Tomorrow's doctors*, London: General Medical Council.

General Medical Council (2009) *Tomorrow's doctors: Outcomes and standards for undergraduate medical education*, London: General Medical Council. Online. Available HTTP: www.gmc-uk.org/New_Doctor09_FINAL.pdf_27493417.pdf_39279971.pdf (accessed 10 June 2014).

Hafferty, F.W. (1998) 'Beyond curriculum reform: Confronting medicine's hidden curriculum', *Academic Medicine*, 73(4): 403–7.

Harden, R.M. (2000) 'The integration ladder: A tool for curriculum planning and evaluation', *Medical Education*, 34(7): 551–7.

Harden, R.M., Crosby, J.R. and Davis, M.H. (1999) 'AMEE guide no. 14: Outcome-based education: Part 1 – An introduction to outcome-based education', *Medical Teacher*, 21(1): 7–14.

Heifetz, R.A. (1994) *Leadership without easy answers*, Cambridge, MA: Belknap Press of Harvard University Press.

Heifetz, R.A., Grashow, A. and Linsky, M. (2009) *The practice of adaptive leadership: Tools and tactics for changing your organization in the world*, Boston, MA: Harvard Business Press.

Hodges, B. (2013) 'Assessment in the post-psychometric era: Learning to love the subjective and collective', *Medical Teacher*, 35(7): 564–8.

Kauffman, S. (1993) *The origins of order: Self-organization and selection in evolution*, New York, NY: Oxford University Press.

Kaufman, A. (ed.) (1985) *Implementing problem-based medical education: Lessons from successful innovations*, New York, NY: Springer.

Kaufman, A., Mennin, S., Waterman, R., Duban, S., Hansbarger, C., Silverblatt, H., Obenshain, S.S., Kantrowitz, M., Becker, T., Samet, J. and Wiese, W. (1989) 'The New Mexico experiment: An educational innovation and institutional change', *Academic Medicine*, 64(6): 285–94.

Mennin, S. (2010a) 'Self-organization, integration and curriculum in the complex world of medical education', *Medical Education*, 44(1): 20–30.

Mennin, S. (2010b) 'Sustainability of PBL and innovation in medical education at Maastricht University'. In: H. van Berkel, A. Scherpbier, H. Hillen and C. van der Vleuten (eds) *Lessons from problem-based learning*, Oxford: Oxford University Press.

Mennin, S. and Petroni-Mennin, R. (2006) 'Community-based medical education', *The Clinical Teacher*, 3(2): 90–6.

Miller, G.E. (1990) 'The assessment of clinical skills/competence/performance', *Academic Medicine*, 65(9 Supp): S63–7.

Morcke, A., Dornan, T. and Eika, B. (2013) 'Outcome (competency) based education: An exploration of its origins, theoretical basis, and empirical evidence', *Advances in Health Sciences Education*, 18(4): 851–63.

Motola, I., Devine, L.A., Chung, H.S., Sullivan, J. and Issenberg, S.B. (2013) 'Simulation healthcare education: A best evidence practical guide. AMEE guide no. 82', *Medical Teacher*, 35(10): e1511–30.

Neufeld, V.R. and Barrows, H.S. (1974) 'The 'McMaster philosophy': An approach to medical education', *Journal of Medical Education*, 49(11): 1040–50.

Norcini, J. and Burch, V. (2007) 'Workplace-based assessment as an educational tool: AMEE guide no. 31', *Medical Teacher*, 29(9): 855–71.

O'Sullivan, H., van Mook, W., Fewtrell, R. and Wass, V. (2012) 'Integrating professionalism into the curriculum: AMEE guide no. 61', *Medical Teacher*, 34(2): e64–77.

Papa, F.J. and Harasym, P.H. (1999) 'Medical curriculum reform in North America, 1765 to the present: A cognitive science perspective', *Academic Medicine*, 74(2): 154–64.

Patterson, J.W. (1956) 'Weston Reserve interdepartmental and departmental teaching of medicine and biological science in four years', *Journal of Medical Education*, 31(4): 521–9.

Patterson, L., Holladay, R. and Eoyang, G.H. (2013) *Radical rules for schools: Adaptive action for complex change*, Circle Pines, MN: Human Systems Dynamics Institute.

Schmidt, H.G. (1993) 'Foundations of problem-based learning: Some explanatory notes', *Medical Education*, 27(5): 422–32.

Schuwirth, L.W.T. and van der Vleuten, C.P.M. (2004) 'Changing education, changing assessment, changing research?', *Medical Education*, 38(8): 805–12.

Schuwirth, L.W.T. and van der Vleuten, C.P.M. (2006) 'A plea for new psychometric models and educational assessment', *Medical Education*, 40(4): 296–300.

Schuwirth, L., Colliver, J., Gruppen, L., Kreiter, C., Mennin, S., Onishi, H., Pangaro, L., Ringsted, C., Swanson, D., van der Vleuten, C. and Wangner-Menghin, M. (2011) 'Research in assessment: Consensus statement and recommendations from the Ottawa 2010 conference', *Medical Teacher*, 33(3): 224–33.

Simpson, J.G., Furnace, J., Crosby, J., Cummings, A.D., Evans, P.A., Friedman Ben-David, M., Harden, R.M., Lloyd, D., McKenzie, H., McLachlan, J.C., McPhate, G.F., Percy-Robb, I.W. and MacPherson, S.G. (2002) 'The Scottish doctor – learning outcomes for the medical undergraduate in Scotland: A foundation for competent and reflective practitioners', *Medical Teacher*, 24(2): 136–43.

Stacy, R.D. (1996) *Strategic management and organizational dynamics*, London: Pitman Publishing.

Stepien, K.A. and Baerstein, A. (2006) 'Educating for empathy: A review', *Journal of General Internal Medicine*, 21(5): 524–30.

Stillman, P.L., Swanson, D.B., Smee, S., Stillman, A.E., Ebert, T.H., Emmel, V.S., Caslowitz, J., Greene, H.L., Hamolsky, M., Hatem, C., Levenson, D.J., Levin, R., Levinson, G., Ley, B., Morgan, J., Parrino, T., Robinson, S. and Willms, J. (1986) 'Assessing clinical skills of residents with standardized patients', *Annals of Internal Medicine*, 105(5): 762–71.

ten Cate, O. (2005) 'Entrustability of professional activities and competency-based training', *Medical Education*, 39(12): 1176–7.

van der Vleuten, C.P.M., Dolmans, D.H.J.M., de Grave, W.S., van Luijk, S.J., Muijtjens, A.M.M., Scherpbier, A.J.J.A., Schuwirth, L.W.T. and Wolfhagen, I.H.A.P. (2004) 'Education research at the Faculty of Medicine, University of Maastricht: Fostering the interrelationship between professional and education practice', *Academic Medicine*, 79(10): 990–6.

West, B.J. (2010) 'Homeostasis and Gauss statistics: Barriers to understanding natural variability', *Journal of Evaluation in Clinical Practice*, 16(3): 403–8.

Worley, P., Silagy, C., Prideaux, D., Newble, D. and Jones, A.H. (2000) 'The parallel rural community curriculum: An integrated clinical curriculum-based in rural general practice', *Medical Education*, 34(7): 558–65.

Wrigley, W., van der Vleuten, C.P.M., Freeman, A. and Muijtjens A. (2012) 'A systematic framework for the progress test: strengths, constraints and issues: AMEE guide no. 71', *Medical Teacher*, 34(9): 683–97.

Zimmerman, B., Lindberg, C. and Plsek, P. (2001) *Edgeware: Insights from complexity science for health care leaders*, Irving, TX: VHA Publishing.

14
IMPLEMENTING INTERPROFESSIONAL EDUCATION
What have we learned from experience?

Dawn Forman and Betsy VanLeit

> *There are significant advantages and lessons to be learned from sharing educational experiences between the different healthcare professions.*

The changing demographics of healthcare demand a significant reassessment of the ways in which healthcare is delivered (Crisp 2010). Interprofessional education (IPE) is an important strategy to address these issues (McPherson et al. 2001; Thompson and Tilden 2009; World Health Organization (WHO) 2010). The WHO (2010) *Framework for Action on Interprofessional Education and Collaborative Practice* mandated all higher-education institutions to embed IPE in their curricula. Actions proposed to achieve this included:

- agreement on a common vision and purpose for IPE;
- development of interprofessional curricula according to principles of 'good' educational practice;
- creation of frameworks for clear interprofessional outcomes.

A number of definitions of IPE and practice are in use. This chapter incorporates the WHO (2010) definitions.

- *IPE* occurs when two or more professions learn about, from and with each other to enable effective collaboration and improve health outcomes.
- *Professional* is an all-encompassing term that includes individuals with the knowledge and/ or skills to contribute to the physical, mental and social well-being of a community.
- *Collaborative practice* in healthcare occurs when multiple health workers from different professional backgrounds provide comprehensive services by working with patients, their families, carers and communities to deliver the highest quality of care across settings.
- *Practice* includes both clinical and non-clinical health-related work, such as diagnosis, treatment, surveillance, health communications, management and sanitation engineering.

Barr (2005) provides an overview of the development of IPE, and more recently Forman et al. (2014) provide a review of how international interprofessional developments have been led.

The present chapter provides case studies from around the world to exemplify how IPE and practice are being taken forward internationally and examines selected interprofessional developments in a wide range of socio-economic and political conditions. The chapter concludes by stating where advice can be gained for anyone introducing IPE and collaborative practice in their own environment.

Where did interprofessional education begin?

There is much debate about where IPE first began and, indeed, even more debate in the early years of IPE development about whether the best place to start IPE is at undergraduate or postgraduate level. Tope (1996) provides examples of innovative health professional education with aspects of shared learning or IPE from across Europe, Cameroon, Sudan, Mexico, Africa, Canada and the USA.

Linkoping University in Sweden is, however, widely acknowledged as an institution which, having initiated an undergraduate interprofessional, problem-based programme for healthcare professions in 1996, has the longest and most sustained history in this field. Their programme has been continuously evaluated and refined over the years; and recently, to ensure that changes in health and social care nationally and internationally as well as changes in politics, emerging technologies, demographics and health indices, have been taken into account, a renewed framework has been designed. This new curriculum incorporates four domains of interprofessional collaborative practice competencies:

1 values/ethics for interprofessional practice;
2 roles/responsibilities;
3 interprofessional communication;
4 teams and teamwork.

Linkoping seeks to develop leaders of change, and to ensure students strive for quality improvement and have strong ethical values (Abrandt Dahlgren et al. 2012). A problem-based, interprofessional learning methodology has been maintained, ensuring the students work together to resolve an issue, thereby learning with, from and about each other but also knowing more about each other's role, and when and how to hand on to another professional. The overall aim is to ensure that at graduation students have the skills and competencies they will require in their future professional roles with a focus on the patient or client in all aspects.

Many institutions have chosen to provide a medical curriculum in which problem-based learning (PBL) is key. On the other side of the world, Notre Dame University in Australia utilises PBL as a means to incorporate interprofessional activities.

The review of interprofessional education in Australia

Recent reviews of healthcare in Australia identified the need for a new model of service delivery. It is clear that an integrated and interprofessional health service is required to meet the challenges of the future (Garling 2008; Commonwealth of Australia 2009, 2011; Government of

Dimension Four: SUPPORTING INSTITUTIONAL DELIVERY. This dimension focuses on the impact of local university structure and culture on the shaping of curriculum design and delivery, such as timetabling, logistics and entry requirements.

Dimension Three: TEACHING, LEARNING & ASSESSMENT. This dimension pertains to the development of appropriate learning, teaching and assessment experiences, all of which have been guided by the messages inherent within D1 and D2.

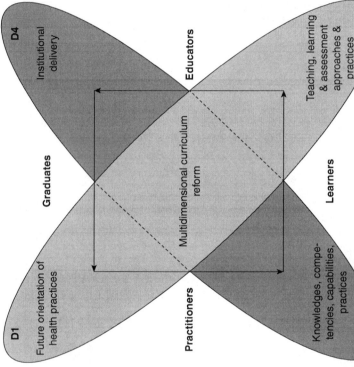

Dimension One: IDENTIFYING FUTURE HEALTHCARE PRACTICE NEEDS. This dimension seeks to connect health professionals' practice needs to new and changing workplace demands in all health sectors. Curriculum considerations take into account global health and educational reforms; how these link to the development of knowledges, competencies, capabilities and practices; as well as local institutional delivery conditions.

Dimension Two: DEFINING AND UNDERSTANDING CAPABILITIES. This dimension describes the knowledges, capabilities and attributes health professionals require. This component addresses how changing health services impact on expertise, identities and practice, which ultimately impacts upon the training and preparation of future health professionals.

Figure 14.1 The four-dimensional interprofessional framework of Lee et al. (2013). Australian and New Zealand Association for Health Professional Educators (ANZAHPE) has freely granted permission to use the image, originally published in *Focus on Health Professional Education*, 14(3):70–83.

Western Australia 2009; Health Workforce Australia 2011). The ability to practise collaboratively is necessary to deliver safe and appropriate client-centred care, effectively and efficiently (Meads et al. 2009).

Australia has recently undertaken a national review of IPE efforts and is in the process of developing a national curriculum framework to guide the implementation of the approach by educational institutions. The framework will utilise a four-dimensional model for health professional curriculum development, expounded by Lee et al. (2013) (Figure 14.1). The methodology recognises the real potential for organisational and logistical barriers to impede the implementation of IPE (Dimension Four) and provides the impetus for overcoming these problems by reconnection with the high-level societal purpose for change (Dimension One). Teaching, learning and assessment are viewed as key in ensuring appropriate learning takes place (Dimension Three). But perhaps the most interesting aspects, as we look at the difference that IPE and collaborative practice makes to the client, are the capabilities that we develop in our students and practitioners (Dimension Two). Key to the development of these capabilities is the collaboration or partnership arrangements that are developed between the higher-education institution and the service or community in which the students and practitioners are working.

Case study 14.1   Weaving interprofessional education into the medical curriculum at the University of Notre Dame, in Western Australia

Carole Steketee and Donna B. Mak

Traditional medical courses have a discipline-based curriculum in which content is presented and learned in relative isolation (e.g. pharmacology, immunology, anatomy). However, patients, as human beings, function as an integrated whole; the University of Notre Dame's medical curriculum recognises this and simultaneously provides students with learning experiences that enable them to encounter knowledge and skills from a wide range of disciplines in the context of authentic patient cases. Cases are delivered via a PBL programme in the first 2 years of the course and via contact with genuine patients in a variety of clinical settings in the final 2 years.

IPE therefore is not teased out and delivered as a discrete subject. Instead, it is co-embedded with the curriculum and integrated within the fabric of patient cases. Nevertheless, at the broad learning outcome level (each unit is 1 year in length), there is a distinct focus on interprofessional healthcare practice. For example, in the first year of the course students will demonstrate an understanding of the importance of interprofessional healthcare of patients. In the second year, students will participate in opportunities of interprofessional learning and healthcare. In the third year, students will work effectively within an interprofessional healthcare team and in the final year, students will work collaboratively as integral members of an interprofessional healthcare team to provide high-quality patient-centred care.

Some examples of activities and learning experiences that enable students to address these learning outcomes are multidisciplinary panel discussions based on hypothetical cases, e.g. a 15-year-old girl seeking contraception from the school nurse; and a married, middle-aged man who feels sexual attraction to a work colleague of the same sex. These panels usually comprise a patient or health consumer representative with first-hand experience of the condition being discussed and a variety of relevant health professionals, each contributing to the discussion on an equal footing.

(continued)

(continued)

During clinical rotations in the final 2 years of the course, students attend team meetings and observe the functioning of a multidisciplinary team. In the final year, students are expected to present at these meetings. Lectures are provided by a range of healthcare professionals in relation to the patient-based problem of the week (e.g. lecture by a dietician with regard to changes in nutritional requirements throughout the life cycle, particularly as it pertains to the elderly and groups with neurological conditions such as Parkinson's disease). Rural and remote community placements take place, where students learn with, and from, local residents in non-clinical settings about health and other issues they face in the bush. In these encounters, the local resident is an equal in the team and directs student learning around issues of importance.

The UK Centre for the Advancement of Interprofessional Education (CAIPE) defines IPE as occurring when 'two or more professions learn with, from and about each other to improve collaboration and the quality of care' (CAIPE 2002). In light of this definition, many of the activities above are not 'pure' IPE. While students learn about and from other health professionals, they do not collaborate with other health professional students to do so. The logistics of coordinating multiple complex timetables has been expressed as the primary reason why this has not occurred to date.

Freeth et al. (2005: 8) suggest that IPE is:

> a learning process that prepares professionals through interdisciplinary education and diverse fieldwork experiences to work collaboratively with communities to meet the multifaceted needs of children, youth and families.

The activities delivered in the School of Medicine at Notre Dame are more aligned to this definition of IPE in that their focus is on helping students understand the role of the patient in their care, particularly in the light of increasing chronic disease and an ageing population. For example, students on placement in the Kimberley (a remote region in Western Australia) are immersed in the community and learn primarily from the locals about the health and societal issues they face. In this context, students learn from Aboriginal language interpreters and are exposed to the role of the Aboriginal health workers and environmental health workers. They examine the functions and dynamics of multidisciplinary teams and other health professionals, and their contributions to health and disease prevention/management in this setting.

An integrated curriculum in medical education has the advantage of providing students with rich, purposeful and contextualised learning opportunities. However, it is not without its challenges. This is evident in the case of IPE, where it would be much easier (and a lot less expensive) to provide students with a discrete unit on the topic. However, integration requires IPE (and other topics) to be woven together with patient problems in an authentic and purposeful way, and then to be resourced accordingly. The School of Medicine at the University of Notre Dame, Australia, does this by way of patient-centred problems. The outcome of this approach could be described as interdisciplinary learning rather than IPE. The curriculum developers will continue to address this issue during review cycles. Participation in a national project on curriculum review in IPE has been instrumental in informing this endeavour.

Two case studies, one from the Philippines and one from Kenya, provide examples of how the partnership between the higher-education institution and the community environment where the students and practitioners are working has enabled interprofessional collaboration (IPC) to be developed to the benefit of the community.

Case study 14.2 Developing community-engaged interprofessional education in the Philippines

Reproduced from *Leadership Development for Interprofessional Education and Collaborative Practice*, edited by Dawn Forman, Marion Jones and Jill Thistlethwaite, published 2014 by Palgrave Macmillan, reproduced with permission of Palgrave Macmillan.

Elizabeth R. Paterno, Louricha A. Opina-Tan and Dawn Forman

In 2007, the Community Health and Development Program (CHDP) was inaugurated as a unit of the University of the Philippines (UP) Manila. It was mandated to forge partnerships with rural municipalities, to set up and maintain community-based health programmes that would benefit both the municipality and the university, and to provide the site for student immersion programmes of all UP Manila academic units, namely the Colleges of Medicine, Nursing, Public Health, Dentistry, Pharmacy, Allied Medical Professions (occupational therapy, physical therapy and speech therapy) and the Arts and Sciences. Two colleges of UP Diliman (another UP campus in Quezon City), the College of Social Work and Community Development and the College of Home Economics, specifically the Department of Nutrition, also joined the programme.

The two objectives of the CHDP agreed upon by all participating units were to provide learning opportunities for the faculty and students of UP Manila in the principles and practice of community healthcare; and to assist communities to attain increasing capacities in their own healthcare and development through the primary healthcare approach.

All the participating colleges agreed upon a common conceptual framework, that genuine improvement in community health and development should be one of the most important outcomes of the partnership. Figure 14.2 graphically explains this conceptual framework.

Development of collaborative patient care and interprofessional education

Prior to 2007, each UP Manila college had its own community immersion site and therefore the colleges had developed their own protocols on community health work. Though the interdisciplinary approach had been articulated as one of the principles that would guide the work in the common community, in practice there were no guidelines on how this would actually be done. In the initial year of programme implementation at the common site, each discipline managed patients independently but referrals to other disciplines were done when deemed necessary according to the patient's needs. As such, patients were often managed by different disciplines at the same time. However, there were no clear guidelines for coordination. Patient management was not streamlined, and was often repetitive. Patients and their families often became fatigued having to entertain different sets of students several times within a day or week, and it was not uncommon, after a few weeks of treatment, for patients to refuse to entertain students.

The evaluation

An evaluation of the programme was done at the end of the first year of implementation where the observations stated in the previous paragraph were documented. The assessment meeting was followed by a study of available literature from other countries where interdisciplinary learning had

(continued)

(continued)

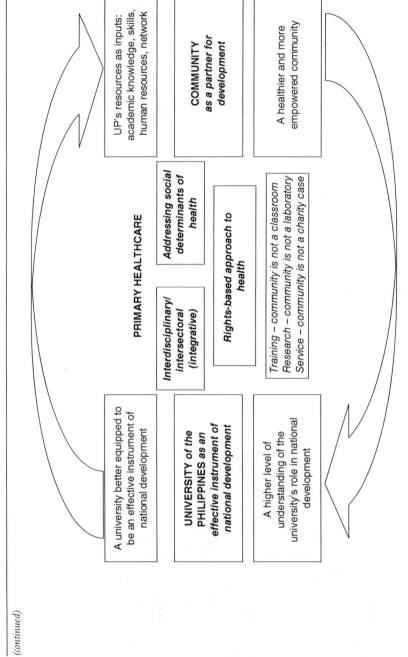

Figure 14.2 Conceptual framework of the Community Health and Development Program, University of the Philippines (UP). (Reproduced from *Leadership Development for Interprofessional Education and Collaborative Practice*, edited by Dawn Forman, Marion Jones and Jill Thistlethwaite, published 2014 by Palgrave Macmillan, with permission of Palgrave Macmillan.)

been taking place for some time. Important lessons gathered from the literature review and affirmed by our experiences included the following:

- Equality and collegiality among the different disciplines are necessary characteristics of a successful collaborative practice. The existing hierarchical relations among the disciplines in the university hospital setting therefore had to be overcome.
- Professionals working together should share common goals, objectives and activities relevant to their practice.
- Understanding and valuing the roles played by other professionals facilitate the development of IPC.
- Having time to interact as well as sharing common working space reduce professional territoriality.
- Good communication among the different disciplines should be an active work, and the value of group discussions among students of different disciplines should be emphasised. Having common documents facilitates communication.

With members of faculty staff working with community representatives, guidelines were developed, agreed upon and implemented. This led to the university being able to implement its framework and improve interprofessional collaborative community practice.

Case study 14.3 COBES at Moi University, Faculty of Health Sciences, Eldoret, Kenya

Reproduced from *Leadership Development for Interprofessional Education and Collaborative Practice*, edited by Dawn Forman, Marion Jones and Jill Thistlethwaite, published 2014 by Palgrave Macmillan, reproduced with permission of Palgrave Macmillan.

Simeon Mining and Dawn Forman

IPE at the College of Health Sciences began in 1996 when the first class of environmental health students joined the medical students for community-based education and services (COBES). This first class was developed following discussions which had taken place through the partnership with Linkoping University, beginning in 1989. This partnership was the initiative of the Ministry of Health in Kenya and a formal agreement was signed in 1990. The partnership is still continuing and evolving, and offers opportunities for both staff and student exchange. The initial joining of environmental health and medical students was quickly followed by the addition of nursing students, and now dentistry, physical therapy and medical psychology are also included.

> Community-based education and service (COBES) gives students a chance to practise what they have learned at various levels in the community ... it enables learners, teachers, health workers and the community to form partnerships early in the students' career.
>
> (Godfrey et al. 2000)

(continued)

(continued)

This quote provides a good illustration of the advantages of the community-based training programmes at Moi University in Eldoret, Kenya. Students from these programmes cooperate on site in the COBES programme and thus practise community-based, multiprofessional education.

The COBES programme is divided into five phases:

1 introduction to the community;
2 community diagnosis;
3 writing a research proposal;
4 investigation – executing the research plan;
5 district health service attachment.

The research projects designed and implemented in Phases 3 and 4 have resulted in the most fascinating reports. The projects in Phase 3 are designed on the faculty's premises, with students then going out into the community again to collect data during Phase 4. The research topics addressed are diverse, ranging from *Women's self-help groups as change agents in alleviating malnutrition among under-fives*, to *Knowledge, attitude and practice of hygienic food handling among kiosk food vendors in Eldoret*.

Attaining the skills required as a healthcare professional

In each of the case studies it is clear that the universities recognise the need to ensure that graduates entering the profession apply and practise knowledge and skills beyond the theoretical knowledge learned at university, and implement newly acquired competencies (Higgs et al. 2004). As this learning is context-based in the community of practice (Dahlgren et al. 2004), peers, role models, mentors and supervisors can significantly influence the quality of learning (Goldenberg and Iwasiw 1993; Ajjawi and Higgs 2008; Johnsson and Hager 2008). Successful adaptation relies on social learning and active participation in reflection, and feedback from reliable others to judge actions and decisions (Regehr and Eva 2007). Self-directed learning, critical thinking, reflective practice, adaptability and flexibility are highlighted as skills for lifelong learning (Barr 2002; Smith and Pilling 2007); development of these skills in the practice environment during this critical transition time facilitates graduates' successful transition to the workforce (Smith and Pilling 2007; Johnsson and Hager 2008).

Assessing collaborative practice

A recently published systematic review identified an inventory of 128 quantitative tools relevant to IPE or collaborative practice (Canadian Interprofessional Health Collaborative (CIHC) 2012). The inventory was designed to assist in making the challenging decision about which tool to use for various contexts, as each tool has different strengths. IPE is difficult to deliver in the clinical setting and there are limitations in the way it is evaluated (Barr et al. 2000; Hammick et al. 2007; Gillan et al. 2011). Quantitative data collected frequently evaluate learners' responses to the programme on the basis of self-assessment of changes in skills. Qualitative data are predominantly students' satisfaction with the experience. This reliance on self-reported data is a weakness of many studies (Hammick et al. 2007). There is a need to include qualitative methods to provide insight about collaboration and how this contributes to changes in outcomes (Reeves et al. 2009).

It is much more difficult to measure changes in behaviour, impact on the community and benefits to the client resulting from the IPE experience, and it is done much less often (Barr et al. 2000). There is no single tool that has been adopted as the 'gold standard' (Gillan et al. 2011). Gillan and colleagues concluded it is not feasible for one comprehensive tool to cover all IPE outcomes, and a toolkit is needed rather than a single instrument.

Tailoring your interprofessional programme to your environment

The context and circumstances in which IPE and collaborative practice take place vary, and lead to the need for different types of leadership, development and sustainability.

The following case studies from New Zealand, Egypt and the USA provide examples of three different international interprofessional environments.

Case study 14.4   Interprofessional education in a rural clinical setting – a quick-start innovation for final-year health professional students, University of Otago, New Zealand

Sue Pullon, Eileen McKinlay, Peter Gallagher, Lesley Gray, Margot Skinner, and Patrick McHugh (with acknowledgements also to Rachael Vernon, Ruth Crawford, Jennifer Roberts, James Windle, Lyndie Foster Page, John Broughton, Bridget Robson, Louise Beckingsale, Rose Parsons, Maaka Tibble, Hiki Pihema, Anne Pearce, Natasha Ashworth, Marty Kennedy, David Edgar and Christine Wilson)

New Zealand (NZ) is a small country with increasing cultural and ethnic diversity. Māori (indigenous peoples) make up 16 per cent of the population. The University of Otago offers health professional degrees in dentistry, medicine, pharmacy, physiotherapy and dietetics. An IPE programme for final-year health professional students was called for by Health Workforce NZ to address educational objectives relating to interprofessional practice, *hauora Māori* (Māori health), rural health and chronic conditions management. The programme involves six health disciplines: those mentioned above plus nursing, in collaboration with the Eastern Institute of Technology (EIT).

The chosen programme site is an isolated, largely rural area. There are high levels of unemployment and socio-economic deprivation. Forty-nine per cent of the population is Māori, who are young with low age of first birth (Dew and Matheson 2008; Statistics NZ 2010). Health need in the region is high, with an undisputed requirement to increase the rural health workforce and to ensure that health professional work is collaborative and well coordinated.

The University of Otago programme was developed from an initial business case and implemented as one of two parallel rural sites – the other being run by the University of Auckland. Common learning outcomes were agreed across both sites; however, institutional and local variables required separate set-up and implementation strategies. An interdisciplinary group of senior academic teachers worked together to devise a 5-week rotational programme. The group reports to a multi-stakeholder governance group and developed relationships with a local Tairāwhiti steering committee, a local Māori advisory group and a local education provider. The programme has a local academic leader, a local administrator and a part-time clinical supervisor/teacher in each of the disciplines and in *hauora Māori*.

During the programme, groups of ten to 12 students from four to six disciplines at a time come to the region and live together in shared accommodation. The intended learning outcomes are met

(continued)

(continued)

with a mix of 'clinical home' placements, interprofessional clinical placements and group activities, including a summatively assessed group community education project. The project topic is chosen by a local community or health provider involved in the development of a community resource and is an important reciprocal gesture. Clinical placements are most often in the community – e.g. general practices, community pharmacies, rural Māori health service providers – but some are at the local rural hospital, e.g. community physiotherapy clinic.

The short set-up time frame was challenging and improvements were needed in each successive block during Year One. There is no curricular or temporal alignment between each participating degree programme, thus making agreed dates, commonly agreed learning outcomes and assessment difficult to achieve. For most, this was the first opportunity for academic course leaders to participate in an interprofessional programme. Providing adequate resources and support for new, distant clinical teachers and clinical provider organisations has been an additional challenge, especially for those unfamiliar with e-learning environments.

The project is being independently evaluated over 3 years. First-year results indicate significant community commitment and very positive student feedback in relation to local hospitality, feeling part of the healthcare team, learning from students of other disciplines and much greater appreciation of the rural health environment. Students report greatly increased confidence in working with Māori, and enjoy producing their community projects. Some students were concerned that they were missing out on their discipline-specific clinical experience, and changes were needed to ensure continuity in a 'clinical home'. Capacity to take students on clinical placements is limited in areas with small populations. Providers and staff need continued support and 'rest periods' for sustainability.

The set-up of a new interprofessional programme is complex. From the outset, all disciplines need to be involved in governance, planning and curricular design to remain engaged and committed. Without this there is no commitment to student supply or ongoing staff support. Temporal course alignment is not possible when quick set-up is required. Adaptations are required from all disciplines. Clinical teachers need guidance to develop an 'interprofessional identity' to support students' learning in new ways. Clinical capacity needs active management, and excellent administration and coordination. Roll-out to multiple sites needs interprofessional leadership, local flexibility, well-developed resources and skill acquisition for local clinicians in the use of IPE methods and e-learning tools.

Another example of interprofessional community education can be seen in Ismailia, Egypt, where the focus has been on developing the interprofessional programme with a focus on the needs of the community and working with the community to address this issue.

Case study 14.5   Applying interprofessional education in primary care facilities for fourth-year students at the Faculty of Medicine, Suez Canal University, Egypt

Somaya Hosny and Mohamed H. Shehata

Community-based education (CBE), with its focus on integrative learning, provides a very appropriate environment for introducing IPE activities. To improve students' learning experiences, an integrated module on infection control was implemented in 2010–11 for the fourth-year medical students. Students were expected to develop their competencies in infection control, leadership, quality improvement and IPE/IPC.

Instead of receiving didactic lectures about the subject, students were assigned a group task to improve one area of performance related to infection control (for example, hand hygiene among providers of care). Students were trained to do the task in a systematic way using the Challenge Model (Galer and Vriesendorp 2001), to observe the current situation, analyse the root causes, identify the key obstacles and provide a solution. They used Ministry of Health infection control standards to observe the compliance of workers with hand-washing steps. They worked with multidisciplinary teams in the primary care facilities (nurses, physicians, dentists and manual workers) to analyse the reasons for the lack of compliance. This was followed by brainstorming sessions to suggest simple solutions to improve the compliance of the healthcare team. The experience of working with a multidisciplinary team to improve the compliance of the healthcare team with hand hygiene was highly valued by students and teachers (Hosny et al. 2013). Difficulties encountered included: the need to train all field tutors on this particular model of improvement, and involving other professions without the required background for the Challenge Model. In addition, the limited time for the task precluded students from going through the monitoring and evaluation of outcomes of their efforts.

In spite of these obstacles, the feedback was excellent from all parties:

- Healthcare providers appreciated this simple approach and valued the mutual learning experience with the students.
- Tutors thought that the best outcomes of this experience were motivating students to be future leaders, increased sense of responsibility among students about the quality of care provided and, more importantly, being able to work with multidisciplinary teams.
- Most of the students enjoyed working in this practising environment where they could express their thoughts and apply their ideas for improvement.
- What students valued most was working with their peers in a real professional context on real-life problems. They said this experience would definitely help them overcome obstacles in the future.

CBE is an effective medium for integrated learning and application of IPE. Tutor training is crucial for successful implementation of such models. A more elaborate programme evaluation would be beneficial. Medical schools should allow more time for such activities and design specific IPE modules.

In New Mexico, USA, the context of working with a rural community and addressing their needs has also played an important part in the design of the interprofessional programme.

Case study 14.6 Interprofessional education to prepare health professionals for rural practice in underserved New Mexico communities, USA

Betsy VanLeit

New Mexico is a vast, rural state with significant inequities in access to healthcare. Most of the counties in the state are underserved, lacking health professionals or accessible systems of care. This

(continued)

(continued)

is particularly problematic in regions of the state that have large Hispanic and American Indian populations. In this context, the University of New Mexico Health Sciences Center (UNMHSC) has a vision of working with community partners in order to help New Mexico make great strides in health and health equity. The mission of the UNMHSC is to provide an opportunity for all New Mexicans to obtain an excellent education in the health sciences, and to advance health sciences in the most important areas of human health with a focus on the priority health needs of regional communities.

The UNMHSC has spearheaded many initiatives over the past few decades to build a strong healthy workforce that is committed to serving communities throughout the state. This case study describes one of those initiatives, called the Rural Health Interdisciplinary Program (RHIP), created and sustained for many years with federal training grant dollars. The intent was to provide health professions with training that prepared students for teamwork and introduced them to rural practice in a manner that was attractive and compelling. The RHIP operated from 1991 until 2008. Unfortunately, we were not able to keep the programme going without additional resources. RHIP was time-intensive for the academic instructors, and without salary support the academic instructors were unable to maintain their involvement. In addition, the loss of financial support for rural coordinators, student housing and travel made it impossible to maintain the rural component of the programme. Repeated attempts to obtain institutional support and/or support from the state legislature were unsuccessful and RHIP closed its doors in 2008.

The RHIP initially involved the academic instructors and ten students from the fields of medicine, nursing, pharmacy and physiotherapy. The programme, at its peak, annually involved over 100 students from 12 health-related disciplines – dental hygiene, public health, medical laboratory sciences, medicine, nursing, occupational therapy, pharmacy, physical therapy, physician assistant, respiratory therapy, social work and speech language pathology.

There were two major phases to the RHIP each year. In January, students and faculty were divided into interprofessional teams that spent several months together on campus engaged in interprofessional weekly PBL sessions. Teams typically consisted of eight to 12 students, and one or two academic instructors, and most groups had representation from four to six professions. Teams were assigned according to the community where they would complete clinical rotations later in the year.

The first PBL case was developed and facilitated by academic instructors. After that, students took the lead in developing and facilitating PBL cases, with academic instructors playing more of a supportive role. The PBL scenarios were designed to require interprofessional teamwork to evaluate and address complex health issues. The cases highlighted the multidimensional nature of community-based healthcare problems, including cultural, ethical, regional, financial and legal issues. The cases reflected a wide variety of conditions commonly seen in rural New Mexico, and they dealt with the full continuum of care (acute care, rehabilitation, chronic management, prevention and health promotion).

During the months of June and July, student teams completed the off-campus component of RHIP in selected rural communities. Teams lived rurally while completing clinical training that was specific to their own profession. Our original goal was to offer students opportunities to do clinical training in teams; however, this rarely reflected the reality of practice. For example, a pharmacy student might train at the local pharmacy, while the medical student trained at a local clinic, and the nursing student and the occupational therapy student trained at the local hospital in different departments. Living and working in rural communities provided the students with experience and appreciation for rural health practice and the culture of the region. In addition, this gave rural communities an opportunity to recruit graduating students as healthcare providers. Student groups in the communities were also responsible for completing a small interprofessional health project identified by the community. An on-site rural coordinator helped the students to connect with community leaders and organisations and to facilitate student integration with community life. Faculty from UNMHSC drove to the communities on a weekly basis to participate with students during this phase.

The RHIP evaluation, completed annually, consistently found that participants increased their positive perceptions of working in rural and underserved communities, and increased their confidence and intent to engage in interprofessional practice. Many of the students commented that RHIP was the highlight of their educational experience and that they thought all students should participate. A longitudinal follow-up study indicated that 36 per cent of all participants chose to practise in rural communities, and 46 per cent practised with underserved populations after graduating. A qualitative study using extensive interviews and reflective logs highlighted the many ways that students came to appreciate the complexity of health and healthcare needs in rural and remote communities as a result of participating in RHIP.

Although the RHIP was highly valued by academic instructors, students and rural communities, it was expensive and logistically complex to administer. It required extensive academic instructor involvement during all phases of the programme, ongoing involvement on the part of community coordinators all around the state, a full-time administrator to oversee day-to-day operations and funding to support student housing and travel. This is why, when the federal funding disappeared, UNMHSC was unable to keep the RHIP operating as a coherent initiative. Currently, we offer some interprofessional PBL on campus, and new innovations include the use of team assessments of standardised patients. In addition, some students are still able to engage in interprofessional service learning in community settings, but it is more sporadic than it was in the past.

We have learned that key elements to assuring the ongoing success of this type of curricular innovation include:

- active support of the top leadership in the institution;
- buy-in from academic instructors and administrators in multiple professional programmes;
- coordinated schedules between multiple professional programmes;
- financial support that reflects the costs of travel, housing, academic instructors' time and administrative support.

This chapter highlights how IPE and practice are now being seen as important internationally. It is only right that different countries, communities and organisations develop interprofessional activities in ways which are appropriate to their context. What is equally important, however, is that internationally we share experiences and learn with and from one another.

Useful websites for information for interprofessional education and collaborative practice

- American Interprofessional Health Collective: http://www.aihc-us.org/
- Australasian Interprofessional Practice and Education Network: www.aippen.net
- Canadian Interprofessional Health Collaborative (CIHC): www.cihc.ca
- Centre for the Advancement of Interprofessional Education: www.caipe.org.uk/
- European Interprofessional Practice and Education Network: http://www.eipen.eu/

- Higher Education Academy Health Sciences and Practice Subject Centre: www.health.heacademy.ac.uk/
- Intered: www.interedhealth.org
- Japan Association for Interprofessional Education: www.jaipe.jp
- Nordic Interprofessional Network: www.nipnet.org

Take-home messages

- Interprofessional education and collaborative practice are now taking place internationally.
- There is literature now available on this topic and a number of websites can be consulted for further advice and information (see above).
- There is, however, still a lot of work needed in this area to ensure that interprofessional activities are evaluated.
- A greater evidence base is required to demonstrate the difference that IPC can make both to individuals and to their community.

Bibliography

Abrandt Dahlgren, M., Dahlgren, L.O. and Dahlberg, J. (2012) 'Learning professional practice through education'. In P. Hager, A. Lee and A. Reich (eds) *Practice, learning and change*, New York, NY: Springer.

Abrandt Dahlgren, M. Richardson, B. and Sjostrom, B. (2004) 'Professions as communities of practice'. In J. Higgs, B. Richardson and M. Dahlgren (eds) *Developing practice knowledge for health professionals*, Edinburgh: Butterworth Heinemann.

Ajjawi, R. and Higgs, J. (2008) 'Learning to reason: a journey of professional socialisation', *Advances in Health Sciences Education: Theory and Practice*, 13(2): 133–50.

Barr, H. (2002) *Interprofessional education: Today, yesterday and tomorrow*, London: LTSN Health Sciences and Practice.

Barr, H. (2005) *Interprofessional education today, yesterday and tomorrow: A review* (revised ed), London: Higher Education Academy: Health Sciences and Practice.

Barr, H., Freeth, D., Hammick, M., Koppel, I. and Reeves, S. (2000) *Evaluating interprofessional education: A UK review for health and social care*, London: British Educational Research Association and CAIPE.

Canadian Interprofessional Health Collaborative (2012) *Inventory of quantitative tools to measure interprofessional education and collaborative practice*, Vancouver: Canadian Interprofessional Health Collaborative.

Centre for the Advancement of Interprofessional Education (CAIPE) (2002) *Interprofessional education – A definition*, London: CAIPE.

Commonwealth of Australia (2009) *A healthier future for all Australians: Interim report December 2008*, Canberra: National Health and Hospitals Reform Commission.

Commonwealth of Australia (2011) *National Health Reform Agreement: National partnership agreement on improving public hospital services*, Canberra: Department of Health and Ageing.

Crisp, N. (2010) *Turning the world upside down*, Boca Raton, FL: RSM Press.

Dew, K. and Matheson, A. (2008) *Understanding health inequalities in Aotearoa New Zealand*, Dunedin: Otago University Press.

Forman, D., Jones, M. and Thistlethwaite, J. (eds) (2014) *Leadership development for interprofessional education and collaborative practice*, London: Palgrave Macmillan.

Freeth, D., Hammick, M., Reeves, S., Koppel, I. and Barr, H. (2005) *Effective interprofessional education development, delivery and evaluation*, Oxford: Blackwell Publishing.

Galer, J.B. and Vriesendorp, S. (2001) 'Developing managers who lead. The manager (Boston)', *Management Science for Health*, 10(3): 2.

Garling, P. (2008) *Final report of the Special Commission of Inquiry: Acute care in NSW public hospitals, 2008 – Overview*, Parramatta, New South Wales: Department of Police and Justice (NSW).

Gillan, C., Lovics, E., Halpern, E., Wiljer, D. and Harnett, N. (2011) 'The evaluation of learner outcomes in interprofessional continuing education: A literature review and an analysis of survey instruments', *Medical Teacher*, 33(9): e461–70.

Godfrey, R., Odero, W. and Ettyang, G. (2000) *Handbook of community based education: Community Based Education and Services (COBES)*, Faculty of Health Sciences, Moi University, Eldoret, Kenya: Network Publications.

Goldenberg, D. and Iwasiw, C. (1993) 'Professional socialisation of nursing students as an outcome of a senior clinical preceptorship experience', *Nurse Education Today*, 13(1): 3–5.

Government of Western Australia (2009) *WA health clinical services framework 2010–2020*, Perth, Western Australia: Department of Health.

Hammick, M., Freeth, D., Koppel, I., Reeves, S. and Barr, H. (2007) 'A best evidence systematic review of interprofessional education: BEME guide no. 9', *Medical Teacher*, 29(8): 735–51.

Health Workforce Australia (HWA) (2011) *National health workforce innovation and reform strategic framework for action 2011–2105*. Online. Available HTTP: http://www.hwa.gov.au/sites/uploads/hwa-wir-strategic-framework-for-action-201110.pdf (accessed 15 July 2014).

Higgs, J., Andresen, L. and Fish, D. (2004) 'Practice knowledge – Its nature, sources and contexts', in J. Higgs, B. Richardson and M. Dahlgren (eds) *Developing practice knowledge for health professionals*, Edinburgh: Butterworth Heinemann.

Hosny, S., Hany Kamel, M., El-Wazir, Y. and Gilbert, J. (2013) 'Integrating interprofessional education in community-based learning activities; case study', *Medical Teacher*, 35 (Supp 1): S68–73.

Johnsson, M.C. and Hager, P. (2008) 'Navigating the wilderness of becoming professional', *Journal of Workplace Learning*, 20(7/8): 526–36.

Lee, A., Steketee, C., Rogers, G. and Moran, M. (2013) 'Towards a theoretical framework for curriculum development in health professional education', *Focus on Health Professional Education*, 14(3): 70–83.

McPherson, K., Hendrick, L. and Moss, F. (2001) 'Working and learning together good-quality care depends on, but how can we achieve that?', *Quality in Health Care*, 10 (Supp 2): 46–53.

Meads, G., Jones, I., Harrison, R., Forman, D. and Turner, W. (2009) 'How to sustain interprofessional learning and practice: Messages for higher education and health and social care management', *Journal of Education and Work*, 22(1): 67–79.

Reeves, S., Zwarenstein, M., Goldman, J.M., Barr, H., Freeth, D., Hammick, M. and Koppel, I. (2009) 'Interprofessional education: Effects on professional practice and health care outcomes (review)', *Cochrane Database System Review(1):* CD002213.

Regehr, G. and Eva, K.W. (2007) 'Self-assessment, self-direction, and the self-regulating professional', *Clinical Orthopaedics and Related Research*, 449: 34–8.

Smith, R.A. and Pilling, S. (2007) 'Allied health graduate program: Supporting the transition from student to professional in an interdisciplinary program', *Journal of Interprofessional Care*, 21(3): 265–76.

Statistics NZ (2010) *Demographic trends: 2010*. Government Statistics NZ. Online. Available HTTP: http://www.stats.govt.nz/browse_for_stats/population/estimates_and_projections/demographic-trends-2010/chapter2.aspx (accessed 18 July 2014).

Thompson, S.A. and Tilden, V.P. (2009) 'Embracing quality and safety education for the 21st century: Building interprofessional education', *Journal of Nursing Education*, 48(12): 698–701.

Tope, R. (1996) *Integrated interdisciplinary learning between the health and social care professions: A feasibility study*, Aldershot: Avebury.

World Health Organization (2010) *Framework for action on interprofessional education and collaborative practice*, Geneva: World Health Organization.

PART 4

Teaching and learning

15

HOW CAN LEARNING BE MADE MORE EFFECTIVE IN MEDICAL EDUCATION?

Stewart Mennin

Contemporary practices and practical approaches have been designed to enhance the effectiveness of learning.

The thesis of the present chapter is that effective learning is already within the grasp of contemporary medical educators. The assumption is that how we think about learning affects what we do to enhance it. Accomplishing effective learning requires learners and teachers to diminish the gap between actual day-to-day practices in medical education and what is known, understood and believed about the underlying assumptions of those practices. Three themes are explored and discussed to promote more effective learning:

1. the importance of a continuous co-evolution between practice and theory (theory, in this context, refers to the underlying assumptions and beliefs that inform how we understand the world);
2. the implications of understanding learning as a complex adaptive process;
3. the necessity of matching the continuum of dimensions (number of factors involved that make a difference) among tasks, situations, conditions and pedagogy.

Three case studies are incorporated to illustrate these three themes at work in effective relationships between practice and theory and in the match of dimensions of tasks and teaching across different orders of magnitude: student–teacher–curriculum; patient and physician; and between two different institutions. Learning as a complex adaptive process is woven throughout the discussions.

Several ideas and concepts are presented that may be new to the reader and may involve new and perhaps unfamiliar terminology related to learning that challenges contemporary thinking about the importance of understanding the nature of learning as it relates to becoming a physician. This chapter intentionally seeks to disturb the status quo of some areas of medical education, to promote rethinking and to extend our understanding of the essential nature of interdependence and, in so doing, take medical education to an expanding frontier of effective learning practices. Sometimes it is necessary to see the familiar from different perspectives to realign practices and adapt understanding to changing circumstances.

Practice and theory: a praxis for learning

Innovative and effective educational practices and theories emerge complete and fully as an integrated whole. After a while, practice and theory begin to separate, to move further apart in time and space. They begin to age, to lose their sensitivity to variability, and their interdependence with each other diminishes as they are repeated, passed on from teacher to teacher, from school to school, and from generation to generation. Practice disconnected from its underlying assumptions and theory tends to metamorphose into habits, steps and procedures without the benefit of the insight, curiosity and understanding that made them interdependent and attractive as innovations in the first place. Problem-based learning is an example of a strong initial practice in medical education that, over time, became more and more disconnected from its underlying theory, promoting a decline in the understanding about its use and adaptability by practitioners (Schmidt 1993; Moust et al. 2005). As practice can lose its relationship to theory, so too can theory become an ineffective abstraction without practice. The challenge of achieving more effective learning is to reunify, strengthen and enhance the nature of the relationship between practice and theory across the spectrum of medical education and professional practice; to restore the coherence of learning practices that are respectful of variability and, at the same time, true and useful in that they promote action that remains fit for function.

Practice informed by theory and theory in practice is known as praxis. The word praxis comes from Greek and Latin roots meaning 'doing': 'where patterns of learning emerge as individuals take action based on theories they hold about the world. Their theories about how the world works change as their experiences give them new insights' (Teaching-Learning Collaborative 2011) and as they learn individually and collectively. Praxis is an educational experience in which both practice and theory co-evolve as an interdependent pair; they are complementary (Kelso and Engestrom 2006; Sullivan and Rosin 2008; Teaching-Learning Collaborative 2011; Eoyang 2012; Patterson et al. 2013).

A useful description of praxis comes from the Human Systems Dynamics Institute (2011) Teaching and Learning Collaborative. At any given moment, the capacity of the learner lies at the intersection between ongoing practice (activities and actions that make up their day-to-day life) and learners' underlying assumptions, knowledge and beliefs that inform how they see the world. Learners come to new challenges in either place; i.e. if they are asked to do something they don't know how to do, for example a new clinical skill (a practice challenge), or if they encounter a theory or idea that is new to them, for example the concept of the social determinants of health (theory/understanding challenge). Learners try something new; they change what they are doing and/or how they are thinking about what they are doing. They think about what will work and try it out – testing both their new skill and the underlying assumptions that are informing the trial. Then they see how it works. The trial and test help them know whether the new way of acting or the new way of seeing the world is more or less effective than where they stood before the trial. That answer informs their next step. If the new 'theory' provides better insight and generates more effective action, they continue to use those new ideas as they plan next steps. If not, they abandon the ideas or try to adapt them to fit what they experienced. They continue the cycle of observing, testing and reflecting around new ideas and new skills until eventually a higher level of performance or action emerges as their way of 'doing' – it becomes their praxis (adapted from the Human Systems Dynamics Institute 2011).

That practice and theory should be inseparable and embodied in teaching and learning may seem obvious and the vast majority of medical schools will surely claim to aspire to it. If you could visit all the medical schools in the world and observe how, and under what conditions, learning is actually occurring, chances are you would find it to be fragmented, overly stressful and distant from the practical realities and necessities of local and regional health needs. The learning process and environment would appear to be dominated by transmission and repetition with little time for understanding; and by an imbalance favouring the description and the naming of things more than an exploration of underlying assumptions, knowledge and beliefs. At the same time, you would find a variety of innovative learning practices in play: organ system modules, small-group problem-based and team-based learning (TBL), longitudinal clerkship experiences, entrustable professional activities, progress testing, formative assessment, simulation, assessment in authentic settings, community-oriented education, ethics and professionalism, social responsibility, permanent education, distance education, online 'learning' and complementary medicine, to name a few.

Concepts and theories of learning vary from transmission, behaviourism and cognitivism to constructivism and constructionism. Newer ideas expanding our understanding of the dynamics of interactions involved in learning are gaining traction: cultural historical activity theory, complex adaptive systems and adaptive action (Doll 1993; Davis et al. 2008; Engestrom 2008; Daniels et al. 2010; Bleakley et al. 2011; Dornan et al. 2011; Dent and Harden 2013; Eoyang and Holladay 2013; Swanwick 2014).

Nevertheless, medical education practices remain largely disconnected from each other and from explanations based on underlying assumptions and theory. The two seem to exist as parallel lines that may rarely meet, if at all. Bits and pieces of methods are added together in an 'educational alchemy' in the hopes that something effective happens. In contrast, understanding that emerges from praxis promotes learning and coherence. Coherence refers to the degree to which patterns of praxis present across the whole of any given education programme are similar, without losing the richness of difference at the same time (Eoyang and Holladay 2013). The increased attention to outcomes and outcome-based medical education reflects recognition of the need for a sustainable praxis (Harden et al. 1999; Smith 2009).

Some might attribute the absence of coherence as a norm to the massively entangled socio-economic and political realities of healthcare, health professions education and the systems in which they are embedded; to the autonomy given to the professions by society; and to an incomplete understanding of the similarities and differences between the medical expertise necessary for patient and healthcare and the educational expertise necessary for a praxis of teaching, assessing, learning, planning, leading and evaluating across the full spectrum of medical education. Add to this the fluidity of global travel and high-speed communication and collectively we may have invented comparative medical education, lived by many, recognised by few. It becomes important to consider that learning practices together with 'learning theories have histories and are culturally grounded' (Bleakley et al. 2011: 46).

Learning as a complex adaptive process: for whom and for what?

Learning is essential for life. We learn all the time, in different places, under different circumstances and in different ways. Learning in medical education embraces much more than medical students, residents and fellows because they interact and are co-embedded in the lives of teachers, patients, healthcare professionals, administrators, policy makers, institutions, healthcare systems and societies. All of them are co-evolving as they adapt to continuously changing circumstances. There are many definitions of and perceptions about learning. A clear and useful definition is:

> Learning is the social process through which ideas (experiences, knowledge, perceptions, and movements, etc.) interact so that system-wide patterns emerge, and those

patterns (concepts principles, hypotheses, new questions, etc.) influence subsequent thought and action.

(Patterson et al. 2013: 22)

This is consistent with the thesis that learning is situated not as an experience specific to education in a school or institution, but rather instead as part of the day-to-day life of the learner (Dewey 1910): 'education in order to accomplish its ends both for the individual learner and for society must be based upon experience – which is always the actual life-experience of some individual' (Dewey 1938: 89).

The present chapter posits that human thought and learning are complex adaptive processes (Kelso 1995, Tschacher and Dauwalder 2003; Edelman 2006; Friedenberg 2009). Complex adaptive systems consist of many interdependent, semi-autonomous agents (e.g. students, teachers, patients, clinics, laboratories, libraries, groups, committees) held together by physical, cultural and conceptual boundaries. Local interaction of agents has system-wide effects that, in turn, affect local agents. For example, a student may discuss a patient issue with her preceptor or tutor and arrive at an understanding of a particular practice and its related concepts, which in turn changes the way she thinks about many other related situations. Many non-linear, short-feedback loops exist, i.e. a small change in a single event or activity can make a big difference and a big change in policy can make little or no difference. Members of a complex adaptive system (CAS), i.e. people, things and the environment, act interdependently; what one does effects the other and the response of the other affects the one, i.e. they co-evolve. Co-evolution is characteristic of highly effective groups and teamwork (Arrow and Henry 2010; Voogt and Roblin 2010; Bleakley et al. 2011; Hofstadter and Sander 2013; Mennin 2013; Patterson et al. 2013). Complex self-organising systems follow simple rules and are sensitive to small changes in local condition. Well-known properties of the nervous and immune systems and relationship-centred care are examples (Suchman et al. 2011; Patterson et al. 2013; Sturmberg and Martin 2013).

Accepting the premise that learning and thought are complex, emergent phenomena (Patterson et al. 2013), it becomes important to examine the dynamics of the interrelationships that determine the conditions of and for learning (Bruner 1960; Doll 1993; Kelso and Engestrom 2006; Davis et al. 2008; Patterson et al. 2013). Learning emerges from the internal dynamics among thoughts, perceptions and past history without the need for external direction, hence the idea of self-organisation (Prigogine and Stengers 1996; Cilliers 1998). Effective learning is learning that is fit for purpose, i.e. learning that is emergent and makes a useful difference.

Promoting more effective learning requires attention to perceiving, understanding and influencing how we set the conditions for learning (Patterson et al. 2013). This is not a new idea and has been expressed in the medical education literature as critical thinking, deep, significant, meaningful learning (Mann et al. 2011) and deliberate practice (Ericsson 2004). Similar ideas are part of relationship-centred care (Suchman 2006) and entrustable professional activity (ten Cate et al. 2004; ten Cate 2005; ten Cate and Scheele 2007). Praxis, as practical reasoning informed by theory, is the new agenda for higher education, including the health professions (Sullivan and Rosin 2008; Cooke et al. 2010).

Three case studies create a framework of praxis with examples of what works in action followed by discussion of concepts, principles and theories related to and embedded in them. The Primary Care Curriculum (PCC) experiment in medical education (1979–94), from the University of New Mexico School of Medicine, illustrates an innovative approach to learning organised around praxis, expressed as a core set of values that informed the actions and choices of participants (implicit simple rules). It was relationship-centred and inquiry-based across multiple authentic settings for learning.

Case study 15.1 The Primary Care Curriculum at the University of New Mexico School of Medicine

S. Scott Obenshain

The state of New Mexico in the USA is geographically large and sparsely populated with a high proportion of medically underserved and culturally diverse citizens. Access to healthcare services is, and has been, a major challenge. Responding to a request from the state government to address these challenges, the University of New Mexico School of Medicine, with the support of the WK Kellogg Foundation, created in 1979 an experimental, community-oriented, small-group, problem-based, student-centred parallel curriculum track, the PCC. Twenty students learned in PCC and 53 students learned in the parallel traditional curriculum track during the first 2 years of medical school (from 1979 to 1994), after which time students learned together during their final years of study (4-year curriculum) (Kaufman 1985).

Students began learning in a fully integrated curriculum from the first day, working in small-group problem-based tutorials, learning core clinical skills and the relevant sciences basic to medicine. They accepted significant responsibility for their own learning based on questions they developed during their exploration of clinical cases and early clinical and community experiences. Students found this to be highly motivating and rewarding (Kaufman et al. 1989), learning by understanding rather than memorisation (Regan-Smith et al. 1994).

Learning was fully self- and group-directed, without summative grades or formal lectures. Formative assessments, like the curriculum itself, approximated what students would be doing for the remainder of their professional lives, i.e. seeing patients, communicating, acquiring information about the patient's problems, conducting relevant inquiries such as screening history and physical examinations, writing their findings, ordering laboratory and or imaging studies, defining and refining their understanding of the patient's problem(s) based on new information, developing and pursuing learning questions, presenting their approach to the patient's problem to professors, explaining their reasoning and discussing the relevant sciences basic to medicine. This approach was very empowering for students and teachers.

Students were prepared for their clinical experiences early in the first semester and during the second semester with a full-time 16-week longitudinal immersion in a rural primary care setting. Living in a rural community, working in the office of a primary care physician and interacting with their preceptor and patients proved to be one of the most powerful learning experiences in their 4 years of medical school. To help keep both practical and theoretical issues in perspective, faculty members did 'circuit rides', visiting the community and interacting with the student and preceptor once each month during the community attachment. They observed and discussed the student's performance with the preceptor, discussed with students how their relationship with their preceptor was developing, observed students during a patient encounter, observed how they were defining and studying learning questions and derived experiences with patients and community, and how they were getting to know the community (Voorhees et al. 1985). Students designed, completed and presented a community project.

(continued)

(continued)

Students returned to the medical school for a second year of study eager and ready to learn – to extend their experiences in the community. An important lesson for students was the value of taking more and more responsibility for their own learning. They continued to learn self- and peer-assessment skills in small-group tutorials. Students arriving for their third-year clinical rotations were already familiar with this form of assessment.

Another unique aspect of PCC was early role modelling. Students learned clinical skills from their peers who were 1 year ahead of them and teamed with a clinician and a basic scientist. Clinical skills were integral to problem-based tutorials, the sciences basic to medicine and to half-day per week clinical attachments with primary care physicians. The PCC culture embodied authentic human relationships among students, teachers, patients and communities.

What stands out the most is the students' curiosity and motivation to learn and to keep learning. The culture of learning was grounded in inquiry, the need to know, learning in practice and practice for understanding. They learned to recognise uncertainty as an invitation to inquiry. The programme had a lasting impact on everyone it touched and reached far beyond the borders of New Mexico.

Practice with understanding, simple rules

The PCC programme was designed and conducted to be fit for function, i.e. relevant to the healthcare needs of students and the citizens of New Mexico. Students were expected to explain their thinking, choices and practices to build habits of praxis. The designers of PCC were aware that the life history of the learner, and groups of learners, through which their instrumentality was formed (Royson 2002) framed how, and the extent to which, they were predisposed to learn from their interactions with other learners, teachers, patients, objects and the environments they co-habited (Royson 2002; Kelso and Engestrom 2006).

A palpable culture of learning infused students and teachers in PCC. In retrospect, PCC had implicit simple rules: shared values and beliefs that informed the individual actions of a diverse group of people working and learning together as a coordinated whole (Patterson et al. 2013). These broad guidelines became PCC's identity as they functioned across multiple levels for students, teachers, preceptors, community, the medical school and the university. The implicit simple rules guided participants' choices and expectations, shaped how they treated one another and influenced their professional identity and practices. They provided 'coherence among the parts that gives rise to the whole' (Kelso 1995: 252). Coherence of learning derived from implicit simple rules that occurred in diverse environments, activities and tasks encountered by PCC students in communities and classrooms. Early and sustained authentic learning experiences were motivating and effective in promoting readiness to learn (Voorhees et al. 1985) and implicit simple rules guided choices and decisions at the individual level, leading to system-wide patterns and changes (Eoyang and Holladay 2013; Patterson et al. 2013). Three examples of implicit simple rules (Eoyang and Holladay 2013: 99) in PCC were:

1   'Teach and learn in every interaction'. This simple rule perfused experiences in problem-based tutorials for teachers and students, formative assessments, peer teaching, preceptor–student interactions, student–patient interactions, circuit rider (medical school faculty) visits to students and preceptors in the community, and community–medical school relationships all the way up to the state government. The quality of inquiry and the thoughtfulness of the questions asked informed both teachers and students about their continued learning.

2. 'Give and get value for value' was evident in the way students exchanged ideas, and discussed and elaborated on learning questions developed collaboratively at the frontiers of their understanding; in the regular self, peer and teacher feedback sessions; and in the formative assessments with standardised patients. Interpersonal relationships were highly valued. Teachers in PCC treated students the way they wanted them to treat their patients and each other.

3. 'Attend to the whole, the part and the greater whole' refers to seeing the similarities and differences in what was being learned at different levels and orders of magnitude. Problem-based cases embraced multiple levels and scales of biological, social, policy and ethical issues. Authentic early clinical and community experiences functioned as the whole into which relevant aspects of basic clinical skills and principles of sciences basic to medicine were woven. The greater whole was New Mexico's public health system, policies and practices. Learning was enhanced and sustainable when students saw the whole, the part and the greater whole; when they learned to zoom in and out of different perspectives, levels and dimensions of a patient's problem.

Learning: matching dimensions, praxis and causality in medical education

Learning at all levels of professional life is grounded in observation, sense making and action. It involves working with a continuous flow of information, collecting and sorting through data and looking for patterns. Patterns are fundamental to thinking and to the ability to recognise and adapt to situations (Kelso 1995; Eoyang and Holladay 2013). They are essential for learning, caring, diagnosing and treating health problems and issues (Groopman 2007; Hofstadter and Sander 2013). Enhancing learning requires an awareness and sensitivity to matching the dimensions of the tasks and challenges learners face with the dimensions of the surrounding environment, with the dimension of the approach taken by the teacher and practitioner, and with the learner's predisposition to learn. The learner's predisposition to learn is critical because if students, patients and practitioners are not curious, not ready or interested in learning, the school, curriculum, diagnosis and treatment may not matter. The best we have to offer may not be good enough.

The case study of Mrs B and Dr Sweeney involves a mature practitioner dealing with certainty, uncertainty and human relationships as the doctor struggles to match dimensions of attention and communication with Mrs B. The take-home messages from this case are generalisable to learners and practitioners at all levels.

Case study 15.2   Jack's dead and the boys have gone

Sweeney (2006: 3–4)

Some years ago our practice nurse asked me to see Mrs B, an 85-year-old widow, who, as I recall, at the time of consultation had been registered as a patient with me for about 15 years. I knew her well. Her husband, a pleasant chap who had been a builder, had died 5 years previously. Mrs B was pretty much estranged from her two grown sons, who were recurrent petty criminals, both serving prison sentences at the time of the consultation. Box 15.1 shows the conditions from which Mrs B suffered, and Box 15.2 shows her test results, which the nurse wanted me to review with her.

(continued)

(continued)

Box 15.1   Mrs B's comorbidity

Diabetes
Hypertension
Osteoarthritis
Macular degeneration
Hallus valgus

Box 15.2   Mrs B's test results

Glycosylated haemoglobin	9.7%
Blood pressure	180/96 mmHg
Total cholesterol	8.0 mmol/l
Body mass index	29 kg/m^2

When we met, at the practice nurse's request, I rehearsed the abundant evidence supporting interventions to lower blood pressure, to improve the control of her diabetes and reduce her lipid levels. I remember even thinking where the references for this all lay (with a résumé in clinical evidence). I confess to feeling just a shade confident as I explained the abnormalities and how we could 'help' to reduce her risk. After a few moments I stopped – resting my case, as a barrister might say.

Mrs B remained silent for a moment or two. Then she said, 'Well, Jack's dead and the boys have gone'.... At the simplest level, one can say that the consultation, at the point when Mrs B made this contribution, moved from being doctor-centred to patient-centred. It moved, one could say, from the biomedical domain to the biographical domain, or from clinical, evidence-based medicine to a consultation predicated on narrative-based evidence. But the shift was profound. When the consultation moved from its biomedical phase, it shed its parameters of P-values, absolute risk and numbers needed to treat. These were replaced by the parameters of the biographical phase of the consultation led by Mrs B. Here despair, hopelessness, regret, guilt perhaps, and defeat were the parameters. Physical parameters had been replaced by metaphysical ones – two intellectual worlds seem to have collided. ... It is clear that when Mrs B offered her contribution, the consultation took off in another direction. Up until that point, a fairly straightforward consultation was proceeding, drawing on scientific evidence gleaned from good clinical trials, many of them randomised and controlled, in the great tradition of scientific medicine. The remainder of the consultation, led by Mrs B, had nothing to do with that way of thinking and arose from her lived experience. Yet in that context Mrs B's narrative evidence had more impact on the outcome of the interaction between Mrs B and myself than the clinical evidence-based observations with which I led the consultation. There were, one could argue, two ways of explaining things which were competing for influence – two explanatory models which at first sight did not seem to overlap much. At a deeper level, there were two types of knowledge jostling to influence. Two different types of viewing and making sense of the world were at stake.

Indeed, there are at least two explanatory models are at play in this case. One is best practice and evidence-based medicine that rely on certainty, reproducibility and a linear additive logic of causality. Given this problem plus that problem, this pattern of data plus that pattern of data, the best-evidence literature says treat this way. Dr Sweeney's initial view of the pattern of Mrs B's problems was best practice; her problems were known, her lab values given and useful literature available to guide his decisions and advice. When the answer is known, best practice prevails.

The second explanatory model came into play at the speed of thought when Mrs B said, 'Jack is dead and the boys are gone.' The number of factors at play increased dramatically to a high degree of uncertainty about the appropriate course of action. The consultation became complex, uncertain and unpredictable. Linear and additive logic was no longer fit for function as causality was now emergent and non-linear. Dr Sweeney and Mrs B had to collaborate to find a solution to try and then together see and learn what would happen.

What is significant is Dr Sweeney's shift from linear best practice based on biological data to non-linear adaptive action (Eoyang and Holladay 2013) based on biographical data during his relationship with Mrs B. Moving from moderate to high dimensionality, switching from linear to non-linear thinking requires a lot of experience. We teach, and students learn, the linear (certain and known) aspects of healthcare very well, especially in the early phases of medical education. We're not as good with teaching the non-linear (uncertain and unpredictable) aspects of healthcare, nor are we comfortable with non-linear emergent causality because uncertainty means not knowing and medical students are taught to know and to act with certainty. Students learn early in medical education to avoid admitting they 'don't know'. Patients too are uncomfortable with uncertainty and want specific answers. Studying and learning to become a physician require a healthy tolerance for uncertainty because every day brings something new to be learned.

Many teachers and learners try to linearise non-linear complex situations so that they think they can know what to do and to avoid appearing not to know something. Not knowing is culturally uncomfortable in the practice of medicine and in medical education. When there is no correct or known answer, when what worked in the past is no longer effective, the strategy is to formulate questions that focus inquiry and lead to action that is fit for function. Learning to recognise and differentiate between certainty and uncertainty and to match the dimensionality of teaching with the conditions of the tasks at hand enhances the effectiveness of inquiry, learning, patient care and the health system.

Praxis at an international level

The felt need of Singapore to develop basic medical research capabilities and to invest in the development of a new medical school to support that goal is explored in the next case study. International institutional collaboration between the National University of Singapore and Duke University in the USA illustrates how praxis can be fit for function between institutions and countries.

Case study 15.3 Addressing the educational needs for the 21st century – the Duke-National University of Singapore experience

Sandy Cook and Robert Kamei

In 2000, Singapore's strategic mission was to develop a biomedical research hub in Southeast Asia. Singapore noted a lack of local researchers who could fill research roles in this industry,

(continued)

(continued)

lead research initiatives and bridge the gap between the practice of medicine and the latest research findings. To fill this gap, Singapore chose to partner with the Duke School of Medicine to establish the first US-style postgraduate medical school in the area. Duke was chosen because of its success in biomedical research and its unique medical school curriculum, with a third year dedicated to research. The education team that came to Singapore to set up the new school had an opportunity to explore ways to improve traditional medical educational strategies, keeping in mind the need to deliver the Duke content while honouring local context and working within limited existing faculty resources. TBL (Michaelsen et al. 2002; Parmelee et al. 2012) was chosen as the educational strategy to deliver and enhance the Duke-National University of Singapore (Duke-NUS) pre-clinical science curriculum while ensuring appropriate Singapore context with local faculty.

We had 17 months to recruit and train faculty in TBL, recruit students and develop the TBL modules. We created over 70 TBL modules in the first year to address the core Duke curriculum. Duke provided videos of core content which helped to keep our two schools' curricula aligned. Duke-NUS faculty developed the TBL tests and application questions. In the first year, we administered the same assessments to both Duke and Duke-NUS students to ensure they were learning the basic science foundation needed to perform well on the United States Medical Licensing Examination (USMLE), Step 1 (Kamei et al. 2012). We enhanced the TBL structure by engaging students in crafting team questions and facilitating in-class discussions. Further engaging students with the content helped students to pursue a deeper understanding and develop important lifelong learning skills (Duke-NUS 2011).

This strategy is now well integrated into our programme, well received by students and faculty, and has achieved the desired outcomes. Our success has motivated the Duke School of Medicine to take on the difficult task of introducing TBL into its pre-clinical curriculum. Changes in education are always difficult, and our success was helped by:

- an administration willing to provide the opportunity to develop a new learning paradigm (TBL);
- an office of education that provided comprehensive support to faculty to learn effective TBL design and implementation, mentoring in the development of quality TBL material and the provision of all-inclusive administrative support in preparation of materials, assessments and in-class implementation;
- faculty willing to be student-centric and step out of their comfort zone in teaching;
- students tolerant of early mistakes in our implementation of TBL and willing to take charge of their own learning.

The Duke-NUS case study illustrates awareness at the national level of the need to bring the practice of medicine closer to research-based inquiry. Praxis was evident in the development of a curriculum valuing inquiry with understanding. They thought about how TBL fit with their needs, modified it based on their understanding of the underlying assumptions and worked to use both theory and practice to improve their curriculum over a period of years. The video in the case study illustrates how the culture of practice and understanding perfused learning and was complementary to the development of the Duke-NUS partnership. The learning relationship within Duke Medical School and Duke-NUS was held together (bounded) by shared interests and values, setting the conditions for self-organisation such that the Duke-NUS programme remained fit for function as it evolved. The relationship between the two schools followed an implicit simple rule, give and get value for value; Duke Medical School learned about TBL from Duke-NUS and Duke-NUS learned about the relationship of inquiry-based learning to research and practice.

We can begin to improve learning effectiveness when we move away from the concept of learning as content acquisition, input–process–output, 'banking of information' and storage and retrieval models of cognition. Models of learning that embrace uncertainty, that recognise the complex adaptive nature of thinking and its interdependence with the learner's life history, are more appropriate (Davis et al. 2008; Friedenberg 2009; Doll and Trueit 2010; Mennin 2010; Suchman et al. 2011). Inquiry-based medical education is fit for function in all dimensions (low to high) of practice and understanding. It enables learners to perceive the patterns of data and information, and to answer the question, what is going on?; to understand the meaning and significance of the patterns of information observed, i.e. to answer the question, so what does this mean for me, for the patient, for the group?; and to take action to influence the conditions that influence the emerging patterns, i.e. to ask the question, now what will we do? What? So what? and Now what? constitute adaptive action as three very important questions that shape inquiry-based learning (Eoyang and Holladay 2013).

Learning is always a complex adaptive process, the essence of which is experiential and uncertain. Praxis is action that combines practice and theory. The three case studies illustrate a similar pattern of praxis that enhanced learning for students, teachers, curriculum, medical school and the state of New Mexico; in a doctor–patient relationship between Mrs B and Dr Sweeney; and for an international collaboration between the Duke-NUS and the Duke Medical School. The praxis patterns are those of practice with understanding, 'patterns that connect' (Bateson 2002: 7), through 'similarities, differences, and connections that have meaning across space and time' (Eoyang and Holladay 2013: 43).

Standing in inquiry in which there is a match among the dimensions of activities, tasks and conditions (low, moderate and high) promotes the emergence of learning, i.e. new patterns of thought and ideas that are fit for function. When learners are curious, when they examine and question the assumptions about what they see and do at the edge of certainty and uncertainty, at the intersection of the familiar and novel, rich and generative learning emerges. Practice, together with an understanding of underlying assumptions, knowledge and beliefs that inform how we see the world, enhances learning in medical education.

Take-home messages

- More effective learning is readily accessible by combining practice and theory (praxis) in what we already know and do.
- More effective learning is more about praxis and less about needing more methods, techniques and tools for medical education.
- Situations, tasks and conditions of learning can be understood along a continuum of low to high dimensionality depending on the number of factors involved that make a difference.
- Learning is always a complex, adaptive process regardless of the dimensionality involved in the situation.
- More effective learning occurs by matching the dimensions of the tasks and challenges for learning with the dimensions of the environment and teaching approaches, and matching the predisposition of students, patients and practitioners to learn.

- Coherence in medical education exists when the patterns of practice and understanding are similar across the whole of the curriculum while preserving the richness of differences among individuals and groups.
- Implicit and explicit simple rules preserve individual choice and lead to system-wide changes that enhance learning.

Acknowledgements

The author thanks Regina Petroni Mennin, Glenda Eoyang and Royce Holladay for critical commentary and thought-provoking challenges during the composition of this chapter.

Bibliography

Arrow, H. and Henry, K.B. (2010) 'Using complexity to promote group learning in healthcare', *Journal of Evaluation in Clinical Practice*, 16(4): 861–6.
Bateson, G. (2002) *Mind and nature: A necessary unity*, Cresskill, NJ: Hampton Press.
Bleakley, A., Bligh, J. and Browne, J. (2011) *Medical education for the future: Identity, power and location*, Dordrecht: Springer.
Bruner, J. (1960) *The process of education*, Cambridge, MA: Harvard University Press.
Cilliers, P. (1998) *Complexity and postmodernism: Understanding complex systems*, London: Routledge.
Cooke, M., Irby, D.M. and O'Brian, B.C. (2010) *Educating physicians: A call for reform of medical school and residency*, San Francisco, CA: Jossey-Bass.
Daniels, H., Edwards, A., Engestrom, Y., Gallagher, T. and Ludvigsen, S.R. (eds) (2010) *Activity theory in practice: Promoting learning across boundaries and agencies*, London: Routledge.
Davis, B., Sumara, D. and Luce-Kapler, R. (2008) *Engaging minds: Changing teaching in complex times*, New York, NY: Routledge.
Dent, J.A. and Harden, R.M. (eds) (2013) *A practical guide for medical teachers*, Edinburgh: Churchill Livingstone, Elsevier.
Dewey, J. (1910) *How we think*, Boston, MA: D.C. Heath.
Dewey, J. (1938) *Experience and education*, New York, NY: Touchstone.
Doll Jr, W.E. (1993) *A post-modern perspective on curriculum*, New York, NY: Teachers College Press.
Doll Jr, W.E. and Trueit, D. (2010) 'Complexity and the healthcare professions', *Journal of Evaluation in Clinical Practice*, 16(4): 841–8.
Dornan, T., Mann, K., Scherpbier, A. and Spencer, J.A. (eds) (2011) *Medical education: Theory and practice*, Edinburgh: Churchill Livingstone, Elsevier.
Duban, S. and Kaufman, A. (1985) 'Clinical skills: Enhancing basic science learning'. In: A. Kaufman (ed) *Implementing problem-based medical education: Lessons from successful innovations* (pp. 89–105). New York, NY: Springer Publishing.
Duke-NUS (2011) *TeamLEAD at Duke-NUS*. Online. Available HTTP: https://www.youtube.com/watch?v=BlVPLYGdBLg&feature=youtube (accessed 9 October 2014).
Edelman, G. (2006) *Second nature: Brain science and human knowledge*, New Haven, CT: Yale University Press.
Engestrom, Y. (2008) *From teams to knots: Activity-theoretical sides of collaboration and learning at work*, Cambridge: Cambridge University Press.
Eoyang, G.H. (2012) *Sir Isaac's dog: Learning for adaptive capacity*, H.D. Institute. Online. Available HTTP: http://www.hsdinstitute.org/learn-more/library/articles/newtons-dog-2012-12-20.pdf (accessed 29 September 2014).
Eoyang, G.H. and Holladay, R. (2013) *Adaptive action: Leveraging uncertainty in your organization*, Stanford, CA: Stanford University Press.
Ericsson, A.K. (2004) 'Deliberate practice and the acquisition and maintenance of expert performance in medicine and related domains', *Academic Medicine*, 79(10 Supp.): s70–81.
Friedenberg, J. (2009) *Dynamical psychology: Complexity, self-organization and mind*, Litchfield Park, AZ: ISCE Publishing.
Groopman, J. (2007) *How doctors think*, Boston, MA: Houghton Mifflin.
Harden, R.M., Crosby, J.R. and Davis, M.H. (1999) 'AMEE guide no. 14: Outcome-based education: Part 1 – an introduction to outcome-based education', *Medical Teacher*, 21(1): 7–14.

Hofstadter, D. and Sander, E. (2013) *Surfaces and essences: Analogy as the fuel and fire of thinking*, New York, NY: Basic Books.
Human Systems Dynamics Institute (2011) *The learning triangle: Seeing learning as a complex adaptive system*. Online. Available HTTP: http://www.hsdinstitute.org/learn-more/online-learning-and-products/learning-triangle.pdf (accessed 9 October 2014).
Kamei, R., Cook, S., Puthucheary, J. and Starmer, F., (2012) '21st century learning in medicine: traditional teaching versus team-based learning', *Medical Science Educator*, 22(2): 57–64.
Kaufman, A. (ed.) (1985) *Implementing problem-based medical education: Lessons from successful innovations*, Springer series on medical education, New York, NY: Springer.
Kaufman, A., Mennin, S., Waterman, R., Duban, S., Hansbarger, C., Silverblatt, H., Obenshain, S.S., Kantrowitz, M., Becker, T., Samet, J. and Wiese, W. (1989) 'The New Mexico experiment: an educational innovation and institutional change', *Academic Medicine*, 64(6): 285–94.
Kelso, S.J.A. (1995) *Dynamic patterns: The self-organization of brain and behaviour*, Cambridge, MA: MIT Press.
Kelso, S.J.A. and Engestrom, D.A. (2006) *The complementary nature*, Cambridge, MA: MIT Press.
Mann, K., Dornan, T. and Teunissen, P. (2011) 'Perspectives on learning', in T. Dornan, K. Mann, A. Scherpbier and J. Spencer (eds) *Medical education: Theory and practice*, Edinburgh: Elsevier.
Mennin, S. (2010) 'Teaching, learning, complexity and health professions education', *JIAMSE*, 20(2s): 162–5.
Mennin, S. (2013) 'Health professions education: Complexity, teaching and learning'. In J.P. Sturmberg and C. Martin (eds) *Handbook of systems and complexity in health*, Heidelberg: Springer.
Michaelsen, L.K., Knight, A.B. and Fink, L.D. (2002) *Team-based learning: A transformative use of small groups in college teaching*, Sterling, VG: Stylus Publishing.
Moust, J.H.C., van Berkel, H.J.M. and Schmidt, H.G. (2005) 'Signs of erosion: Reflections on three decades of problem-based learning at Maastricht University', *Higher Education*, 50(4): 665–83.
Parmelee, D., Michaelsen, L.K., Cook, S. and Hudes, P.D. (2012) 'Team-based learning, AMEE guide no. 65', *Medical Teacher*, 34(5): e275–87.
Patterson, L., Holladay, R. and Eoyang, G.H. (2013) *Radical rules for schools: Adaptive action for complex change*, Circle Pines, MN: Human Systems Dynamics Institute.
Prigogine, I. and Stengers, I. (1996) *The end of certainty: Time, chaos, and the new laws of nature*, New York, NY: The Free Press.
Regan-Smith, M., Obenshain, S.S., Woodward, C.A., Richards, B., Zeitz, H.J. and Small, P.A. (1994) 'Rote learning in medical school', *The Journal of the American Medical Association*, 272(17): 1380–1.
Royson, H.A. (2002) Personal communication to Mennin, S., June 30.
Schmidt, H.G. (1993) 'Foundations of problem-based learning: Some explanatory notes', *Medical Education*, 27(5): 422–32.
Smith, S.R. (2009) 'Outcome-based curriculum'. In J.A. Dent and R.M. Harden (eds) *A practical guide for medical teachers*, Edinburgh, Churchill Livingstone: Elsevier.
Sturmberg, J.P. and Martin, A. (eds.) (2013) *Handbook of systems and complexity in health*, New York, NY: Springer.
Suchman, A.L. (2006) 'A new theoretical foundation for relationship-centered care: Complex responsive processes of relating', *Journal of General Internal Medicine*, 21(Supp 1): S40–4.
Suchman, A.L., Sluyter, D.J. and Williamson, P.R. (eds.) (2011) *Leading change in healthcare: Transforming organizations using complexity, positive psychology and relationship centered care*, London: Radcliffe.
Sullivan, W.M. and Rosin, M.W. (2008) *A new agenda for higher education: Shaping a life of the mind for practice*, San Francisco, CA: Jossey-Bass.
Swanwick, T. (ed.) (2014) *Understanding medical education: Evidence, theory and practice*, Chichester: John Wiley.
Sweeney, K. (2006). *Complexity in primary care: Understanding its value*, Oxford: Radcliffe.
Teaching-Learning Collaborative (2011) 'The learning triangle: Learning as a complex adaptive system'. Online. Available HTTP: http://wiki.hsdinstitute.org/learning_triangle (accessed 20 April 2014).
ten Cate, O. (2005) 'Entrustability of professional activities and competency-based training', *Medical Education*, 39(12): 1176–7.
ten Cate, O. and Scheele, F. (2007) 'Competency-based postgraduate training: Can we bridge the gap between theory and clinical practice?', *Academic Medicine*, 82(6): 542–7.
ten Cate, O., Snell, L., Mann, K. and Vermunt, J. (2004) 'Orienting teaching toward the learning process', *Academic Medicine*, 79(3): 219–28.

Tschacher, W. and Dauwalder, J.-P. (eds) (2003) *The dynamical systems approach to cognition: Studies of nonlinear phenomena in life science*, Hackensack, NJ: World Scientific.

Voogt, J. and Roblin, J.P. (2010) *21st century skills*, discussion paper, Universiteit Twente, The Netherlands: Universiteit Twente Faculty of Behavioral Sciences.

Voorhees, J.D., Bennett, M.D. and Counsellor, A. (1985) 'Extended community preceptorship: Problem-based learning in the field'. In A. Kaufman (ed.) *Implementing problem-based medical education: Lessons from successful innovations*, New York, NY: Springer.

16

NEW TECHNOLOGIES CAN CONTRIBUTE TO A SUCCESSFUL EDUCATIONAL PROGRAMME

John Sandars

> *Learning technologies have moved from being esoteric tools used by a few pioneering faculty to mainstream applications integrated into the medical school educational enterprise.*

The last decade has seen an increasing global availability and use of a wide range of new technologies, especially social media and mobile devices. These new technologies have become almost ubiquitous and are an integral part of daily life for many people, especially the younger generation who have grown up using these technologies at home and school (Lenhart et al. 2010). The internet has had a major impact on the delivery of educational programmes, increasing their accessibility to students in terms of content, resources, and when and where they can study. Social media is a wide term and includes social networking sites (such as Facebook and Twitter), blogs and wikis (such as WordPress and MediaWiki), media sharing sites (such as Flickr and YouTube) and communication technology for instant messaging and live chat (such as Skype). The original distinction between different social media has become increasingly blurred, with the integration of several functions within each site. For example, Facebook comprises blogs (an easily updated webpage for sharing with others on the network) with media sharing (photographs and videos) and live chat. Mobile devices have also become increasingly integrated, with smartphones and tablet computers (such as iPads) enabling users to take and share photographs and videos, and have access to the many social media sites at a time and place that are convenient for them.

Most readers of this chapter will have experience of using some or all of the above new technologies in their personal lives and many will also have used the same technologies in their professional or clinical practice. New technologies provide unrivalled opportunities to create content, provide a link to existing content, share content with other people and facilitate communication between people, either one to one or one to many. However, the potential for the use of these technologies to enhance teaching and learning will only be fully realised and effective if there is careful attention to integrating the needs of the learner, the opportunities that can be offered by the technology and the context within which the technology is to be used. This integration requires an essential 'learning-centric' focus, which is underpinned by educational principles to provide a structure to the learning experience, instead of a 'technology-centric' focus, that introduces a new technology without consideration of how it provides value to the educational process.

Responding to the needs of the learner

There is increasing focus on the learner being at the centre of the learning process, with the essential recognition that all learners have their own unique needs. An important aspect is the learner's preferred approach to learning, since meeting the needs of the learner improves motivation and engagement with the learning process, resulting in a more effective learning experience. The South African case study and the Dundee, UK case study highlight how the needs of the learner were recognised and used to inform the development of an innovative and effective learning experience with technology.

Case study 16.1   Digital story telling (DST) to enhance reflection on service learning, University of Pretoria, South Africa

Jannie Hugo

One response to the challenge of serious inequity in health in South Africa has been to engage students in service learning in rural district healthcare. At the University of Pretoria, students had a 7-week block in district health in the final 18 months of the course. Students worked in maternity, emergency unit and district clinics across 15 different districts distributed in Mpumalanga, a large rural province. Rural service learning is costly and labour intensive. It was therefore important to ensure that optimum learning was taking place. Reflection is an important component of this learning and students performed several reflection tasks during the block, including a daily learning journal, reflections about obstetric deliveries and written reflection on patient care.

Students regarded reflection tasks as an added responsibility that bores some and frustrates others. As with South African society, the MBChB class of 240 students was also very diverse, with students coming from different ethnic and cultural backgrounds, from rural or urban areas, and from at least 11 different home-language groups. Although English was the language of instruction and working, it was a second language to most students, and students were encouraged to speak the patient's language as much as possible. Writing narrative in English did not come naturally to these students.

The aim of the DST task was to integrate reflection and learning at the end of the district health block. This task was compulsory: all students received orientation and guidance on how to prepare the story, but it was not formally addressed. Students were expected to identify important learning experiences and provide a picture to represent these experiences. The pictures could be obtained from the internet but most students would take a series of photographs during the block, mainly using their own mobile phone. For ethical reasons, no pictures of staff or patients were allowed.

During the last week of the block, students returned to the campus in Pretoria where they went through all of their reflections and pictures to integrate them into a reflective digital story. This story of their experience and learning during the block was presented to the group in the form of a PowerPoint presentation of five to seven pictures.

In a focus group evaluation, students reported overwhelmingly positive experiences of using DST. During the block, students consciously thought of their experiences 'in pictures': they remembered their experiences and the learning of the block as pictures about people and not in academic terms. Some reflection appeared to happen while taking the photograph, and then it was relived when the pictures were reviewed and chosen for the presentation. There was also an opportunity to work through negative experiences, share and come to terms with these experiences. Further reflection occurred while doing the presentation and watching the other presentations and even continued afterwards by reminding the student about experiences related to pictures.

For tutors the DST was enjoyable, time efficient and very informative as to what students really experience and learn during the block. Teachers regarded DST as that part of the block that provided most job satisfaction!

As a learning task, students preferred DST to written and more structured reflective assignments. It was experienced as non-judgemental and pictures made it possible to say things that were difficult to say in words, especially when English was a second language. The opportunity to reflect also appeared to be enhanced, with numerous points for reflection both during the creation of the DST and after the presentation.

There is research on present-day medical students that suggests that there is a preference for a more active and visual approach to learning rather than the more traditional text-based approaches to teaching (Sandars and Homer 2008). This is likely to be more important in cultures that have an oral narrative tradition and also where English is a second language. Active learning usually has a collaborative component, with 'one-to-one' or 'one-to-many' interactions. Information and opinion are shared to create a mutual and deeper understanding. The South African case study utilised group presentations to enhance the learning from reflection and the Dundee, UK case study (see below) offers several opportunities to collaborate, including the development of content and networking between students and with their teaching staff.

Case study 16.2 Using blogs to engage students and teaching staff in a medical school, University of Dundee, UK

Natalie Lafferty

Medical schools have been early adopters of educational technologies yet have faced challenges in delivering an integrated spiral curriculum in traditional virtual learning environments (VLEs), such as Blackboard and Moodle. With a focus on how they want to teach and support learning, medical educators are increasingly exploring the potential of social media tools, including blogging platforms such as WordPress and microblogs such as Twitter, to support their teaching. Inspired by medical blogs such as *Life in the Fast Lane* and *Clinical Cases and Images* hosting growing medical education libraries of cases and resources, Dundee Medical School explored the potential of the WordPress blogging platform to support undergraduate teaching.

The Medical School set up its own WordPress server (MedBlogs) and teaching leads began to explore, using it as an alternative to the VLE to deliver their teaching. Students were also engaged in this process, helping staff to develop sites in different specialties. Blogs were initially piloted in the respiratory and musculoskeletal system teaching blocks to supplement core teaching resources delivered via the VLE. Teaching staff found MedBlogs straightforward to use and used their blogs to link to journal articles and websites, comment on topical news stories and embed videos. Patient scenarios were also posted which

(continued)

> *(continued)*
> students discussed via blog comments, and at the end of the week a post from teaching staff provided a detailed explanation of each case. The response from students to the blogs was positive and enthusiastic, and analytics showed students made extensive use of them both during the teaching blocks as well as in revision periods. Students found them easy to use and to post questions, which were promptly answered by teachers, and they asked for more to be set up for other teaching blocks. Students reported higher levels of engagement with learning resources and repeatedly highlighted that the blogs supported more self-directed learning and increased their engagement, enthusiasm and motivation for learning than when resources were delivered via the VLE.
>
> Further teaching blocks were added to MedBlogs and feedback from staff and students continued to be positive, with both sets of users finding the emerging MedBlogs learning portal more intuitive and easier to use than the VLE. There was increased teaching staff engagement to support online learning, with a new level of autonomy to personalise their online teaching space through links to journals, specialist organisations and embedding Twitter feeds in their blogs. There was also improved support for integration of themes, systems and specialities across the curriculum.
>
> Ongoing positive evaluation and feedback from staff and students has led to the decision to migrate online delivery of the medical curriculum from the original VLE to a new Dundee MBChB MedBlogs learning portal built in WordPress. The flexibility and usability of blogs have been recognised, with increased engagement of both students and teaching staff.

It is interesting that the Dundee case study used a 'formal' institutionally provided blogging platform instead of asking students to use more familiar social media (such as Facebook). Previous studies have noted that students prefer to use technologies that are familiar but wish to keep social and university activities separate (Joint Information Systems Committee (JISC) 2007). This may sound contradictory, but it is important for teaching staff to respect the privacy of students. However, students may set up their own 'informal' networks using social media and there are increasing numbers of doctors and students worldwide using social media to support personal development and reflective practice as well as collaborative learning across specialties. The accessibility, social nature and ease of use of social media have supported the development of global online communities of practice across the continuum of medical education. Their use is very much learner-centred and driven by the desire to engage in regular learning conversations. There are several open medical education blogs that are remixing open content from around the web. This approach has become known as free open-access medical education – FOAMed. Content from social media sites, such as YouTube, Vimeo and Flickr, can be surrounded by learning conversations via blog comments and Twitter. An example of the FOAMed approach is *Gasclass*, an anaesthetics blog, where a case scenario is posted as a blog post and then discussed by anaesthetists around the world on Twitter using the hashtag #gasclass, with additional information introduced over the course of the week.

Responding to the needs of the community

New technologies have provided an unrivalled opportunity to respond to health workforce shortages in rural and remote locations by enabling the development of decentralised medical education programmes and distance learning. The US case studies from Idaho State University and the University of Washington present two models of decentralised medical education, one using video and audio connections to deliver classroom-based teaching and the other in-person delivery supported by VLE.

Case study 16.3 Two models of decentralised medical education, United States

Ruth Ballweg, David Talford and Jared Papa

Two physician assistant (PA) programmes in the US Pacific Northwest rural states have responded to health workforce shortages by developing decentralised medical educational models to serve their region better. The University of Washington's (UW) MEDEX Northwest PA Program and Idaho State University's (ISU) PA Program share common goals in developing their decentralised educational sites; however, each institution chose a different model of delivery to respond best to the needs of their specific service area.

Both programmes are required to meet the educational standards of their accrediting body – the Accreditation Review Commission on the Certification of Physician Assistants (ARC-PA), which requires that decentralised educational sites demonstrate educational equivalency between campuses. This includes curriculum, facilities, faculty, staff and university oversight.

By creating decentralised sites, both the UW and ISU sought to provide opportunities which would not otherwise be available to 'place-bound' students in rural and widely dispersed geographic areas. These decentralised expansions assured the delivery of proven high-quality curricula without the expensive 'start-up' costs of newly established programmes. They also allowed for utilisation of local-community resources (clinicians practising in the communities) and previously unused clinical training facilities.

Idaho State University case study

Idaho is one of America's most rural states and ranks 49 out of 50 US states in physician-to-population ratio. As the designated health education institution in Idaho, ISU is located in Pocatello, Idaho, 250 miles away from Boise, the main population centre. In deciding to establish an additional site, the PA programme chose a technologically unified classroom approach with both video and audio connections.

Major factors in the ISU implementation included assuring adequate internet bandwidth between the two sites, the inclusion of annual equipment maintenance/upgrade expenses, consideration of classroom acoustics and provision for one full-time audio/visual technician per site. The start-up costs were US$40,000 per classroom. Technical issues included camera considerations and planning for open microphones. Planning for teaching needed to include the engagement of the distant site, developing plans for managing interactive delays and the acquisition of new presentation tools for this type of delivery.

ISU reported positive outcomes and findings. Data revealed high levels of student satisfaction between campuses with continued increase in satisfaction over time. There was equality between the two sites in clinical and written exam scores as well as high National Certification Exam results. The programme is now in the process of expanding to a third training site.

ISU pearls and pitfalls

- *Pearls* – It is important to maintain an adequate faculty-to-student ratio at all physical sites. Technology inevitably does occasionally fail, so an audio/visual technician at each site is critical to resolve glitches and maintain backup recordings.

(continued)

(continued)
- *Pitfalls* – The central campus can easily be perceived by faculty and students as being superior to the other sites. Engaging faculty at satellite sites in leadership roles can help avoid this.

University of Washington case study

The University of Washington and its MEDEX Northwest PA Program serve as the medical education resources for multiple rural states in the Pacific Northwest. Since the Washington, Wyoming, Alaska, Montana, Idaho (WWAMI) Regional Medical Program was created in 1971, the institution has offered Year 1 of medical education – and some clinical training opportunities – in the states it serves. The expanded need for PAs as a result of health reform generated requests from states, hospitals and local communities to train PAs closer to home as a strategy for building the rural health workforce:

- Central Washington (Yakima) geographic isolation of Central Washington created barriers for students to become PAs. The community was interested in a partnership (1993–2013).
- Eastern Washington (Spokane) is also distant from a medical school: this economic centre needed PAs to provide care in the surrounding rural communities and refer them into Spokane's regional and tertiary care hospitals (opened 1996).
- Alaska (Anchorage) PAs had become a major fixture of healthcare in Alaska; however it was a hardship for Alaskans to be in Seattle, a large urban centre so far from home (opened 2008).
- Western Washington (Tacoma) is a military town where returning military members sought additional training slots in their home community (opened 2013).

As compared to the ISU technology model, the UW chose an 'in-person' delivery model combined with electronic tools (e.g. Moodle) for curriculum management.

Faculty requirements for each distant site (24 students per site) include three full-time PA faculty, and one full-time staff person per site. A large cadre of faculty and staff at the programme's 'home' in Seattle support teaching and administrative needs of all sites. The Seattle site on the UW campus admits 40 students per year. The programme leadership (Program Director and Medical Director) serves all sites. Other faculty rotate across sites to allow students to benefit from their individual expertise.

All courses are 'chaired' by a PA faculty member who 'hires', orients and monitors teaching by community-based faculty. PA faculty serve as advisors, mentors and role models for students at their sites. An overarching Student Progress Committee reviews student performance regularly. Faculty representatives of all sites serve on this committee. Annual faculty retreats for each course result in updates and modifications, which are implemented across all sites.

In terms of outcomes, student characteristics – upon admission – are similar across all sites (32 years of age and 8 years of clinical experience prior to entry). Students in rural sites appear more likely to enter primary care employment. Students in decentralised sites tend to choose employment in their home communities. Student performance varies little across sites with respect to grades or board performance.

UW pearls and pitfalls

- *Pearls* – It is important to recruit stable faculty who are willing to integrate themselves fully into their new community. Similarly, it is important to create systems in the community as a substitute for those usually found in a larger academic setting.

- *Pitfalls* – The coordination of faculty and students takes time – and commitment – from programme leadership. Flexibility in response to crises is the key to success.

Two PA programmes have successfully developed and implemented decentralised medical educational programmes in two very different models. Both programmes have been successful in increasing student throughput and expanding access in remote and rural communities.

Similarly, the case study from Uganda demonstrates how communication technologies can be used to support teaching effectively across international boundaries. This case study, it may be argued, offers a vital opportunity for medical schools to share expertise and support work in less well-resourced communities and countries.

Case study 16.4   Using communication technology for surgical skills teaching in Uganda – a pilot study among intern doctors at Mulago National Referral and Teaching Hospital

Josaphat Byamugisha, Yosam Nsubuga, Mark Muyingo, Amy Autry, Sharon Knight, Felicia Lester, Gerald Dubowitz and Abner Korn

Mulago National Referral and Teaching Hospital in Kampala, Uganda, delivers babies for 32,000 mothers annually. Interns rotate through obstetrics, medicine, paediatrics and surgery every 3 months. Given such a large service demand, it made sense to explore the use of technology such as the internet to augment instruction in basic skills such as suturing.

Video internet communication through Skype to teach and evaluate basic surgical skills was explored for intern physicians rotating in obstetrics and gynaecology. A selected group had three video teaching sessions with the University of California San Francisco (UCSF) faculty via Skype. We found an improvement of 50 per cent or more for interns who participated in online suture session. Participation in the sessions improved two-handed knot tying significantly and was found to be helpful. The interactive nature of the online teaching was enjoyable, equal to in-person teaching. All UCSF faculty involved in the teaching sessions enjoyed participating and thought the interns improved their knot-tying skills.

Remote teaching is feasible, effective and well accepted by both learners and teachers. Repetitive remote teaching sessions may encourage more independent learner practice of skills. In under-resourced settings, where faculty time is limited and visiting faculty are not always possible, this technology can improve surgical skills teaching and retention, even for basic skills.

The opportunities offered by new technologies

The Dundee and Singapore case studies highlight how new technologies can offer new and innovative opportunities for learning compared with existing technologies, especially VLEs and organisational information repositories that archive material.

Case study 16.5 An online hyperlinked radiology case repository to facilitate postgraduate training in diagnostic radiology, National University of Singapore

Goh Poh Sun

The Department of Radiology has both a clinical and academic role, with 30–40 residents in radiology following the residency guidelines of the Accreditation Council for Graduate Medical Education International (ACGME-I 2013). The 24 clinical radiologists in the department have a subspecialty focus and share teaching duties. The objective of building up an online radiology case repository was to develop a collection of clinical cases that present the major and important diagnostic categories encountered in clinical practice, to allow residents in training the opportunity to be exposed to a wide variety of cases in each category, with a standardised and comprehensive exposure to cases representing the full clinical spectrum (from typical, to less typical, and atypical cases, and clinical examples with confounding features and multiple diagnoses) and to provide authentic radiology cases for exemplar teaching for postgraduates.

The neuroradiology case repository has over 2,000 online cases accumulated over the last 2 years. Every day the clinical radiologists used a mobile device to photograph all cases with potential teaching value. The photographs were taken directly off reporting workstations and then anonymised and uploaded on to the case repository. These cases were displayed via an online blog which presented radiology cases thematically, as unknown cases for quiz and drill exercises, and as a hyperlinked index for self-study (Figures 16.1–16.3; Goh 2013). The online case repository closely mirrored the range and complexity of actual clinical radiology practice, with authentic case material. Reusability of material was possible without the need for copyright considerations as the material has been selected and authored in house.

The popularity of the neuroradiology teaching blog was reflected in viewership statistics (over 25,000 views since its inception 2 years ago). Feedback from residents showed that they valued the efficiency of case presentation via online blogs, as well as opportunities for revision and self-study. They also valued online case material to supplement their daily supervised clinical practice since it broadened their clinical exposure. The teaching staff used the online cases to provide a uniform exposure of the core spectrum of case material in neuroradiology for the residents. Having a large and continually developing online repository of cases allowed a written curriculum to be elaborated with the actual spectrum of clinical case material that residents are expected to have reviewed. This has been used for daily case review and discussed in topic-focused tutorials, and in assessments. The case repository has also facilitated peer review of teaching and assessment case material.

The major challenge was to convince fellow departmental teaching staff that this method was the most efficient way of archiving material, as compared to making a note of interesting cases and coming back on another day. The process of building up and utilising the online case repository provided evidence via a working prototype that this process was an efficient and effective method of building up a collection of case material, which was of sufficient quality for teaching purposes.

The online repository provided the wide variety of different cases for drill and practice that is required for mastery training in radiology. Developing a working prototype has demonstrated the value of using instructional technology to users and the development process fostered collaboration amongst students and teachers.

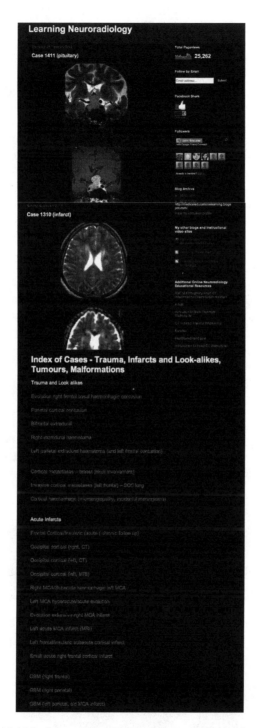

Figures 16.1, 16.2 and 16.3 Selected pages from our neuroradiology teaching blog, which presents radiology cases thematically, and as a hyperlinked index for self-study.

The Dundee case study appeared to be successful, since the blogging platform was not only more intuitive to use but also offered increased functionality that was not possible within current VLE platforms. The usability (ease of use) of a technology is an important, but often neglected, aspect of using technologies in medical education because it determines the motivation of both learners and teaching staff to engage with technology (Sandars and Lafferty 2010). Any new technology may be potentially useful for learning but will never achieve its intended potential unless it has high usability.

Technology is becoming increasingly used in healthcare organisations for information management systems and an important aspect of these systems is the storage of vast amounts of information, both text and images. The complexity of existing systems and their information governance controls, to ensure confidentiality of stored clinical information, limit their potential use for learning. The Singapore case study used a blogging tool to archive radiographical images that were selectively obtained by teaching staff using their own mobile devices. The online images were shared between learners and with their tutors by the use of the social networking capability of the blogging platform to create effective online learning communities.

Both the Dundee and Singapore case studies describe the essential opportunity for personalised learning that new technologies can offer learners. Central to personalised learning is the recognition that the learning needs for an individual learner are unique and there is no 'one size fits all' approach to meeting these needs. In response to an identified need, the learner proactively meets these needs by selectively integrating a range of different learning resources, such as content on blogs or from interactions on social networks. This approach is in marked contrast to more traditional didactic approaches.

The context of the use of new technologies

The Leeds, UK, case study highlights how the context in which new technologies are used can produce innovative opportunities for teaching and learning, but also highlights the challenges that have to be overcome if the potential benefits are to be realised. The main advantage of workplace-based assessment is that actual performance of learners in authentic situations can be achieved. These authentic contexts are usually busy clinical environments and the use of mobile devices has great potential; clinical procedures and encounters with patients can be observed by assessors and assessment templates can be completed and uploaded to electronic portfolios (e-portfolios) for both formative and summative assessment.

Case study 16.6 Mobile devices for learning and assessment in clinical settings, University of Leeds, UK

Gareth Frith

Learning through clinical practice is an increasingly important part of the undergraduate curriculum, with students in Years 4 and 5 spending the majority of their time in a range of primary and secondary care clinics and hospitals. It is important that students can effectively learn from this experience by getting prompt assessment of their performance and good-quality feedback from the medical and healthcare professionals with whom they are working.

Since 2010, undergraduate medical students at the University of Leeds have been part of a mobile learning programme (MLP) which has provided students with an iPhone that has both 3G and wireless data connection. The students had the device from the beginning of Year 4 until they graduated at the end of Year 5.

In order to support students' placement learning, they were provided with access to specific medical content through the *Medhand Dr Companion* app with copies of medical texts such as the *British National Formulary, Oxford Handbooks of Clinical Medicine, Clinical Specialties,* and other titles. These interactive books are resident on students' phones so that they are not dependent on network connectivity. As further support, a website with guidance on suitable medical apps relevant to their learning was provided.

Students were encouraged to seek timely 'near-patient' feedback on their clinical work through multiple feedback exercises with clinical and other healthcare professionals who had observed them working with patients. Students were provided with a workplace-based assessment iPhone app (MiniCEX/WPBA) to record the assessments and these were synchronised with their progress file (e-portfolio). The accumulated records supported their reflection on their progress through the curriculum to identify strengths and areas for improvement.

Feedback from students was positive about the MLP, but not all students appeared to be technically savvy and a few struggled with the experience. The student response to the use of mobile devices for assessment was tentative at the start, with few assessments undertaken in the first 2 weeks but with a flurry of activity towards the end of the rotation. Interviews with students noted that this was due to lack of confidence in both using a new approach to assessment and also a new technology. Students had to be confident in asking for feedback from a busy clinical team and there was some reticence with appearing unprofessional by using a phone in a clinical environment. As the MLP developed, however, there was increasing confidence and this was partly due to more engagement with the clinical teams by the school taking time to explain the MLP to the professionals and letting them know what to expect from the students. The students were given iPhone cases with the school logo and a text, 'This is a learning tool provided by the University of Leeds, School of Medicine', on the back so they could show professionals and patients. Over the long term, students became increasingly engaged with the MLP and many became fully engaged with all aspects of the work, including actively seeking out professionals to provide assessment and feedback.

Also popular was the provision of the mobile content and e-books. Because these were loaded on to the device and not dependent on the networks, they were more usable than internet-based resources. Clinicians also became more engaged with the students in terms of prescribing and challenging the student to use the device and material to look up content.

Some Year 4 students have started to develop their own apps. A series of Objective Structured Clinical Examination (OSCE) toolkit apps were developed by students as part of a research component of the curriculum. The objective was to help students revise for this important clinical assessment exam.

The MLP appeared to be successful in engaging students in both learning and also workplace assessment and feedback.

The Leeds, UK, case study describes the use of mobile devices for both assessment, with MiniCEX templates, and also learning, with a range of apps that can be used as learning resources. This combination offers innovative approaches to teaching and learning, such as the 'assessment sandwich'. Students can use one of the learning resources on the mobile device prior to a clinical experience, their competence can be assessed and further learning can occur by returning to the learning resources in the device. An educational advantage of such an approach is the situated learning that is more meaningful for the learner. However, the Leeds case study also reveals the difficulties of using new technologies, especially in authentic clinical settings. These difficulties include overcoming misconceptions from both teaching staff and patients ('students are playing with their phones when they should be learning'), concerns about protecting confidential patient information when entering identifying information or taking photographs and institutional firewalls that block access to cellular networks.

How to ensure the potential for teaching and learning

A new range of digital competences will need to be developed by both teaching staff and learners if social media are to be used effectively to enhance teaching and learning (Sero Consulting 2007). These digital competences include enquiry, production, participation and digital literacy.

Enquiry

Finding information in the first place and then critically evaluating what is found is essential if effective learning is to be obtained from the vast number of websites and other internet resources, such as podcasts.

Production

Activities related to the production of content, including multimedia resources, are becoming increasingly important in teaching and learning, especially if teaching staff and learners are to become active contributing members of online communities.

Participation

Successful online networks and collaborative learning do not occur by chance. The new technologies can easily link widely dispersed learners but there is still the necessary human aspect and this is often forgotten. New competences in communicating and participating online need to be developed so that mutual trust and respect can allow individuals to share information and opinions.

Digital literacy

This is an essential competence since there are rights and responsibilities that need to be considered when publicly sharing information, opinions and support. Confidentiality and respect for privacy are essential components of medical practice but several studies of the Facebook entries made by medical students and junior doctors have highlighted the public nature of most comments and many entries often contain identifiable patient information (Guseh et al. 2009). There have also been several high-profile cases where inappropriate comments have been made about tutors or other students.

It is easy to be cynical about the contribution of new technologies in the provision of effective teaching and learning across the continuum of medical education. Much of this concern is the perception that most of the learning is superficial, yet the South African case study highlights the depth of reflective learning that can be facilitated. There are also important aspects related to the nature of knowledge required for professional practice that need to be critically considered. All healthcare professionals require both information (explicit knowledge) and opinion (tacit knowledge) to answer many of their identified learning needs that arise from dealing with the complex 'messy' problems of professional practice. The explicit knowledge can be answered through information sources but the tacit knowledge requires opportunities to network and share experiences with other professionals. This online networking is central to social media and is highlighted in the Dundee and Singapore case studies.

The role of the 'teaching' with social media has to be redefined, from a 'sage on the stage' to 'the guide on the side'. A shift from a simple provider of content, including entries on blogs, to that of an educational facilitator that is more concerned with the process of learning is required. This facilitation function requires an understanding of some educational theories that may be less familiar to medical educators, such as ecology of learning and connectivism (Sandars and Haythornthwaite 2007). These theories can inform the medical educator to use approaches that either externally scaffold the learning, such as by providing or suggesting a range of resources within a learning landscape (as in the Dundee case study), or by developing the internal scaffolding of learners through opportunities to reflect on the process of learning, in which the various resources can be connected to construct learning that is personally relevant, and not simply on whether learning outcomes have been met (as in the Singapore case study). These insights of meta-learning are essential for the development of lifelong learners.

The introduction of new technologies can lead to transformational changes in the curriculum (as in the Dundee, Singapore and Leeds case studies), but often the changes are of a lesser degree. The important aspects of connectivity to cellular networks, as well as competence and confidence in using the new technologies, are essential basic requirements that need to be met. There may be poor connectivity in rural and remote areas, and even in urban areas there is often blocking of access due to firewalls in healthcare organisations. The Leeds case study highlights the paradox that is often seen with the so-called net generation of students that have grown up with technology: these students are often only confident and competent in using a small range of familiar technologies (Bennett et al. 2008). Making major changes to existing approaches to educational provision can be highly disruptive and one approach is to blend new teaching and learning approaches supported by new technologies with existing approaches (as in the South Africa case study). One innovative blended approach is the 'flipped classroom', in which a phase of online learning deliberately occurs before the face-to-face teaching (Ash 2012).

There appears to be little evidence base to show whether new technologies do produce more effective learning than alternative approaches, but this is typical of other aspects of using technology for teaching and learning, such as more traditional linear learning packages or podcasts. However, all of the case studies identified increased staff and learner satisfaction and motivation to learn, leading to improved engagement with the wider endeavour of teaching and learning across the medical education continuum. It is interesting that the Uganda case study showed improved skills, possibly because of the high interactivity between tutors and learners.

The six case studies have clearly shown that new technologies can contribute to a successful educational programme with increased engagement and contribution by both teaching staff and students. These innovative changes can have transformative aspects with major changes in programmes and the case studies offer useful illustrative examples of the potential impact on teaching and learning. However, there are often barriers to be overcome before the potential of new technologies can be fully realised and these are mainly related to the healthcare and institutional context within which the new technologies are introduced. Future research on the impact of new technologies on teaching and learning is required, especially to identify the critical factors that lead to an impact on learning, such as the design of approaches to learning and the relative potential benefits of different types of new technology, including blended learning.

Take-home messages

- New technologies, such as the internet, have had a major impact on the accessibility and delivery of educational programmes.
- For new technologies to enhance teaching and learning, careful attention needs to be paid to integrating the needs of the learner, the opportunities offered by the technology and the context in which the technology will be used.
- This integration requires a 'learning-centric' rather than a 'technology-centric' approach.
- The effective use of social media and other new technologies to enhance teaching and learning requires the development of a new range of digital competencies by staff and learners: enquiry, production, participation and digital literacy.
- Used well, social media and new technologies can contribute to increased student engagement and reflective and active learning.

Bibliography

ACGME-I (2013) *Accreditation Council for Graduate Medical Education International.* Online. Available http://www.acgme-i.org (accessed 24 March 2015).

Ash, K. (2012) 'Educators evaluate flipped classrooms', *Education Week*, 32(2): s6–8.

Bennett, S., Maton, K. and Kervin, L. (2008) 'The 'digital natives' debate: A critical review of the evidence', *British Journal of Educational Technology*, 39(5): 775–86.

Goh, P.S. (2013) *Learning neuroradiology blog.* Online. Available http://learningneuroradiology.blogspot.sg (accessed 12 March 2013).

Guseh, J.S., Brendel, R.W. and Brendel, D.H. (2009) 'Medical professionalism in the age of online social networking', *Journal of Medical Ethics*, 35(9): 584–6.

Joint Information Systems Committee (JISC) (2007) *In their own words: Exploring the learner's perspective on e-learning*, Newcastle: Joint Information Systems Committee.

Lenhart, A., Purcell, K., Smith, A. and Zickuhr, K. (2010) *Social media and mobile internet use among teens and young adults*, Washington, DC: Pew Internet and American Life Project.

Sandars, J. and Haythornthwaite, C. (2007) 'New horizons for e-learning in medical education: Ecological and Web 2.0 perspectives', *Medical Teacher*, 29(4): 307–10.

Sandars, J. and Homer, M. (2008) 'Reflective learning and the net generation', *Medical Teacher*, 30(9–10): 877–9.

Sandars, J. and Lafferty, N. (2010) 'Twelve tips on usability testing to develop effective e-learning in medical education', *Medical Teacher*, 32(12): 956–60.

Sero Consulting (2007) *Next generation user skills: A report for digital 2010 and the SQA: Sero Consulting.* Online. HTTP: www.sqa.org.uk/sqa/files_ccc/HNComputing_NGUSReport_NextGenerationUserSkills.pdf (accessed 8 May 2014).

PART 5

Assessment

17
HOW TO IMPLEMENT A MEANINGFUL ASSESSMENT PROGRAMME

Lambert Schuwirth

> *Assessment is central to medical education and has come to be understood as co-embedded with learning.*

Assessment is not what it used to be. Where normally such a phrase is uttered in a nostalgic tone, here it is meant in a more positive vein. Assessment used to be a reasonably straightforward issue; it was mainly a problem of correctly measuring the students' traits, as there were knowledge, skills, problem-solving ability and attitudes. The goal was to produce the optimal instrument for each of these four and the combination of those results would add up to medical competence. The typical discussions in the literature about whether open-ended questions are superior to MCQs and the various comparisons of standard-setting methods are all examples of that line of thinking.

Things have become more complex since then. First, the idea took root that every assessment instrument would have its advantages and disadvantages and that building a high-quality assessment programme was mainly about optimally combining instruments rather than trying to find a holy grail for each trait (van der Vleuten 1996). Second, the notion of competencies was developed (e.g. Frank 2005). Competencies embody a clear integration of knowledge, skills, abilities, attitudes and reflection rather than a separation of each of them (Albanese et al. 2008). Assessment programmes that rely on a reductionist approach can therefore not achieve a valid evaluation of students' competence. Simply adding up a patient's responses to history taking, findings on physical examination and lab values does not automatically – or by some arithmetic formula – result in a good evaluation of the equally holist and integrated notion of 'health'. It is fair to say that this has created a landslide in our thinking about, and literature on, the quality of assessment. Publications on assessment to promote student learning (Shepard 2009) or the acquisition of academic values (Boud 1990), on assessment *for* learning (Schuwirth and van der Vleuten 2011), programmatic assessment (van der Vleuten and Schuwirth 2005) and on quality frameworks for programmes of assessment have filled the literature since.

The first case study demonstrates how this line of thinking has led to improvements in assessment programmes to broaden the scope of competencies being captured by such programmes.

Case study 17.1 Assessment in family medicine rotation, College of Medicine, King Saud University, Saudi Arabia

Eiad AlFaris, Hussain Saad Amin and Naghma Naeem

King Saud University (KSU) College of Medicine undergraduate family medicine curriculum consists of a 6-week rotation in the fourth year of medical school (Al-Faris 2000). Assessment in this course has evolved over the last 20 years, steadily moving towards a more authentic assessment that targets the upper level of Miller's pyramid (Miller 1990).

In the beginning, the focus of assessment was knowledge, which was assessed by context-free multiple-choice questions (MCQs), modified essay questions (MEQs), practice profiles and oral examinations. There were two summative assessments, over the 6-week period, 40 per cent continuous assessment and 60 per cent final examination.

As assessment evolved, a 'blueprint' was developed to ensure content validity. In addition, critical reading questions were included in the continuous assessment and the oral examination was discontinued because of time requirement and concerns regarding its reliability and validity. The next reform in assessment was the inclusion of Objective Structured Clinical Examination (OSCE) to assess the psychomotor and communication skills. The use of MEQs was discontinued. The continuous assessment (40 marks) included single best context-rich MCQs, student-led seminars, case-based (CbD) discussion and evidence-based medicine (EBM) presentations with reports. The final assessment (60 marks) included MCQs, OSCE and evaluation in community centres. In addition, faculty development workshops were conducted to improve the quality of MCQs and OSCEs. More recently, the quality, diversity and number of OSCE stations have been improved, and a data interpretation paper has been added. The blueprint has been further developed and a committee of course teachers at departmental and central levels has been formed to review all assessment items.

Challenges and proposed solutions

The upper level of Miller's triangle is not well covered

This needs to be covered in the form of workplace-based assessment (WPBA) tools, such as the mini-clinical evaluation exercise (mini-CEX) and/or a simple portfolio that includes self- and peer-assessment and professionalism questionnaire with reflection. A recorded student consultation with a patient using one of the consultation models, such as the Calgary-Cambridge Consult scale, would be added to the portfolio package.

There is little emphasis on formative assessment

More emphasis should be placed on formative assessment in the form of mock examinations with reflection and the use of self-assessment questions on the blackboard. Bilateral 'student and teacher' feedback should be strongly encouraged.

Clinical assessment in community centres is not discerning enough

Currently, most of the students' scores are 9–10 out of 10. Annual meetings with the community centre supervisors are being planned, and university teachers will accompany students in the community centres to conduct experiential teaching and encourage more appropriate and insightful assessment that covers professionalism using WPBA tools.

Assessment of students' assignments and presentations varies a lot between teachers (hawk and dove effect)

A calibration exercise will be conducted. Video-taped student presentations will be used for this purpose with the aim of improving inter-rater reliability.

The development of a blueprint that includes the objectives, content and methods of assessment is the first step towards achieving a valid course assessment

The Miller's pyramid of competence is the framework that should be followed for achieving high validity in teaching and assessment. This requires the use of multiple methods, particularly WPBA tools, and the provision of frequent and constructive feedback. All the teachers who participate in the course should be either involved or informed about the course details (Al-Faris and Naeem 2012).

What is clear from this example is that assessment is no longer *merely* a measurement – reliability and construct validity – problem but has become increasingly an educational design, organisational and staff-development problem. So the attention has shifted towards the influence assessment has on the motivation for learning (and not just on study behaviour), the influence acceptability has on whether the theoretical curriculum, the enacted curriculum and the hidden curriculum align, and the cost efficiency of the programme to make it sustainable.

The next case studies in this chapter serve as illustrations for the broad palette of factors that determine the quality of an assessment programme.

The second case study, from Austria, addresses issues of efficiency and cost-effectiveness in relation to assessment.

Case study 17.2 Implementing a meaningful assessment programme, Medical University of Vienna, Austria

Michael Schmidts and Michaela Wagner-Menghin

Until 2009 at the Medical University of Vienna the entire cohort of 720 second-year students routinely took a practical clerkship entry exam on basic clinical skills (two stations), physical examination (two stations) and history taking (one station). With only five stations, the exam's reliability was only 0.50.

In 2009 we gained additional resources, but still not enough to reach the minimum recommended reliability of 0.7 for summative examinations (Downing 2004). So, instead of adding additional stations to increase the precision of the test globally, we decided to focus on improving reliability for the pass/fail decision and piloted a sequential testing approach.

(continued)

(continued)

Since 2010 all students take an initial eight-station practical exam. Despite a still low reliability of 0.61, students can be separated into a clear pass, a clear fail and a borderline group performing close to the pass/fail criterion. Only the 'borderliners' (about 25 per cent of the cohort) take an additional six stations to increase the reliability and better justify their pass/fail decision ($r = 0.74$). The borderline group can be estimated by counting the number of candidates below the score distribution within the limits of a confidence interval round the pass/fail score (Harvill 1991; Downing 2004).

This sequential approach requires only 6,840 student–examiner contacts compared to the 10,080 that would have been required in a conventional 14-station OSCE. Despite the low number of screening stations, we regard content validity as acceptable, since the number of assessable procedures is still limited in the second year.

As the resources of the faculty usually have to be allocated prior to the exam, the number of borderline students who will need further testing has to be estimated in advance, either based on a pilot study or by analysing data from previous examinations. This is necessary because the size of the borderline group is influenced by many factors, such as the cohort's ability, reliability, pass/fail criterion's distance to the score mean, score variance and score distribution skewness. Fortunately, the borderline group sizes have remained very stable in Vienna in recent years.

For logistical reasons there is about a week between screening and further testing in our setting. As sequential testing starts from the assumption of an unchanged object of measurement, one might argue whether it is correct to add up the results from screening and further testing to an overall score. However from an educational point of view, this time between screening and further testing makes a virtue out of a necessity. The weak performers receive feedback and are allowed to visit our skills lab for remedial action.

The decision about the pass/fail criterion is also challenging. In the second phase the borderline regression method does not work as all candidates tested here are already borderline candidates. Stations used for further testing have to be criterion-referenced in advance.

As it is not possible to distinguish justifiably between 'excellent', 'good' and 'average' students within the 'clear pass' group – since the screening's reliability is low – no grades other than 'pass' or 'fail' should be given in this type of assessment.

Student acceptance of the sequential assessment can be increased when the exam is announced as a 14-station OSCE, which is shortened for students with better test results, instead of pronouncing that students with weaker results have to take a longer test.

It is important to keep in mind that sequential testing is more challenging to implement than a classical assessment. This assessment format requires careful piloting and psychometric assessment during the implementation phase. One has to decide the number of stations for the screening as well as further testing by taking reliability and validity issues into account. Although we acknowledge concerns about the violation of measurement assumptions, we established a very objective and structured 'double-spot' assessment that is formative for those students who probably most urgently need remediation. This fills the gap between single-spot summative and continuous assessment. Similar to recently reported results (Muijtjens et al. 2000; Smee et al. 2003; Cookson et al. 2011), the success of introducing sequential testing at Medical University of Vienna lies in saving resources by cutting down on student–examiner encounters and still having justifiable pass/fail decisions with acceptable reliability in the vicinity of the pass/fail criterion (Wagner-Menghin et al. 2011).

Assessing 720 students with an OSCE in a context with limited resources is a challenge. This case study is important in this chapter. Not because of its focus on optimising a single test of competence. Nor is it chosen because of the measurement issue it addresses; this is theoretically simple: if you want higher reliability, you simply include more cases, and if you cannot or won't do this for the whole group of students, do it for those for whom it matters most. This would be neither new nor exciting. What is important is the approach the authors took.

First, they made a clear analysis of the local problem: huge student numbers, restrictive boundary conditions in terms of staff time and financial resources and a requirement to optimise the pass/fail decision at a certain point in the curriculum were at the core of the problem. Second, they consulted carefully the literature to find the best solutions that could and would work in their own context. Third, they adapted the findings to their local situation. And finally, they redesigned the OSCE and trialled and evaluated it.

If we want to put this problem in a broader context, it is helpful to look at validity from the perspective of Kane (2006). Kane describes validation as a stepwise process of generating supportive arguments or plausible evidence for the inference from observation of behaviour to conclusions about the construct of interest. If, for example, we want to draw conclusions about a student's clinical reasoning skills, we can observe the student during simulated or real patient consultations. In order to draw such conclusions a series of inferences have to be made. First, the observation has to be translated into a score or verbal summary; for example, 85 per cent or 'good'. Second, an inference has be made as to how generalisable this score or summary is (the so-called 'universe generalisation' inference). Third, an inference has to be made to the so-called target domain (this could be clinical decision making) and, finally, to the construct of interest (clinical reasoning).

The second, universe generalisation, inference was central in the case example, and the authors have focused on reliability. But, reliability in the classical test theory sense is only one argument we could make for the universe generalisation, and there are others. Saturation of information is another type of argument. This is a methodological strategy often used in qualitative research. It differs conceptually from the notion of reliability. Reliability is firmly rooted in the assumption that all observations need to agree on the ability of the candidate. If in a panel viva the judges of the panel disagree about the competence of the candidate, this disagreement is seen as a source of unreliability. Saturation of information is based on the notion that generalisation is optimal if no *new* disagreement arises. So, if the panel in this viva disagree, this does not automatically mean that the assessment has poor generalisation, but that more judges are needed, and when adding new judges does not lead to *new disagreements,* the whole kaleidoscope of the candidate's competence has been judged and therefore universal generalisation has occurred. Of course, just adding random opinions does not suffice in this case, but adding *expert* opinions does. Therefore, teacher training, clear rules and regulations, communities of practice and prolonged engagement are processes to ensure that opinions are based on sufficient exposure and expertise. Furthermore, a structure of evaluation and adding information needs to be in place, so benchmarking, stepwise replication, second opinion and transparency (audit trails) are organisational elements to ensure universe generalisation (Driessen et al. 2005).

It is fair to state that numerical scores (for example, on written or computer-based tests) are better supported by reliability approaches and assessment based on human judgements more on saturation of information approaches. In any case, a choice has to be made and followed through – much like in the case study, by analysing the problem, exploring the literature, applying the most promising solution and evaluating it – to design meaningful assessment.

Case study 17.3   Implementing a meaningful assessment programme, St George's University of London, UK

Jonathan Round

St George's University of London is a graduate and undergraduate medical school in the UK with 270 students per year. The medical school undergoes regular reviews of its medical course and its assessment structure. Prior to 2008 there were a plethora of different assessment tools used to assess skills and knowledge, applied at the end of the second, fourth and final years of the courses.

Following advice from the General Medical Council (GMC) and *Tomorrow's Doctors* (2009), the medical school grouped all summative assessments under a professor of assessment, with an integrated strategy designed to test students' skills in three domains: the doctor as a scholar and scientist; the doctor as a practitioner; and the doctor as a professional. I took responsibility for part of the doctor as scholar and scientist area, and developed end-of-year examinations in knowledge and its clinical application.

As a consultant, parent, patient and tax payer, I wanted a high and increasing standard for medical school graduates. Medical school is arduous and some students can avoid learning that which is not tested and use compensation between testing areas to reduce their own learning load.

At the outset, the principles we developed were:

- Test it once, test it properly.
- Test at the right level.
- Test only what is general practitioner (GP) or F1/2 relevant.
- All questions are clinically situated.
- Use evidence-based methodologies.
- Tell the students what they are being tested on.
- Make it feasible.

We chose to use single best answers (SBAs), testing for 180 minutes each year around subjects covered that year. We used an Angoff method for standard setting. These formats were chosen as being evidence-based, effective and simple.

The first year of testing was 2009–10. We developed a house style and promoted this with writer workshops for clinical academics. We had blueprinting meetings, which were initially stormy. There was much debate about question allocation across the curriculum. A formula was developed to calculate question numbers based on teaching time that year, if it was examined later and GP or F1/2 relevance. As in any spiral curriculum, some subjects are taught in more than one year. The faculty began to appreciate that more questions in one year was a better test than questions spread over two or more years. Once blueprinting had calculated the number of questions for each subject area, it further specified the skill to be tested and the setting of the clinical encounter in the SBA, in order to ensure adequate sampling and spread across the curriculum.

We found that some individuals took quickly to SBA writing and others, despite much assistance, remained poor. Many questions had to be rewritten almost from scratch to ensure quality and consistency of format. Common foibles were negative questions, 'two-step' questions, questions on minutiae, heterogeneous options, backwards questions or clinically implausible scenarios. In 2011 the management structure of the examination strand was changed to develop a small team to assist in this process.

> Students appreciated the fairness of the examination, although felt it was taxing. We had intended to produce rapid feedback, but manpower challenges and lack of pre-planning prevented this initially.
>
> The same format was extended to the fourth year in 2011 and the final year in 2012. For the final year, the medical school asked that multiple SBAs should be nested in 30 patient scenarios, testing aspects of practical patient management, reflecting situations F1s would be likely to encounter. Similar to real life, there would be multiple pieces of information, some irrelevant, to assimilate.
>
> This format posed new challenges – how to sample the entire curriculum adequately, and how to avoid cueing answers by developments further along in the case. We found these questions particularly challenging to write well, and are developing further workshops to address this.
>
> A key part of any assessment strategy is its own evaluation. Systems were put in place to record and review the performance of all questions used, discarding or rewriting poorly performing items. A question bank is currently being installed to facilitate this and to identify pre-written questions to meet future blueprints. The most useful data, however, are an exam's predictive power. We are currently examining the outcome of those students on either side of the pass mark for these exams, both at medical school and beyond.
>
> Evaluation should lead to change (learning). We are happy with the overall performance of this part of our assessment strategy, but believe more can be done to improve the quality of feedback to the students, and we are considering increasing the testing time to make the test more discriminatory for borderline students.
>
> Medical school summative exams are a vital part of the medical course, encouraging excellence and preventing the public being exposed to poorly trained doctors.
>
> By developing clear principles, and with considerable effort, an effective examination can be developed, be respected by the students and be able to distinguish between those students able to proceed and those who need further study and work.

The St George's case study describes the challenges in setting up a new examination for a previously not well-assessed domain. An important aspect in this case study is the focus on the expertise of the faculty staff involved in the process. It starts with a clear statement about the purposes of the assessment and the way to achieve these. The second step is the development of a house style or template, to ensure that all those involved in the production of assessment material are on the same page. The third is the involvement of the faculty in the content or the distribution of the question. Finally, and most importantly, is the faculty development process that was put in place. The review of items by a team was not only used to improve the quality of the items and by this of the assessment, but also with feedback and assistance to raise the expertise of staff members in writing items. In this way the case study illustrates two other assertions in the opening section of this chapter, namely that assessment is as much an educational design and staff development problem.

If my daughters, who are currently almost 6 and 8 years old, were assigned the task of handing out multiple-choice exam papers they could most probably do that without having any impact on the assessment quality of the method. They would not influence the validity or the reliability of the assessment. My eldest would even be able to score the papers (if she sets her mind to it) and produce the results for each candidate. In multiple-choice tests the expertise is needed to produce the questions and not to administer the tests or produce the scores. This being said, I would never dream of asking my daughters to conduct a mini-CEX even if they were given an optimally structured and standardised form. The 'administration' of the assessment is where the expertise is needed and not the production of scores. If we go back to the validity concept by Kane (2006), expertise is needed to make the inference from observation to scores and if you don't have the expertise you cannot make this inference. Actually, the specific form, whether it has nine or 20 criteria, whether it has a nine-point or a three-point scale, is largely irrelevant – an expert could validly conduct a mini-CEX with a blank sheet of paper. It is fair to say that any form of assessment requires expertise and therefore appropriate staff development, but it should be determined very carefully where and how that expertise should be used (or, as is often the case with the use of checklists, stifled) in the process.

The question then remains what this expertise entails. First, it is content expertise. If an assessor does not know what s/he is required to judge or what should be seen as good performance and what as poor performance, s/he cannot come to a valid inference from observation to score. Second, it is assessment expertise. This is not necessarily knowing much about the theory of assessment but more the acquisition of tacit knowledge of acceptable and unacceptable candidate performance (Berendonk et al. 2013), experience to develop adequate performance scripts (Govaerts et al. 2012) and gaining experience with negotiating the organisation, rules and regulations governing the assessment. As such, the required assessor expertise bears remarkable similarities with the development of diagnostic expertise in medicine, which has important implications for staff development programmes.

Diagnostic expertise resides in the ability to solve ill-defined problems through the development of meaningful knowledge networks (semantic networks), aggregating into illness and instance scripts. Through these, experts are not only better at diagnosing but also more efficient, allowing them to manage caseloads that non-experts – even with elaborate analytical reasoning and access to the internet – would not be able to manage. The same applies to expert assessors who develop meaningful networks and performance and person scripts which enable them to 'diagnose' competence in an assessment situation more effectively and more efficiently. It is clear that for such a difficult expertise a single training workshop will never do, like a single workshop does not turn a student into an expert diagnostician. In the case study, the staff development activities such as consensus building on the aims of the assessment, involvement in the content to create engagement, involvement in the review process and the constant feedback and training on the job all recognise the need for an ongoing staff development process focusing on where the expertise is needed.

The three case studies in this chapter illustrate the importance of other aspects of quality of assessment than construct validity and reliability. Currently, quality is no longer seen as a feature unique to the assessment instrument but as a constant interaction between the user and his/her organisation. To use a simplistic clinical metaphor: a surgeon cannot operate with a dull blade, but even with a sharp blade a non-expert can do serious harm to people, and over-reliance on the quality of the instrument without paying attention to the user will invariably produce harm.

When we return to the topic of this chapter – how to implement meaningful assessment – the case examples have illustrated the processes we currently see as unavoidable in achieving this. It starts with a clear analysis of the educational need or problem (and not a 'new' instrument). The second step is to explore the literature carefully for possible solutions, evaluate their quality, select the most promising ones and adapt them to the local situation. As previously highlighted, there is nothing magical about any assessment instrument, but the value lies in the interaction with the user and the organisation. The next step is the implementation of the instrument, involving users and other stakeholders and engaging them in the process. Finally, an ongoing faculty development or expertise development process needs to be in place to ensure an optimal interaction between method, staff and institution.

It is fair to say that such a full process may not always be possible: there may not be the time, there may not be the resources and there may not be the expertise within the organisation, and compromises may have to be made. But, in order to make the best compromise having a clear picture of the whole gamut of factors to consider is helpful, and it is hoped that the case studies with the annotations in this chapter have been helpful.

Take-home messages

- Meaningful assessment involves more than just the measurement of ability and assurances of the reliability and validity of the method. It requires a clear statement of the educational need or problem to be addressed.
- Expertise is essential to ensure that the design and assessment of the measurement tool are adequate to address the educational need or problem.
- The design of the assessment instrument or method requires the careful examination of existing evidence of tools and their quality and their adaptation to the particular case.
- Ongoing faculty development is essential to ensure the engagement of stakeholders in the realisation of meaningful assessment.

Bibliography

Albanese, M.A., Mejicano, G., Mullan, P., Kokotailo, P. and Gruppen, L. (2008) 'Defining characteristics of educational competencies', *Medical Education*, 42(3): 248–55.

Al-Faris, E.A. (2000) 'Students' evaluation of a traditional and an innovative family medicine course in Saudi Arabia', *Education for Health*, 13(2): 231–5.

Al-Faris, E.A. and Naeem, N. (2012) 'Effective teaching in medical schools', *Saudi Medical Journal*, 33(3): 237–43.

Berendonk, C., Stalmeijer, R.E. and Schuwirth, L.W.T. (2013) 'Expertise in performance assessment: Assessors' perspective', *Advances in Health Sciences Education*, 18(4): 559–71.

Boud, D. (1990) 'Assessment and the promotion of academic values', *Studies in Higher Education*, 15(1), 101–11.

Cookson, J., Crossley, J., Fagan, G., McKendree, J. and Mohsen, A. (2011) 'A final clinical examination using a sequential design to improve cost-effectiveness', *Medical Education*, 45(7): 741–7.

Downing, S.M. (2004) 'Reliability: On the reproducibility of assessment data', *Medical Education*, 38(10): 1006–12.

Driessen, E., van der Vleuten, C.P.M., Schuwirth, L.W.T., van Tartwijk, J. and Vermunt, J. (2005) 'The use of qualitative research criteria for portfolio assessment as an alternative to reliability evaluation: A case study', *Medical Education*, 39(2): 214–20.

Frank, J.R. (ed.) (2005) *The CanMEDS 2005 physician competency framework: Better standards. Better physicians. Better care*. Ottawa: The Royal College of Physicians and Surgeons of Canada. Online. Available HTTP: http://www.royalcollege.ca/portal/page/portal/rc/canmeds (accessed 26 July 2013).

General Medical Council (GMC) (2009) *Tomorrow's doctors: Outcomes and standards for undergraduate medical education*. London: GMC. Online. Available HTTP: www.gmc-uk.org/New_Doctor09_FINAL.pdf_27493417.pdf_39279971.pdf (accessed 10 June 2014).

Govaerts, M.J.B., Van de Wiel, M.W.J., Schuwirth, L.W.T., Van der Vleuten, C.P.M. and Muijtjens, A.M.M. (2012) 'Workplace-based assessment: raters' performance theories and constructs', *Advances in Health Sciences Education*, 18(3): 375–96.

Harvill, L.M. (1991) 'Standard error of measurement', *Educational Measurement: Issues and Practice*, 10(2): 33–41.

Kane, M. (2006) 'Validation'. In R.L. Brennan (ed.) *Educational measurement*, Westport, CT: ACE/Praeger.

Miller, G.E. (1990) 'The assessment of clinical skills/competence/performance', *Academic Medicine*, 65: 563–7.

Muijtjens, A.M., van Vollenhoven, F.H., Femke, H.M., van Luijk, S.J. and van der Vleuten, C.P.M. (2000) 'A sequential testing in the assessment of clinical skills', *Academic Medicine*, 75(4): 369–73.

Schuwirth, L.W.T. and van der Vleuten, C.P.M. (2011) 'Programmatic assessment: From assessment of learning to assessment for learning', *Medical Teacher*, 33(6): 478–85.

Shepard, L. (2009) 'The role of assessment in a learning culture', *Educational Researcher*, 29(7): 4–14.

Smee, S.M., Dauphinee, W.D., Blackmore, D.E., Rothman, A.I., Reznick, R.K. and des Marchais, J. (2003) 'A sequenced OSCE for licensure: administrative issues, results and myths', *Advances in Health Sciences Education*, 8(3): 223–36.

van der Vleuten, C.P.M. (1996) 'The assessment of professional competence: Developments, research and practical implications', *Advances in Health Science Education*, 1(1): 41–67.

van der Vleuten, C.P.M. and Schuwirth, L.W.T. (2005) 'Assessing professional competence: From methods to programmes', *Medical Education*, 39(3): 309–17.

Wagner-Menghin, M., Preusche, I. and Schmidts, M. (2011) 'Clinical performance assessment with five stations: Can it work?', *Medical Teacher*, 33(6): 507.

18
WRITTEN AND COMPUTER-BASED APPROACHES ARE VALUABLE TOOLS TO ASSESS A LEARNER'S COMPETENCE

Reg Dennick

With proper attention to key principles it is possible to create accountable and robust written and online assessment procedures.

Aims and objectives

This chapter is concerned with the use of objective written tests in medical education assessment. By 'objective' we mean tests with unambiguous answers that can be dichotomously marked as either correct or incorrect. Objective written tests are predominantly oriented towards the knowledge domain and are mainly of multi-format design using multiple-choice (single best answer), multiple-response (multiple answers), extended matching, fill in the blanks (cloze), drag and drop, script concordance and hotspot image questions. More recently, objective written tests have been created and marked by computers and for the purposes of this chapter they exclude essays or short written answers which cannot yet be marked in this way.

The importance of written objective tests lies in their ubiquitous global use to test knowledge and their increasingly strong association with computer-based assessment systems. There is a common misconception that objective tests can only assess simple recall and understanding, whereas in principle most types of knowledge in Bloom's taxonomy, from recall through application to problem solving, can be assessed by appropriately constructed questions. Nevertheless, the knowledge that can be tested always needs to be mapped ('blueprinted') against the learning outcomes of the course at an appropriate level. Online assessment systems should readily fit into the exam cycle, as shown in Figure 18.1.

Range of assessments

The range of objective written tests that can be marked by computer include:

- multiple-choice questions (MCQs);
- extended matching items (EMIs);
- ranking questions;

- fill in the gap (cloze) and text/number entry;
- script concordance testing;
- image hotspots;
- labelling ('drag and drop');
- video.

The key attributes of each of these will be summarised below.

MCQs

The major objective formats are outlined in the guide produced by Case and Swanson (2002). These formats are employed in most conventional types of assessment and can be readily modified for the online environment by including images, sound and video clips.

These objective tests are structured around the format of a question (stem) followed by a series of possible answers with the correct answer embedded or surrounded by a range of incorrect answers or 'distractors'. For example a 'single best answer' might have the correct answer listed with four distractors (Figure 18.2). It is possible to extend this format into the 'multiple-response' style of question, where more than one item should be selected from the list. In these cases sufficient distractors should be provided to ensure that the probability of answering the question correctly by chance does not become too high.

EMIs

The EMI format is really an extension of the multiple-choice format in which selected items from one list are matched to items in another list. The usual format is that there is a short

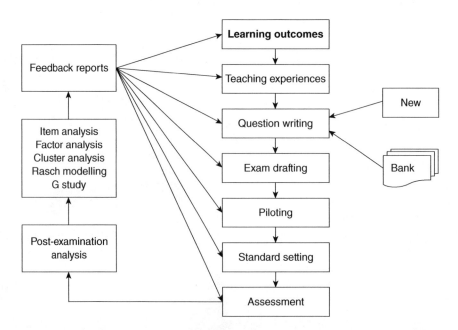

Figure 18.1 The examination cycle. (Reproduced from Tavakol, M. and Dennick, R.G. 'Post-examination analysis of objective tests', *Medical Teacher*, 33(6): 447–58, copyright © 2011, Informa Healthcare. Reproduced with permission of Informa Healthcare.)

> 8. Repeat neurovascular examination of the left hand immediately after treatment shows no change. The patient still cannot flex the interphalangeal joint of the thumb or distal interphalangeal joint of the index finger. There are no sensory defects.
>
> These preoperative and postoperative findings indicate injury to what nerve?
>
> ○ Anterior interosseous, (from median nerve)
> ○ Posterior interosseous (from radial nerve)
> ○ Ulnar
> ○ Radial
> ○ Median
>
> (1 Mark)

Figure 18.2 Example of a 'single best answer' item. A stem provides a clinical scenario and the correct answer is found in a list of incorrect 'distractors'. (Courtesy of Rogo, an open-source program produced by the University of Nottingham.)

list of say two to four clinical scenarios or patient descriptions which must be matched to appropriate items in a longer list of, for example, seven to 12 diagnoses, drugs, organisms, investigations or other clinical entities (Figures 18.3 and 18.4). The format can be extended by the use of images containing items for identification. The advantage of this format is that assessors can test the ability of individuals to differentiate between closely related concepts which potentially identify deeper levels of understanding. Both MCQs and EMIs can be associated with problem-solving or data interpretation stems so that application and problem solving can be tested.

Nevertheless, it has been argued that these types of questions, where the correct answer is essentially given as a choice that can be recognised, are intrinsically easier than having to recall the answer from memory without prompting. Evidence suggests that in the case of single best answer formats there is a significant enhancement in marks between recognition and recall (Newble et al. 1979). There is no doubt that there is a cognitive price to pay but the feasibility of this system has led to its almost universal adoption.

Ranking questions

It is possible to create a question format in which students have to correct the rank or place in order a list of items (Figure 18.5). This might be testing their knowledge of the frequency of occurrence of clinical entities or testing their ability to place a sequence of clinical actions into the correct temporal sequence.

Fill in the gap (cloze) and text/number entry

These are related systems that involve the student entering single words, phrases or numbers into a section of text or a designated text/numerical box. 'Cloze' is the technical term for inserting deleted words into a section of text in order to complete it correctly, and hence for assessing recall of factual information (Taylor 1953). Single words, phrases or numbers can be inserted into designated boxes as answers to a variety of question types (Figure 18.6). The effectiveness of solutions to the problems of error trapping the input and recognising correct answers from all possible inputs is a limiting factor in the use of this question format.

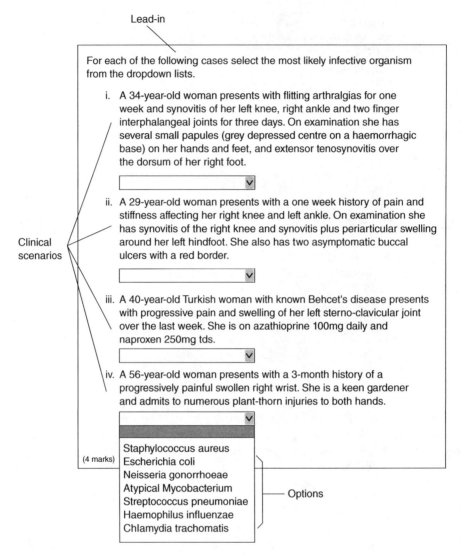

Figure 18.3 An example of an online extending matching question in which the longer list is found in a 'drop-down' menu. (Courtesy of Rogo, an open-source program produced by the University of Nottingham.)

Script concordance testing

Script concordance testing is increasingly being used to design questions that test clinical reasoning. The standard approach is to construct a question based around, for example, the interpretation of history taking, physical examination or investigations and to ask the student if the results of these processes influence differential diagnostic decisions according to a rating scale (Figure 18.7). The student's response is compared to the consensual decision from a panel of experts and marked accordingly.

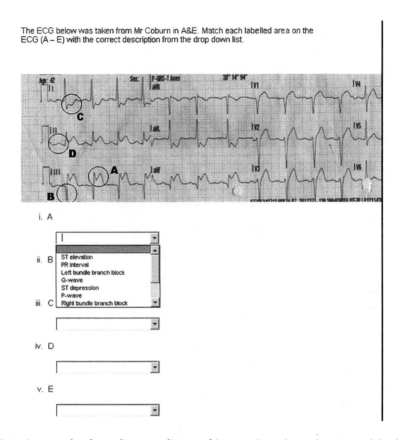

Figure 18.4 An example of an online extending matching question using an image containing items for identification listed in a 'drop-down' menu. (Courtesy of Rogo, an open-source program produced by the University of Nottingham.)

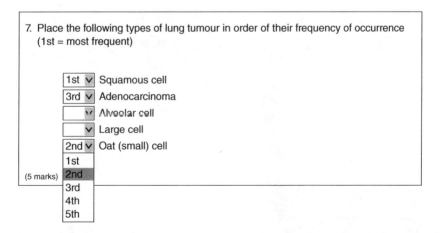

Figure 18.5 A ranking question in which the ranking order is selected from a 'drop-down' list. (Courtesy of Rogo, an open-source program produced by the University of Nottingham.)

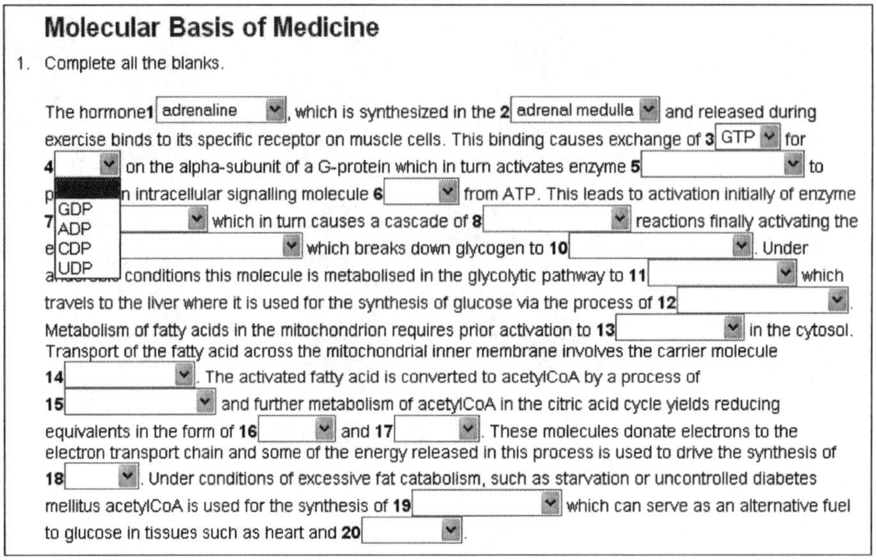

Molecular Basis of Medicine

1. Complete all the blanks.

The hormone **1** [adrenaline ▼], which is synthesized in the **2** [adrenal medulla ▼] and released during exercise binds to its specific receptor on muscle cells. This binding causes exchange of **3** [GTP ▼] for **4** [GDP / ADP / CDP / UDP ▼] on the alpha-subunit of a G-protein which in turn activates enzyme **5** [____▼] to produce an intracellular signalling molecule **6** [____▼] from ATP. This leads to activation initially of enzyme **7** [____▼] which in turn causes a cascade of **8** [____▼] reactions finally activating the enzyme **9** [____▼] which breaks down glycogen to **10** [____▼]. Under aerobic conditions this molecule is metabolised in the glycolytic pathway to **11** [____▼] which travels to the liver where it is used for the synthesis of glucose via the process of **12** [____▼]. Metabolism of fatty acids in the mitochondrion requires prior activation to **13** [____▼] in the cytosol. Transport of the fatty acid across the mitochondrial inner membrane involves the carrier molecule **14** [____▼]. The activated fatty acid is converted to acetylCoA by a process of **15** [____▼] and further metabolism of acetylCoA in the citric acid cycle yields reducing equivalents in the form of **16** [____▼] and **17** [____▼]. These molecules donate electrons to the electron transport chain and some of the energy released in this process is used to drive the synthesis of **18** [____▼]. Under conditions of excessive fat catabolism, such as starvation or uncontrolled diabetes mellitus acetylCoA is used for the synthesis of **19** [____▼] which can serve as an alternative fuel to glucose in tissues such as heart and **20** [____▼].

Figure 18.6 An example of cloze in which the correct word in the sequence is identified from a 'drop-down' list. This solves the problem of error trapping data entry for each word but requires plausible distractors for each word to be found. (Courtesy of Rogo, an open-source program produced by the University of Nottingham.)

Clinical vignette:
A three-year old girl presents to the ER with important sialorrhea, diminished neck movements, and fever for more than 24 hours. Parents report no recent trauma and no episode of foreign body obstruction.

If you were thinking of ...	And then you find ...	This hypothesis				
An epiglottitis	An updated vaccination against Haemophilus influenzae B	−2	−1	0	+1	+2
A retropharyngeal abscess	Widened pre-vertebral soft tissue on a lateral neck x-ray	−2	−1	0	+1	+2

Legend
−2 = ruled out or almost ruled out
−1 = less probable
 0 = neither less or more probable
+1 = more probalbe
+2 = certain or almost certain

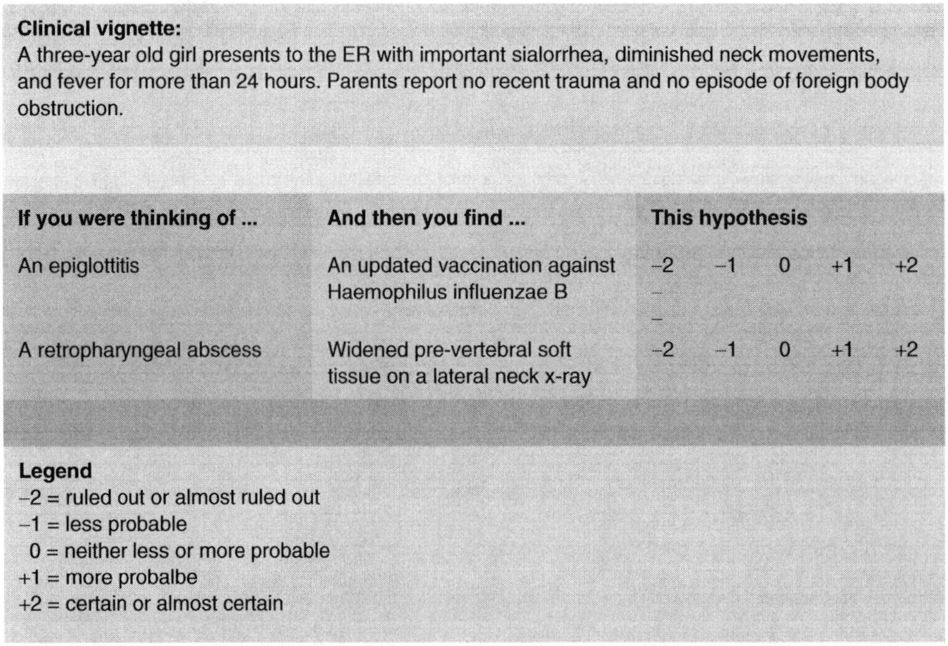

Figure 18.7 An example of script concordance testing. Students must choose the correct number from the list on the right, which is scored according to the consensus of a group of clinical experts. (Courtesy of Rogo, an open-source program produced by the University of Nottingham.)

Image hotspots

Image hotspot questions are good for assessing visual knowledge that would be difficult to achieve though an MCQ or other textual question type. They have a second advantage in that there are no visual cues as to where the correct answer lies, there are no discrete distractors to choose from, and each pixel is a potentially correct or incorrect answer. Questions have to be constructed by outlining the area on an image that must be identified correctly (Figure 18.8). There will inevitably be boundary issues associated with this procedure (what is 'in', what is 'out'), but nevertheless these type of questions can be made highly reliable.

Labelling (drag and drop)

Labelling questions, like image hotspots, are ideally suited to assessing visual knowledge, and differ in the cues they provide. With a labelling question a number of 'place holders', the empty

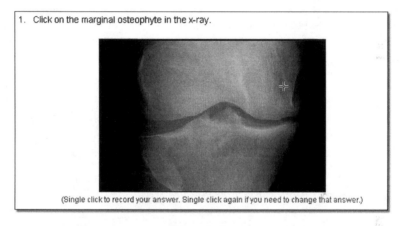

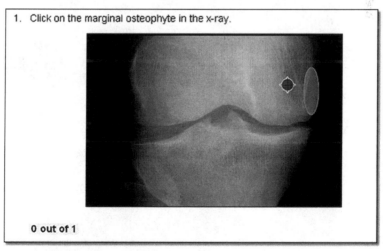

Figure 18.8 An example of an 'image hotspot' question. The top image shows what the student sees and the cursor which must select the correct area of the image. The bottom image shows the area selected by the assessor (large oval) in which the cursor must be placed. (Courtesy of Rogo, an open-source program produced by the University of Nottingham.)

rectangles (Figure 18.9), are pre-displayed over the image of interest. The examinee must drag labels from the left and drop them into the relevant place holders. Sometimes a larger number of labels than place holders, acting as distractors, are used to make the question more difficult.

Video

The ability to deliver video or moving images to a student during an assessment considerably extends the scope of question formats. Videos of patients, doctor–patient interactions, procedures, consultations and communications can all be used to create appropriate assessment scenarios that have high content validity (Figure 18.10). Video can be used to set up a scenario which can be subsequently assessed by means of the formats described above.

Writing questions

The construction of objective written questions requires some skill. The fundamental issue is to ensure that the question is valid and unambiguous and does not contain information that will allow an individual to identify any element of it as either correct or incorrect without using the knowledge constructs that the question is aimed at. Distractors in particular have to be plausibly incorrect and homogeneous with the correct answer, otherwise they can easily be eliminated without the student necessarily knowing the correct answer. There need to be sufficient distractors so that the question cannot easily be answered by chance alone. In the case of single best answers this probability should not usually be greater than 1 in 5 or 20 per cent. With multiple-response questions more distractors are required to maintain this level of probability. (The creation of plausible distractors is often the most difficult aspect of good item writing.)

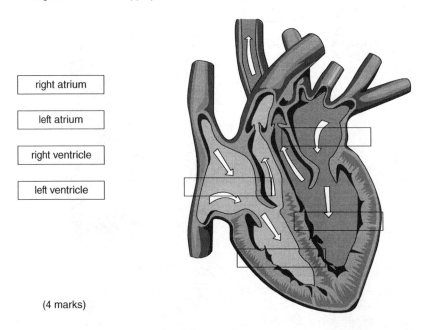

Figure 18.9 A simple 'drag and drop' question. Extra labels may be added as distractors if necessary.

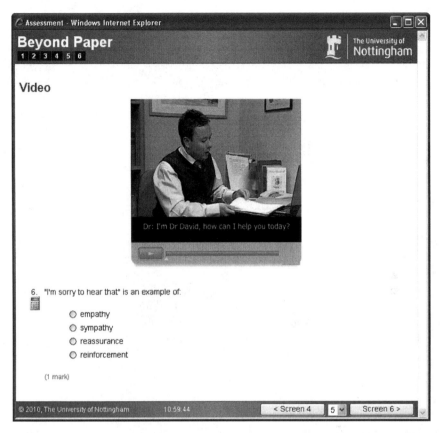

Figure 18.10 A screen shot from a video question in Rogo (http://rogo-oss.nottingham.ac.uk/). The student watches and listens to the video and then answers a series of questions, one of which is shown. (Courtesy of Rogo, an open-source program produced by the University of Nottingham.)

Grammatical issues in sentence construction can also allow the 'test-wise' candidate to identify implausible distractors. Anything that provides inappropriate information will reduce the reliability of the question and the test; it will generate 'noise'. A useful reference work for writing good-quality items is Case and Swanson (2002).

There are a number of key criteria that can be used to characterise assessments, including validity, reliability and feasibility, and these can easily be satisfied by objective written tests.

Validity

In general, assessment validity is concerned with whether an assessment measures what it is designed to measure and can be subdivided into a variety of different types (Dent and Harden 2013):

- Content validity: does the test measure and sample relevant learning objectives or outcomes?
- Construct validity: does the test measure an underlying cognitive trait, e.g. intelligence?
- Concurrent validity: does the test correlate with the results of an established test?
- Predictive validity: does the test predict future performance?
- Face validity: does it seem like a fair test to the candidates?

For the purposes of this chapter the most important elements that might be influenced by being online would be content validity and possibly the related concept of construct validity. However, Schuwirth and van der Vleuten (2006) argue that assessments must also have face validity for students. This is an important issue, particularly when introducing online e-assessment for the first time to students who may be unfamiliar with its processes and may require reassurance.

Certainly content validity can be enhanced and expanded by means of online assessment technology. For example, the following additional features can be added to online questions:

- animations, video and sound (if headphones are used in the examination room);
- 'hotspot' questions which require students to place a mark anywhere on an image or diagram;
- dragging labels directly over an image.

In all these cases the online nature and technological aspects of the assessment can significantly influence the authenticity of questions that can be created in comparison to other forms of paper-based assessment media (Sim et al. 2005). Evidence for increased validity can be found in an evaluation of multimedia online examinations by Liu et al. (2001). They investigated student and staff attitude to multimedia exams and found very strong support for their use. For example they found that:

- assessment more closely matched the material that was being taught;
- the presentation of more than one medium of information seemed to aid the students' recall;
- questions reflected real-world situations more accurately;
- students seemed to learn more in these assessments, which helped them as they continued their studies.

Reliability

The reliability of an assessment refers to its ability to give the same measure of learning consistently when used repeatedly despite sampling error. The most common cause of unreliability in objective testing is poorly constructed questions that are ambiguous, too easy or too hard. In the sort of objective testing we are describing here, where objective criteria are decided beforehand, questions are constructed avoiding the problems described above and questions are marked electronically, this type of reliability problem can be diminished.

A well-known measure of reliability is the internal consistency of the assessment task, usually measured by correlating individual item scores to other items or to the global test score which can be processed to give a value of reliability, such as Cronbach's alpha statistic (Tavakol and Dennick 2011b). Because with online assessments it is possible to supply a different set of questions from a question bank to different individuals in the same examination, or to generate different numerical values for calculations or problem-solving items within a question, the questions delivered to individuals can vary slightly. Provided the range of these variables is within agreed boundaries overall, the reliability of the test should not be greatly compromised.

In the case of computer-based tests reliability can also be influenced how easily individuals are fatigued by using a visual display unit (VDU). Guidance recommends that online tests should last no longer than 2 hours.

Feasibility

Online assessment is not necessarily cheaper than alternative forms simply because a whole cohort can be marked in a matter of seconds. The following costs need to be taken into consideration:

- large numbers of computers are required for a simultaneous start;
- additional invigilators will be required if these machines are located in different computer rooms;
- dedicated assessment servers are required to minimise failure risk;
- assessment software will be required;
- departmental/institutional staff are required to support the system;
- educationalists are required, advising on pedagogic approach and assessment strategies;
- programmers' salaries need to be factored in;
- trainers familiar with the assessment software are required;
- IT support technicians are required.

Some of the costs of online assessment are considerable, for example, server hardware, large computer labs and the licence cost of the assessment software itself. Less tangible costs include members of IT support staff spending more time maintaining systems. However, once the investment is made in online testing it rapidly becomes the most feasible and efficient method of assessing knowledge-based examinations.

Question banks and adaptive testing

Collaboration between medical schools in the UK has produced the Medical School Council Assessment Alliance (MSC-AA), an arrangement between UK medical schools in which questions can be banked and shared. Metadata can be attached to items to provide information on the learning objectives being tested and item difficulty and discrimination. Banked questions can be used to generate adaptive test papers in which questions of increasing difficulty or challenge are presented to learners in response to their answers to previous questions.

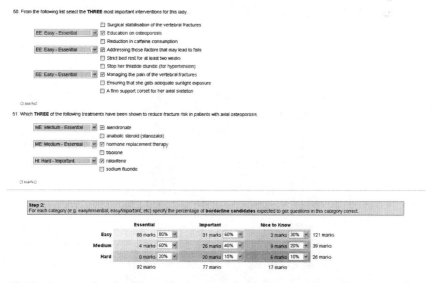

Figure 18.11 An example of online standard setting of objective test items. The questions have been examined by multiple assessors and the consensus scores recorded. (Courtesy of Rogo, an open-source program produced by the University of Nottingham.)

A11CLS: May (2008/09)
Miss G. Brogan Feedback

Key
○ Acquisition of 80–100% of specific objective
■ Acquisition of 50–79% of specific objective
▽ Acquisition of 0–49% of specific objective
[r] **hyperlink** – jump to section in the NLE for further details

Learning Objectives

Below is a list of all the unique learning objectives tested by this paper. Because multiple questions may test the same objective it is possible to have partial acquisition of an objective. Use the results below to concentrate on red ▽ and amber ■ objectives you have not fully mastered.

- ○ Briefly outline the techniques which may be offered during a pregnancy ie CVS, amniocentesis, fetal blood, skin biopsy, USS [r] **CLS/L1/07**
- ○ Compare and contrast the antigen receptors of T cells and B cells. [r] **CLS/L1/26**
- ○ Compare mitosis and meiosis and discuss the importance of recombination and non-disjunction [r] **CLS/L1/02**
- ○ Construct and draw a 3 generation family tree using correct symbols [r] **CLS/L1/05**
- ■ Define the terms hypertrophy, hyperplasia, atrophy, apoptosis, involution, hypoplasia, agenesis and metaplasia, with an example of each [r] **CLS/L1/08**
- ■ List the structure/function of some important molecules of the bacterial cell envelope [r] **CLS/L1/14**
- ■ Outline the classification and structure of medically important fungal organisms [r] **CLS/L1/22**
- ■ Describe the ways in which various categories of infective agents differ [r] **CLS/L1/03**
- ■ Outline the function of cell stress proteins [r] **CLS/L1/08**
- ▽ List the main properties of innate and adaptive immunity [r] **CLS/L1/13**
- ▽ Outline the properties of complement and the pathways off complement activation [r] **CLS/L1/25**
- ▽ Provide an overview of the following as major bacterial targets for antibiotics: 1. Cell wall synthesis; 2. Plasma membrane integrity; 3. Nucleic acid synthesis; 4. Ribosomal function; 5. Folate synthesis. [r] **CLS/L1/15**

Summary Information
Paper title   A11CLS: May (2008/09)
Started at   01/06/2009 10:00
Exam length 02:00:00
Time spent   01:06:47

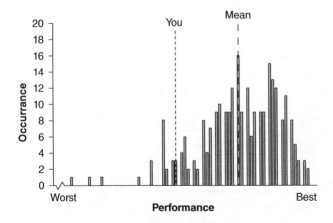

Figure 18.12 An example of a 'traffic-light' feedback system in Rogo that provides students with feedback on how well they scored on the learning objectives associated with each question in the assessment. This enables the questions to be kept and used again. (Courtesy of Rogo, an open-source program produced by the University of Nottingham.)

Standard setting, external examining and online feedback

Online objective test papers can readily be made available to groups of examiners and external examiners so that they can engage in online standard setting (Figure 18.11). For example, using the Angoff method, each question can be evaluated for the probability that a 'borderline' student will answer it correctly (Angoff 1971). By collating the online evaluations a consensus cut score can be obtained.

Online systems mark items immediately, although it is wise to allow some time for moderation and checking before releasing marks to students. Such systems also allow students to be given rapid feedback on their answers (Figure 18.12). When tests are used formatively, students can revisit the online paper and see which questions they answered correctly and which they did not. Feedback to answers can be attached to items, leading to an 'assessment for learning' environment. In the case of high-stakes summative examinations, when items need to be reused, learning objective metadata for each item can be used to generate a more generic form of feedback that does not allow items to be displayed again.

Psychometric analysis

Online objective assessment systems can be configured to process data using a variety of psychometric methods. As well as mean marks, item difficulty and discrimination can be calculated, in addition to Cronbach's alpha statistic (Tavakol and Dennick 2011b).

Computer-based testing in practice

The following case study from India highlights some of the key issues associated with implementing computer-based testing (CBT) and discusses the process undertaken by the National Board of Examiners (NBE) in India.

Case study 18.1   Computer-based testing – a paradigm shift in student assessment in India

Bipin Batra

Billions of examinations and assessments are administered every year across the globe. In recent times, CBT has drawn the attention of assessment institutions as a new approach to deliver tests and assess performance of candidates or rank them on their abilities.

Conventionally, medical entrance examinations have been conducted as paper-based testing (PBT), in which a booklet containing a predetermined number of questions is provided to the candidates. On testing day candidates have to mark their responses on the optical mark reader (OMR) sheets. PBT, though simple in approach and implementation, is plagued with a multitude of problems such as the possibility of leakage of confidential material/information, the unfair use of electronic gadgets, impersonations and cheating by the examinees and logistics-related issues in transporting the question paper.

The NBE, India, is an organisation in the field of medical education that conducts various types of student assessment. Concerned with relative weakness and threats to the PBT, NBE introduced

(continued)

(continued)
computer-based testing for entrance examinations. CBT is an IT-driven process which requires computer labs equipped with servers, secure wide-area network connectivity, firewalls, trained human resources and appropriate software and hardware. A CBT significantly enhances the scope of items to use in the test and enhances the test blueprint. The NBE conducted one of the largest tests using CBT, the National Eligibility cum Entrance Test, with 90,377 examinees in December 2012 and the steps undertaken are outlined below.

Prior to test

- The plan was tested.
- The details of estimated candidates and resources required, especially test centres, IT labs, questions/item bank and faculty support required, were mapped.
- Engagement of all stakeholders towards the impending change from PBT to CBT was undertaken by social media, internet discussions and direct communications.
- The test blueprint was prepared, the size of item bank required was estimated and the requisite numbers of items for use in the test were generated and transferred to the item banking software at specially convened item-writing workshops.
- Candidate registration and test centre scheduling were performed through web-based application.
- Computer labs with predefined technical requirements and hardware specifications were arranged at required locations with appropriate seating capacity.
- Pilot administration was undertaken 2 days before the actual test.

Testing phase

- Test administration was undertaken, with test forms released on the wide-area network immediately before onset of the test.
- Examinee feedback was undertaken on a structured questionnaire.
- After completion of the test, the responses of examinees were uploaded to the server.

Post-test phase

- Items analysis was performed through computation of difficulty and discriminatory index on two parameter models.
- Post-test form validation workshop was undertaken to review the difficulty and discriminatory indices.
- Item response theory and generation of equated score were applied to ensure comparability of different test forms used.
- Equated score was scaled using linear transformation.
- Results were published.

The NBE deployed the latest IT infrastructure to capture examinee biometrics and video record the testing phase. For 58 per cent of examinees this was their first exposure to CBT: 95 per cent of examinees felt the CBT of December 2012 met their expectations.

The conversion from PBT to CBT involved stakeholder acceptance and it was important to engage faculty, students and academic leadership at institutions and universities in the process at all stages. Medical teachers were appropriately sensitised towards use of psychometric tools and underlying principles of assessment. A sound test blueprint and adherence to principles of assessment supported with psychometric tools, ensuring stakeholder confidence and meticulous planning, were the keys to success.

Technical issues

System requirements

When an online exam begins, all the computers that the students are using will send their requests back to a single web server which holds the exam paper. The main drawback of this system is that it introduces a single point of failure, which must be addressed by appropriate security and backup systems. Testing of online exam systems should be routine and, where possible, a dedicated assessment server should be used which is independent of other systems.

Going live

The live delivery of an online summative exam, under conventional exam conditions, is the most crucial phase of the process. There is an international standard produced by the British Standards Institution entitled *A Code of Practice for the Use of Information Technology (IT) in the Delivery of Assessments* (BS ISO/IEC 23988 2007) which covers many aspects of exam delivery in generic terms.

Security

External security risks are possible with any server attached to the internet. Hackers anywhere worldwide are constantly using methods and software systems to root out vulnerable servers. Firewall systems should be robustly utilised to control requests and protocols accepted and transmitted by a server, and all software subsystems should be patched and kept up to date. Internal security should ensure that online test papers can only be accessed by authorised individuals. Segregating groups of students for consecutive sittings of an exam when computer screens are a limiting factor is essential. Preventing cheating by students in online exams requires configuring computers to allow access only to the exam and to provide visual barriers between screens.

For further information the interested reader is referred to Dennick et al. (2009).

Take-home messages

- Objective tests can be used to assess a wide variety of knowledge at different levels of complexity.
- Objective tests must be carefully constructed using valid and unambiguous items with plausible and homogeneous distractors to increase reliability and eliminate 'noise'.
- Images and other media can be added to objective tests to extend the range of knowledge tested using hotspots, drag and drop and video.
- Objective tests are ideally suited to computer-based platforms and a variety of online systems can now reliably and securely deliver high-stakes assessments to individuals.
- Online objective test systems can provide psychometric analysis of exam results which can be mapped to learning outcomes and provide feedback to learners.

Bibliography

Angoff, W.H. (1971) 'Norms, scales, and equivalent scores'. In R.L. Thorndike (ed.) *Educational measurement* (2nd edn), Washington, DC: American Education on Education.

British Standards Institution (2007) *BS ISO/IEC 23988 Information technology – A code of practice for the use of information technology (IT) in the delivery of assessments*, London: British Standards Institution.

Case, S.M. and Swanson, D.B. (2002) *Constructing written test questions for the basic and clinical sciences* (3rd edn), Philadelphia, PA: National Board of Medical Examiners.

Dennick, R.G., Wilkinson, S. and Purcell, N. (2009) Online eAssessment. AMEE guide no. 39. Association for Medical Education in Europe, *Medical Teacher*, 31(3): 192–206.

Dent, J.A. and Harden, R.M. (2013) *A practical guide for medical teachers* (4th edn), Edinburgh: Elsevier.

Liu, M., Papathanasiou, E. and Hao, Y. (2001) 'Exploring the use of multimedia examination formats in undergraduate teaching: Results from the fielding testing', *Computers in Human Behaviour*, 17(3): 225–48.

Newble, D.I., Baxter, B. and Elmslie, R.G. (1979) 'A comparison of multiple-choice tests and free-response tests in examinations of clinical competence'. *Medical Education*, 13, 263–8.

Schuwirth, L.W.T. and van der Vleuten, C.P.M. (2006) *Understanding medical education guides. How to design a useful test: The principles of assessment*, Association for the Study of Medical Education, Edinburgh: ASME.

Sim, G., Strong, A. and Holifield, P. (2005) The design of multimedia assessment objects, *Proceedings for 9th CAA Conference*, Loughborough.

Tavakol, M. and Dennick, R.G. (2011a) 'Post-examination analysis of objective tests', *Medical Teacher*, 33(6): 447–458.

Tavakol, M. and Dennick, R.G. (2011b) 'Making sense of Cronbach's alpha', *International Journal of Medical Education*, 2: 53–5.

Taylor, W.L. (1953) 'Cloze procedure: A new tool for measuring readability', *Journalism Quarterly*, 30: 415–33.

19
MORE ATTENTION IS NOW PAID TO ASSESSMENT OF CLINICAL COMPETENCE AND ON-THE-JOB ASSESSMENT

Vanessa C. Burch

A range of reliable, valued and practical tools are now available to assess a student's clinical competence.

Clinical competence is the bedrock of safe, efficient and effective patient care. Support for this statement is documented in the literature: a well-conducted interview and physical examination lead to the correct clinical diagnosis in more than 80 per cent of patient encounters (Peterson et al. 1992). This holds true even in the face of advanced technology offering a wide range of sophisticated diagnostic tools. Clinical competence is, therefore, the most important outcome of any medical training programme. The responsibility to provide evidence that such expertise has been acquired, and is practised in the workplace, lies with universities and medical licensing bodies.

Over the past 40 years a range of tools for the assessment of clinical competence, in both test settings as well as the workplace, have been developed. This chapter does not provide detailed descriptions of each of these tools since there are many in the literature; three useful references are included for the reader who wishes to pursue the topic in more detail (Norcini and Burch 2007; Kogan et al. 2009; Norcini 2010).

For the purpose of this chapter it is essential to recognise that 'best practices' are always located in real-life (authentic) settings that are subject to context-specific needs and limitations, i.e. 'best practices' are not located in an 'academic vacuum' free of limitations and needs. For the purpose of this chapter the author identifies three key components of 'best practices', as shown in Figure 19.1:

1   the efficient and innovative use of locally available resources;
2   a clear focus on local health needs;
3   optimal use of favourable educational climates to introduce innovations and improve practice.

In this chapter, examples of 'best practices' in the assessment of clinical competence are highlighted using case studies and examples from the literature. The chapter aims to distil the key principles demonstrated by the examples drawn from around the world.

Assessment of clinical competence

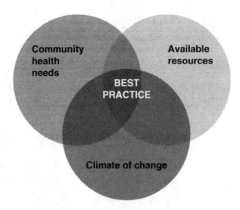

Figure 19.1 Key components of best practice in assessment.

Tools used to assess clinical competence

Over the past four decades a variety of tools have been developed to assess clinical competence. In 1990 George Miller used the figure of a pyramid to describe four categories of assessment of clinical competence: the lowest level of the pyramid tests knowledge (knows) followed by competence (knows how).

The upper levels of the pyramid focus on what trainees are able to demonstrate in a test or examination (shows how) and what trainees actually do in the workplace (does). The literature makes a distinction between these two settings by referring to 'competence' as behaviour observed in a test setting and 'performance' as behaviour in the workplace. This confuses clinicians, who refer to clinical proficiency as 'competence' and only differentiate between the assessment of competence in an artificial setting (test or examination) or in an authentic setting (the workplace). In order to avoid confusion, the author uses the term competence to refer to observed clinical proficiency, which is either assessed in a test setting or in the workplace, more recently known as workplace-based assessment (WPBA).

Strategies assessing clinical competence in a test environment include the objective structured clinical examination (OSCE) and the objective structured long case examination record (OSLER). Tools used for WPBA can be grouped into four broad categories:

1. records reflecting work experience, such as log books or clinical encounter cards (CECs);
2. observed single-patient encounters, such as the mini-clinical evaluation exercise (mini-CEX), direct observation of procedural skills (DOPS) and clinical work sampling (CWS);
3. discussion of clinical cases managed using chart-stimulated recall (CsR), also known as case-based discussions (CbD) in the UK;
4. feedback on routine clinical practice from peers, colleagues and patients collected by survey and collated to provide multi-source feedback (MSF). Information derived from peers is usually captured using the mini-peer assessment tool (mini-PAT) while team feedback and patient surveys provide complementary information to build a holistic picture of the trainee in the workplace.

Designing an assessment system

Before addressing the selection of appropriate assessment instruments the reader should appreciate that any one instrument cannot assess all the competencies required of trainees. A compilation of instruments spanning the spectrum of required competencies is needed (Schuwirth and van der Vleuten 2010). This is the foundation of a balanced, comprehensive assessment system, which limits the impact of error variance due to sampling (number and scope of test items), assessors (leniency, halo effect and shrunken scope of scores), context specificity and other assessment biases embedded in gender, age, ethnicity, language and culture.

The UK case study by Capey and Hays describes a comprehensive assessment system, which forms part of the Foundation Programme used to train new medical graduates in the UK.

Case study 19.1   The use of workplace-based assessment in the UK Foundation Programme

Steve Capey and Richard Hays

The UK Foundation Programme (UKFP) was reviewed and initiated in 2005 as a response to the Modernising Medical Careers (MMC) initiative, whose purpose was to make postgraduate specialty training in the UK both more flexible and potentially shorter (Department of Health 2004).

The UKFP is a 2-year supervised training period undertaken immediately after basic medical education that consolidates and translates learning (knowledge and skills) to the workplace environment, ensuring that entrants to postgraduate speciality training are well prepared for a shorter and more specialty-specific phase. Key to this preparation are the assessments to determine readiness to progress, provide feedback to the trainees (Davies et al. 2009) and identify any 'doctors in difficulty' who require further training and assessment. The UKFP assessments were designed to maximise the amount of feedback that each trainee would receive during the first stages of postgraduate training, through using frequent assessments from multiple perspectives and multiple methods. The onus is on trainees to collate a portfolio of assessments as evidence that they are ready to progress. The individual assessment tools used are WPBA, including the mini-CEX, DOPS, CbD and mini-PAT. All of these individual instruments have been demonstrated to provide a valid measurement of elements related to competence in clinical medicine and were used formatively to provide feedback after each encounter to foster professional development of the trainee.

Despite the theoretical advantages of this approach, some practical issues have arisen during implementation, mainly due to the scale of the change and the substantial logistic challenges involved. A report into the implementation of the UKFP in 2010 found that the WPBA assessments 'have many attractions but [are] time consuming and faculty training ... essential' (Collins 2010: 95). The magnitude of the task of completing the individual assessments was significant, with 250,000 clinical assessments being carried out between August 2008 and August 2009. Clinicians conducting the assessments needed training in the new WPBA methods, as providing mostly constructive feedback to colleagues, with at times decisions that might affect progression, is a complex task that requires specific training in educational supervision and use of the WPBA tools (Carr 2006). Achieving this level of training across such a large system took much longer and consumed more resources than predicted.

Trainees themselves have expressed mixed views about the value of the WPBA instruments used in the UKFP (Bindal et al. 2011). Amidst busy service workloads for all involved, the main issues cited were problems with finding assessors and assessments being completed when required. It was reported that many assessments were completed retrospectively or by more junior and

(continued)

(continued)

relatively untrained colleagues. The view of the trainers was that they had become an onerous tick-box exercise that had little value (Collins 2010).

In conclusion, the individual assessment elements used in the UKFP all have individual validity. The use of these tools as a whole programme of assessment should have provided a well-situated and valid picture of the trainee's clinical competence. However significant implementation issues were encountered and the programme of assessments was trivialised by logistics, training issues and a misunderstanding of the purpose of the assessments by trainees, assessors and employers.

While the assessment system is laudable in many ways, three major limitations were identified when the system was implemented:

1. the extent of the required scale of implementation was not appreciated; for example more than 250,000 assessments were conducted in the first 12 months;
2. there was insufficient resource allocation for faculty training because the scale of implementation was underestimated;
3. there was insufficient time to conduct the assessment events because of a reduction in consultant staff working hours (new European Union regulation) and a failure to allocate time in staff work schedules to perform these assessments.

This resulted in delays in trainee assessment, with a tendency to conduct assessment events retrospectively as well as the need for trainees to ask junior staff to conduct their assessments. Not unexpectedly, trainees' scepticism of the programme is now widely recognised. While assessor training and timely completion of assessment events can be addressed, the issue of adequate time to do so is more complex because the external directive is beyond UK control. Furthermore, these additional demands on working time may impact on clinical service delivery and patient care. How the UK addresses this issue is of international relevance because similar training programmes for junior doctors have been implemented elsewhere, for example, in Australia.

Selecting an assessment tool

The selection of an appropriate assessment tool should be guided by the nine simple questions included in Table 19.1. The order in which these questions are addressed is of secondary importance, because the issues are interrelated and the real task is to strike a balance between assessment purpose and need, available resources, the required quantitative (psychometric) properties of the test scores and the prevailing educational climate. The remainder of this chapter describes, and reflects on, case studies and examples from the literature that describe 'best practices' in the assessment of clinical competence in context-specific settings.

Successes and challenges of achieving 'best practices' in local contexts

The introduction of 'best practice' assessment strategies in novel settings is always a challenge. The process can be likened to using a newly released drug, which has been shown to improve patient outcomes in double-blind randomised controlled trials. In the trial setting all potential dangers and biases are addressed by excluding participants who may negatively influence the

Table 19.1 Questions to guide the selection of tools to assess clinical competence

1	What dimension(s) of clinical competence is/are to be assessed?
2	What are the consequences of the decision to be made?
3	What are the required quantitative properties of the anticipated test scores?
4	What measure of clinical authenticity is required?
5	What resources are available or what can be accessed?
6	Are there identifiable biases to be addressed or avoided?
7	Is the prevailing educational climate open to change and innovation?
8	What is the expected impact on trainee learning and professional behaviour?
9	Are local/regional/national health needs being addressed?

study results. Once benefit has been shown and new 'best practice' has been established, the average doctor is faced with the challenge of using the new drug in real practice, which is fraught with risks, biases and limitations that were specifically excluded during the drug trials. The challenge, to introduce the new drug into routine clinical practice, is akin to the process of introducing novel educational strategies and adapting them for use in local conditions. Indeed, it is at the interface between the adoption and adaptation of assessment practices in new settings that context-sensitive practices emerge, i.e. 'best practices'. The following examples illustrate the point.

Implementing the OSCE: Brazil vs Argentina

The Objective Structured Clinical Examination (OSCE) is widely accepted as a valid, reliable and effective means of assessing clinical competence in a controlled test environment. While OSCEs have been 'best practice' in affluent countries for many years, the use of this resource-intensive assessment instrument is not universal in the developing world. Furthermore, such 'best practice' assessment strategies may not be accepted if introduced in unfavourable educational climates. Two examples from South America are useful to consider.

In 1995 an attempt was made to introduce OSCEs at the Faculty of Medicine of Ribeirão Preto of the University of São Paulo, Brazil (de Almeida Troncon 2004). The initiative was met with much resistance from both faculty and students. A lack of human resources and limited knowledge of contemporary assessment practices were two important reasons why the initiative failed. But, the main reason for the negative reaction was an unfavourable educational climate in a conservative medical school that did not have a tradition of using objective examinations to test clinical skills. Since then the Brazilian government has made major progress in improving population health and modernising medical education (Schmidt and Duncan 2004). Teaching and assessment innovations are now being implemented in many institutions in Brazil, demonstrating the power of changed political will, social reform and economic growth, all of which underpin the educational changes witnessed over the past 25 years (Blasco et al. 2008; De Souza et al. 2008).

In contrast to the Brazilian experience, OSCEs were successfully implemented at the National University of Cuyo in Mendoza, Argentina, in 2003 (Vargas et al. 2007). The key reasons for the success in Argentina were:

- *A favourable educational climate:* the medical school had embarked on a process of curriculum revision and modernisation of assessment practices and so faculty were keen to implement OSCEs.

- *The creative use of existing resources:* locally available pedagogical and assessment experts were consulted; faculty attended locally run workshops on OSCEs and then trained their colleagues at no additional cost; local-community theatrical actors were trained as standardised patients at minimal cost; existing furniture and clinic space were configured to create OSCE stations.
- *A clear idea of needs:* national priority health needs were identified and stations were designed so that clinical skills could be assessed in these scenarios; the psychometric requirements of the assessment results of such a high-stakes examination were recognised and achieved with appropriate test design and faculty training.

The mini-CEX

The mini-CEX is a valuable tool to assess clinical competence in the workplace. Currently it is recommended that this tool be used for formative assessment with an emphasis on feedback and the development of action plans to improve trainee performance. Two case studies demonstrate some of the challenges of introducing this tool in routine clinical practice.

In a study conducted at 17 postgraduate cardiology training centres in Buenos Aires, Argentina, the mini-CEX was very well received in terms of feedback to the trainees, but most trainees failed to obtain sufficient encounters to yield reproducible results (Alves de Lima et al. 2007). This study emphasised the importance of feedback rather than focusing on psychometric rigour that was not achievable in the workplace. As previously stated, the challenge is to strike a balance among authenticity, learning value and psychometric rigour. Ultimately the issue can be reduced to two of the questions previously listed: *What is the key purpose of the assessment event?* and *What are the consequences of the event?* In this example, the assessment tool provided feedback to improve competence in the workplace and not a judgement decision for academic certification.

The case study from Argentina demonstrates a critical issue relevant to directly observed assessment strategies – the impact of examiner-derived inferences on the perceived competence of the trainee.

Case study 19.2   Role of feedback for inference clarification during a mini-CEX encounter at the Instituto Cardiovascular de Buenos Aires, Argentina

Alberto Alves de Lima

This case study took place during my daily teaching rounds with cardiology residents. One morning during teaching rounds, I performed a mini-CEX with a postgraduage Year 3 resident. Initially he presented the patient case in the hallway, followed by an examination (history taking and physical examination). The patient was a 78-year-old female who had presented to the emergency room 24 hours before with symptoms of heart failure. The history was taken appropriately. During the physical examination at the bedside, the resident palpated the lower limbs for the presence of oedema and to assess the femoral and tibial pulses. He did not, however, remove the sheet from the patient. The physical examination technique of the lower limbs was deemed suboptimal by my standards. Before giving my recommendations regarding his examination skills, I asked the resident why he had not removed the sheet during the physical examination. The resident replied that there were six people around the bed and he wished to avoid embarrassing the woman.

High-level inference has the potential to undermine feedback quality because the potential exists for that feedback to be based on faculty assumptions (Kogan et al. 2011). When I, and other doctors, observe a resident during a clinical encounter, we not only make assumptions and inferences about behaviour, but also provide narrative feedback framed as recommendations. Provoking residents' self-reflection and developing plans to undertake and evaluate residents' improvements by the teachers are key factors for effective feedback on clinical performance (Norcini and Burch 2007). Feedback should be more than something exclusively trainer-driven. It has to be a two-way process during which trainers provide comments (recommendations) and trainees reflect on their performance and there is ongoing dialogue that enriches both (Archer 2010). In addition to self-reflection (reflection on action) supported by external feedback (trainers' recommendations), there has to be linkage with personal goals (action plans) in a coherent, coordinated process rather than a series of unrelated events (Archer 2010). Feedback has been shown to reinforce or modify behaviours and to help learners to reconstruct knowledge, change their performance and feel motivated for learning.

Feedback, an integral part of the mini-CEX, has to be specific and based on what was directly observed during the encounter (Alves de Lima 2008). Questioning, discussing and active testing of the inferences drawn from the observation are crucial before starting the feedback process. Conclusions about resident performance require teachers to use real data (actual residents' actions), to select behaviours and give meaning that can lead to actions (rating and feedback) (Kogan et al. 2011). Feedback that includes recommendations, self-reflections and action plans functions as a coherent process rather than as a series of unrelated events. The value of feedback is determined by the participants rather than by the instruments used. Understanding how different factors can affect an assessor's judgements and ratings during direct observation and how they relate to a resident's learning needs is essential and has to be a key element taken into consideration when organising training sessions. The focus is on the participants instead of on the instruments (Alves de Lima et al. 2011; Pelgrim et al. 2012). Now when I observe residents during rounds, I am aware of engaging them in dialogue around feedback rather than telling things to them as recommendations.

An important, often unnoticed, source of observation bias is the inferences made by clinicians while observing trainees in clinical practice. Since experienced clinicians routinely make inferences about information derived from patients during clinical encounters, it is not surprising that they also do so when assessing trainees. In this case study, a trainee's attempt to preserve patient privacy and dignity in front of a large crowd of clinicians at the bedside was misinterpreted as a lack of clinical competence. The message of the case study is clear – assessors must be aware of this tendency, which is best avoided, or at the very least, recognised and directly addressed with the trainee before making decisions about observed clinical competence. Factors which impact on directly observed assessment strategies, such as the mini-CEX, include: (1) the frames of reference used by assessors when translating observations into judgements and ratings; (2) the high levels of inference made during the assessment process; (3) the methods by which judgements are transcribed into numerical scores, and (4) factors external to trainee performance. The latter include context (complexity of the patient used in the assessment process, trainee's prior experience, assessor–trainee relationship) and response to feedback by both the trainee and the assessor (Kogan et al. 2011).

Direct observation of procedural skills

The assessment of procedural skills using DOPS is motivated by the need for safe, effective and cost-efficient patient care. Two case studies highlight issues relevant to using the DOPS assessment tool.

The following case study describes simulation training for surgical skills in a UK setting.

Case study 19.3 Organising and running a simulation training workshop for core surgical trainees in the United Kingdom

T. James Royle and Steve B. Pandey

It is widely acknowledged that full implementation of the European Working Time Directive has had a detrimental impact on surgical training in the UK, in particular elective training opportunities. As a consequence, doctors who have been selected into core surgical training after foundation years have less operative experience and competence relative to their predecessors. In addition, changes in National Health Service (NHS) culture and service expectations are making it increasingly difficult for trainers to take extra time in theatre to facilitate elective training. Therefore there is a need to facilitate surgical training outside of the operating theatre, to help speed up trainees' learning curves to competence, so they maximise their operating opportunities.

A 1-day workshop was organised for rotational core trainees by a hospital with excellent teaching and training facilities in a purpose-built education centre with a fully accredited clinical skills wet laboratory and full-time support staff. The aim of the workshop was to provide trainees with the opportunity to practise and develop their laparoscopic skills, and become competent in deploying bowel-stapling devices in a safe, controlled environment. The workshop was limited to a maximum of 12 trainees with a high trainer-to-trainee ratio led by consultant surgeons and senior registrars.

To keep the cost to a minimum for trainees, industrial support was provided in the form of complimentary stapling equipment with a company representative available for technical advice during the day, and faculty voluntarily gave their time. The workshop was advertised via Deanery email distribution lists to regional trainees with an electronic flyer.

Six weeks prior to the workshop, a pre-course questionnaire was emailed to participants. This learning needs assessment served several purposes:

- Gather information on participants' experience, such as number of operations performed and months in general surgical placements.
- Assess knowledge and encourage relevant study to minimise the requirement for knowledge-based teaching on the day.
- Ask participants why they signed up and to generate their own learning outcomes.
- Enable the faculty to review the participants' responses within the knowledge-based presentations as a way of reflecting on their learning and providing feedback.

During the workshop the participants were encouraged to complete their own assessment forms (self-assessment and reflection). Further written feedback was added by faculty and signed off as the day progressed.

The workshop began with two interactive PowerPoint presentations covering the principles of bowel anastomosis, stapling techniques and a DVD demonstration of the stapling exercises for the afternoon. After this, the remainder of the day was devoted to supervised simulation training. Participants worked in pairs with laparoscopic box trainers, progressing from simple to more complex tasks. In the afternoon, there were two bowel anastomotic stapling sessions, with all participants performing (and assisting their partner with) three or four different stapling tasks using a realistic fresh cadaveric animal model (porcine bowel). The trainers provided tuition and informal feedback throughout the day. A course certificate was presented to each trainee along with the completed assessment form as structured feedback.

Organising such a workshop was challenging and required excellent communication and coordination with administrative staff, industry representatives, catering staff and faculty. Essential tasks included preparation of course materials, faculty training and briefing, and setting up the clinical skills laboratory. For the first workshop the course organiser did most of the above, including setting up the lab for the morning and afternoon sessions. However, a miscommunication with the manager of the local abattoir led to the organiser having to drive to the abattoir to collect the porcine bowel and then prepare it during a lunch break!

The first workshop was very successful and evaluated extremely positively, but for subsequent workshops a laboratory technician was recruited to assist with setting up. This released the course convenor to facilitate the day more effectively. Arrangements with suppliers must be organised well in advance. Faculty training and briefing are also important, particularly to ensure that formal written reflection and feedback are signed off as the day progresses.

The workshop, as demonstrated in the UK case study, has many good features from an assessment perspective.

- The learning needs of the trainees were identified and expected outcomes were clarified before the workshop – an excellent example of alignment between learning needs, expected outcomes and assessment strategies.
- The workshop provided a balance of theory and practical training opportunities.
- The workshop offered both low- and high-fidelity learning opportunities.
- Trainees were required to provide input about their own performance.
- Written feedback was a formal part of the training programme.

The organisers faced challenges related to logistics and the need for adequate technical and administrative support. These are key issues, which, if overlooked, can mean the difference between success and failure.

In the case study from the Pontificia Catholic University of Chile, the authors provide another example of the innovative use of DOPS in a postgraduate training programme.

Case study 19.4 How to assess trainees' clinical competence performing endoscopies in a postgraduate residency programme at the Pontificia Universidad Católica de Chile

Arnoldo Riquelme

The Pontificia Universidad Católica de Chile Medical School (PUCMS) implemented several initiatives in order to improve medical education for undergraduate medical students (Sánchez et al. 2008). Those efforts have been recognised in national and international accreditation processes (Sánchez et al. 2010). However, postgraduate medical education is less developed in our institution, and there has been a significant delay transferring successful teaching and learning innovations or assessment instruments developed in undergraduate level to postgraduate residency programmes (PRPs).

(continued)

(continued)

The Chilean Society of Gastroenterology carried out a Delphi technique consensus, in order to establish the core competencies of the Chilean gastroenterologist (Riquelme et al. 2010). In this consensus diagnostic upper gastrointestinal endoscopy (UGIE) was considered by an expert panel as the most important and essential procedure for the specialty. This case study focuses on an upper gastrointestinal endoscopy basic training programme (UGIETP) of the gastroenterology PRP at the PUCMS.

The gastroenterology PRP is a 2-year programme and the UGIETP takes place in the first 4 months of the first year of this residency programme. During the first 4 weeks, the trainee receives basic information about the endoscope and training process in a simulated environment. During the next 12 weeks, trainees are trained with real patients in the endoscopic room of an outpatient clinic using low-risk patients and only performing diagnostic procedures under supervision of a personal endoscopic trainer (expert).

Trainees who successfully complete the simulated training stage are allowed to continue their training programme with real patients. They start by taking a brief history and gaining informed consent, explaining to the patient what they are going to do during the UGIE. After sedation the trainee starts the procedure under strict supervision and the trainee's performance is assessed with a DOPS developed by the trainers and experts, identifying four key features after each procedure and one complete checklist (33 items) at the end of each session. Additionally, efficiency of movements is assessed using the Imperial College Surgical Assessment Device (ICSAD), allowing objective quantification of movements and the path length travelled by each hand (distance measured in metres) (Aggarwal et al. 2006). The educational activity follows the rules of workplace-based assessment and it is really important to keep it authentic (Norcini and Burch 2007). Therefore, the whole teaching activity takes place in a real environment with real patients.

After each procedure the trainer provides effective feedback, including the strengths and achievements of the trainee and weaknesses that should be improved in future procedures. Effective feedback is a key element in this programme and takes place immediately after the UGIE has been performed by the trainee. UGIE could be considered as a meta-competence because the whole procedure involves clinical skills, patient investigation (taking histological samples or urease test to detect *Helicobacter pylori* infection according to the endoscopic findings), written communication and information-handling skills, ethical aspects and legal responsibilities. For that reason, clinical skills and trainees' progression through the UGIETP are mainly measured with the four-key-feature DOPS and ICSAD measurement. Other competencies related to UGIE are assessed with the 33-items checklist and portfolio activities. Formative assessment also includes a follow-up process for each patient with biopsies. Residents report the final diagnosis, discuss treatment options and follow the patient, including critical appraisal of their endoscopic reports and reflection about selected patients in their portfolio.

Effective feedback has been identified in a meta-analysis as the most important element in WPBA in terms of the educational impact (Miller and Archer 2010). Effective feedback is immediate, accurate and based on the strengths and weaknesses of the trainee. Moreover, trainees establish an action plan with their trainer for the next session in order to acquire knowledge and improve skills and attitudes related to UGIE performance.

Based on the learning curves of the last ten trainees who followed this UGIETP, they are autonomous after 80 procedures and they significantly reduced their travelled path length of each hand (99.7 m to 60 m; distance measured in metres) measured with ICSAD. Second-year residents and experts (trainers) were also measured and their travelled path lengths were 49.7 m and 17.9 m, respectively (González et al. 2012). We observed different levels of performance because some trainees are more skilled than others. It is important to train them, considering their individual achievements based on their strengths, and explain to them how to improve their performance. All trainees construct their own learning curves and we compared them with cumulative curves of previous cohorts of trainees. Summative assessment is based on their progression through the UGIETP and a reflective portfolio about their learning process. If they successfully complete the UGIETP, they are allowed to continue with the next stage, including therapeutic UGIE and colonoscopy in a more complex inpatient endoscopic unit at the hospital.

Learning objectives related mainly to one dimension of a competence, but sometimes competencies relating to a clinical procedure were more complex than we expected. We needed to combine a wide variety of formative and summative assessment instruments, which were suitable (valid and reliable) for evaluating knowledge, skills and attitudes.

The American Society of Gastrointestinal Endoscopy (ASGE) reported that 130 UGIE are needed to be competent (Adler et al. 2012). Our training programme demonstrated that, if you train residents in a simulated environment followed by sessions with real patients in the endoscopic room, following our training system, trainees are autonomous with only 80 procedures. Moreover, we train residents with low-risk patients (American Society of Anesthesiologists (ASA) classification I or II) and have had no endoscopic complications in more than 1,000 UGIEs performed by trainees.

The activity in the simulated environment and the endoscopy room is aligned with the assessment system and the learning outcomes that the trainees must achieve at the end of the UGIETP. What is more interesting is that, according to the results observed in the first ten residents (two cohorts), we learnt more about what is effective in terms of the training process (teaching activities), assessment process (assessment for learning rather than assessment of what was learnt) and feedback (formative assessment) in our training programme. Based on the results obtained using the Postgraduate Hospital Educational Environment Measure (PHEEM) questionnaire, residents perceived there to be a positive educational environment, highlighting trainers' quality, protected time for this educational activity and a safe environment in the endoscopy room (Herrera et al. 2012). The four-key-feature DOPS was easy to use after each procedure, and allowed the construction of learning curves to establish trainees' competence performing UGIE. On the other hand, the 33-item checklist and ICSAD assessed a wider spectrum of competencies and objective quantification of movements, respectively. However, both are time consuming and it is unrealistic to include them after each procedure.

The key learning points of the Chile case study include the following:

- Patient safety is key when teaching procedural skills using real patients. This dilemma often strongly biases training towards simulation settings with little real clinical experience. In this programme, the issue was addressed by allowing trainees to perform endoscopy on low-risk patients identified using an objective risk stratification tool.
- DOPS focused on four aspects of each procedure and a detailed checklist was only completed at the end of each session. This reduced the paperwork between cases and limited the impact on service delivery time.
- DOPS was used in conjunction with another validated procedure-specific rating tool, which improved the quality and objectivity of the assessment process.

The educational impact of workplace-based assessment

The final case study from Saudi Arabia highlights the influence of curriculum change on learning behaviour. At the King Saud University in Saudi Arabia, extensive curriculum innovation was introduced with a focus on integrating WPBA and clinical teaching. Previously, medical students were only allowed to observe patient encounters undertaken by qualified clinical staff and their clinical skills were not assessed in the workplace. Not surprisingly, students placed little value on clinical activities and attendance was poor. Since introducing a suite of WPBA tools, the students have become active participants in the clinical services and appreciate the value of learning and assessment activities in the workplace.

Case study 19.5 Introducing workplace-based assessment in a reformed, undergraduate curriculum at King Saud University, Saudi Arabia

Hamza Abdulghani and Gominda Ponnamperuma

The College of Medicine, King Saud University, was the first medical college in the Kingdom of Saudi Arabia. In line with contemporary changes in medical education, the traditional curriculum of the college has recently undergone many changes to include various innovative strategies in teaching, learning and assessment. For example, clinical teaching has been introduced as early as from the first academic year to make teaching and learning more contextual, interesting and beneficial for the students.

In the past, however, the teachers were more entrenched in the old style of clinical teaching. Usually, clinical teaching took place at the bedside or with students observing clinical teachers at an ambulatory care unit. Thus, objective observation and feedback did not take place. This was contrary to the well-established educational premise that clinical teaching needs good planning, observation of students and continuous feedback (Harden and Laidlaw 2012). Further, the teachers observed that the students gave low priority to attending clinical teaching sessions, as these sessions did not help them in achieving high marks in their final assessment.

In an attempt to find a balance between ensuring that appropriate planning, observation and continuous feedback are practised uniformly throughout all clinical teaching and learning sessions, and that the students take clinical teaching and learning seriously, the college realised that reforming the existing clinical teaching would not be sufficient. In order to remedy this, the college attempted to institutionalise the above good practices of teaching and learning in the clinical setting (i.e. planning, observation and feedback) through assessment. This led to the introduction of WPBA (Carr 2006; Dewi and Achmad 2010).

Three methods of WPBA were agreed by the curriculum committee, to be included in the clinical assessment and teaching: mini-CEX, CbD and DOPS. These methods of assessment and teaching demanded a lot of skills from the tutors to assess and teach their students effectively (Hill and Kendall 2007). Further, the college reckoned that continuous monitoring and evaluation were necessary to prevent the implementation of WPBA being reduced to a tick-box exercise (Bindal et al. 2011).

This situation compelled us to devise methods to improve the faculty skills of applying the above WPBA methods. Many workshops were conducted for faculty to orient them in applying these methods. Feedback from both faculty and students was collected to get their opinion on improving the implementation of WPBA. These feedback and suggestions were applied to upgrade both the ongoing process of workplace-based clinical assessment and teaching, and the faculty development activities on WPBA. The introduction of WPBA also triggered a change in the student perception of clinical teaching and learning. Informal student and staff surveys indicated that students now take clinical teaching and learning much more seriously.

This case study shows how faculty development activities on WPBA, with special emphasis on objective observation and feedback, can be used to institutionalise good practices of clinical assessment and teaching. In addition, it demonstrates that introducing WPBA with the explicit intention of combining assessment with teaching and learning leads to students taking clinical teaching and learning more seriously. Fine-tuning with faculty development activities, based on the continuous evaluation of the implementation of WPBA, is ongoing.

The future of assessment on a global scale

The quantitative properties of assessment scores have been the major focus of attention for far too long. Medical education leaders have made a plea for a broader view of assessment and revision of the traditional measures that are used to determine the quality of assessment practices. In addition, it is also true that the 'big five' – the USA, Canada, the UK, Australia and Western Europe – have dominated medical education practices for far too long.

Global economic and political tides are slowly turning and the BRICS member countries (Brazil, Russia, India, China and South Africa) are likely to lead the way. Currently BRICS member countries are home to almost three billion people or about 43 per cent of the world's population and their combined external trade is worth about $US6 trillion, or 17 per cent of the world total. So, it is plausible that in the coming decade the developing world, led by BRICS, will have a palpable influence on 'best practices' in medical education. This chapter already provides insights into current pockets of regional innovation and excellence. Ultimately, the sharing and exchange of local assessment practices that are responsive to culture, language, available resources and health needs may expand our understanding of 'best practices' in 21st-century medical education.

Take-home messages

To recap, the transversal principles of 'best practices', as demonstrated in this chapter on the assessment of clinical competence, suggest that successful assessment strategies are based on several principles:

- Start planning an assessment event by deciding on the purpose (formative (feedback) or summative (judgement)) and consequence (feedback for improvement or judgement for certification).
- Align assessment practices with learning needs and expected outcomes.
- Attempt to limit biases commonly encountered in WPBA.
- Feedback should:
    - be based on observed behaviour;
    - avoid making inferences;
    - include trainees' perception of their own performance;
    - conclude with an action plan to foster further development.

- The quantitative properties of WPBA scores currently limit their use for high-stakes summative purposes.
- 'Best practices' are achieved when assessment strategies are adapted to suit local circumstances and address local needs.

Bibliography

Adler, D.G., Bakis, G., Coyle, W.J., DeGregorio, B., Dua, K.S., Lee, L.S., McHenry, L. Jr, Pais, S.A., Rajan, E., Sedlack, R.E., Shami, V.M. and Faulx, A.L. (2012) 'Principles of training in GI endoscopy', *Gastrointestinal Endoscopy*, 75(2): 231–5.

Aggarwal, R., Dosis, A., Bello, F. and Darzi, A. (2006) 'Motion tracking systems for assessment of surgical skill', *Surgical Endoscopy*, 21(2): 339–9.

Alves de Lima, A.E. (2008) 'Constructive feedback. A strategy to enhance learning', *Medicina (Buenos Aires)*, 68(1): 88–92.

Alves de Lima, A., Barrero, C., Baratta, S., Castillo Costa, Y., Bortman,, G., Carabajales, J., Conde, D., Galli, A., Degrange, G. and van der Vleuten, C. (2007) 'Validity, reliability, feasibility and satisfaction of the Mini-Clinical Evaluation Exercise (Mini-CEX) for cardiology residency training', *Medical Teacher*, 29(8): 785–90.

Alves de Lima, A., Conde, D., Costabel, J., Corso, J. and Van der Vleuten, C. (2011) 'A laboratory study on the reliability estimations of the mini-CEX', *Advances in Health Sciences Education: Theory and Practice*, 18(1): 5–13.

Archer, J.C. (2010) 'State of the science in health professional education: effective feedback', *Medical Education*, 44(1): 101–8.

Bindal, T., Wall, D. and Goodyear, H. (2011) 'Trainee doctors' views on workplace-based assessments: Are they just a tick box exercise?', *Medical Teacher*, 33: 919–27.

Blasco, P.B., Levites, M.R., Janaudis, M.C., Moreto, G., Roncoletta, A.F.T., de Benedetto, M.A.C. and Pinheiro, T. (2008) 'Family medicine education in Brazil: Challenges, opportunities and innovations', *Academic Medicine*, 83(7): 684–90.

Carr, S. (2006) 'The foundation programme assessment tools: An opportunity to enhance feedback to trainees?', *Postgraduate Medical Journal*, 82: 576–9.

Collins, J. (2010) *Foundation for excellence: An evaluation of the foundation programme*, Medical Education England. Online. Available HTTP: http://hee.nhs.uk/wp-content/uploads/sites/321/2012/08/Foundation-for-excellence-report.pdf (accessed 25 March 2015).

Davies, H., Archer, J., Southgate, L. and Norcini, J. (2009) 'Initial evaluation of the first year of the Foundation Assessment Programme', *Medical Education*, 43: 78–81.

De Almeida Troncon, L.E. (2004) 'Clinical skills assessment: Limitations to the introduction of an OSCE (Objective Structured Clinical Examination) in a traditional Brazilian medical school', *São Paulo Medical Journal*, 122(1): 12–17.

Department of Health (2004) '*Modernising medical careers: The next steps. The future shape of foundation, specialist and general practice training programmes*', London: Department of Health.

De Souza, P.A., Zeferino, A.M.B. and da Aurelio Ros, M. (2008) 'Changes in medicine course curricula in Brazil encouraged by the Program for the Promotion of Medical School Curricula (PROMED)', *BMC Medical Education*, 8: 54. Online. Available HTTP: http://www.biomedcentral.com (accessed 9 September 2014).

Dewi, S.P. and Achmad, T.H. (2010) 'Optimising feedback using the mini-CEX during the final semester programme', *Medical Education*, 44(5): 509.

González, R., Rodríguez, A., Buckel, E., Hernández, C., Tejos, R., Parra, A., Pimentel, F., Boza, C., Padilla, O. and Riquelme, A. (2012) 'Systematization of an upper gastrointestinal endoscopy training program for diagnosis in a simulation-based setting and learning curves in real patients', *Revista Gastroenterologia Latinoamericana*, 23(4): 191–6.

Harden, R.M. and Laidlaw, J.M. (2012) *Essential skills for a medical teacher*, Edinburgh: Churchill Livingstone, Elsevier.

Herrera, C., Olivos, T., Román, J.A., Larraín, A., Pizarro, M., Solís, N., Sarfatis, A., Torres, P., Padilla, O., Le Roy, C. and Riquelme, A. (2012) 'Evaluation of the educational environment in medical specialty programs', *Revista Médica de Chile*, 140: 1554–61.

Hill, F. and Kendall, K. (2007) 'Adopting and adapting the mini-CEX as an undergraduate assessment and learning tool', *The Clinical Teacher*, 4: 244–8.

Kogan, J.R., Holmboe, E.S. and Hauer, K.E. (2009) 'Tolls for direct observation and assessment of clinical skills of medical trainees. A systematic review', *Journal of the American Medical Association*, 302(12): 1316–26.

Kogan, J.R., Conforti, L., Bernabeo, E., Iobst, W. and Holmboe, E. (2011) 'Opening the black box of clinical skills assessment via observation: A conceptual model', *Medical Education*, 45(10): 1048–60.

Miller, G.E. (1990) 'The assessment of clinical skills/competence/performance', *Academic Medicine*, 65(9): s63–7.

Miller, A. and Archer, J. (2010) 'Impact of workplace based assessment on doctors' education and performance: a systematic review', *British Medical Journal*, 341: c5064.

Norcini, J.J. (2010) 'Workplace assessment', In T. Swanwick (ed.) *Understanding medical education: Evidence, theory and practice*, (pp. 232–45), Oxford: Wiley-Blackwell.

Norcini, J. and Burch, V. (2007) 'Workplace-based assessment as an educational tool: AMEE guide no. 31', *Medical Teacher*, 29(9): 855–71.

Pelgrim, E.A., Kramer, A.W., Mokkink, H.G. and van der Vleuten, C.P. (2012) 'The process of feedback in workplace-based assessment: Organisation, delivery, continuity', *Medical Education*, 46(6): 604–12.

Peterson, M.C., Holbrook, J.H., Hales D.V., Smith, N.L. and Staker, L.V. (1992) 'Contributions of the history, physical examination, and laboratory investigation in making medical diagnoses', *Western Medical Journal*, 156(2): 163–5.

Riquelme, A., de la Fuente, P., Méndez, B., Salech, F., Valderrama, S., Méndez, J.I., Oporto, J., Miquel, J.F., Defilippi, C., Soza, A., Sirhan, N. and Sáenz, R. (2010) 'Competencies of the Chilean gastroenterologist: Modified Delphi technique', *Revista Gastroenterologia Latinoamericana*, 21(4): 437–53.

Sánchez, I., Riquelme, A., Moreno, M., Mena, B., Dagnino, J. and Grebe, G. (2008) 'Revitalising medical education: The school of medicine at the Pontificia Universidad Católica de Chile', *The Clinical Teacher*, 5: 57–61.

Sánchez, I., Riquelme, A., Moreno, R., García, P. and Salas, S. (2010) 'International accreditation process at a Latin American medical school: A ten-year experience', *Medical Teacher*, 32(3): 271.

Schmidt, M.I. and Duncan, B.B. (2004) 'Academic medicine as a resource for global health: The case of Brazil', *British Medical Journal*, 329: 753–4.

Schuwirth, L.W.T. and van der Vleuten, C.P.M. (2010) 'How to design a useful test: The principles of assessment'. In T. Swanwick (ed.) *Understanding medical education: Evidence, theory and practice*, (pp. 195–207), Oxford: Wiley-Blackwell.

Vargas, A.L., Boulet, J.R., Errichetti, A., van Zanten, M., Lopez, M.J. and Reta, A.M. (2007) 'Developing performance-based medical school assessment programs in resource-limited environments', *Medical Teacher*, 29: 192–8.

PART 6

The medical school

20
INTERNATIONAL AND TRANSNATIONAL MODELS FOR DELIVERING MEDICAL EDUCATION

The future for medical education

John Hamilton and Shajahan Yasin

Internationalisation is one of the most important forces in higher education today, presenting a powerful challenge and an opportunity for medical school.

As part of a programme to support clinical communication skills development I spent time with Year 1 medical students observing doctor–patient interactions in a small local clinic on the outskirts of a large regional city in Malaysia. These were Malaysian students of the Malaysian-based medical school of an Australian university. The students were observing a consultation between a middle-aged Malaysian doctor and an elderly female Malay patient dressed in the traditional clothes of that region. The doctor I observed was quietly spoken, gentle, caring and seemed to put the patient at her ease. He took time to listen to the patient and reassure her about her concerns. As is the custom in Malaysia when addressing an older person not known to you, he addressed the patient as 'auntie'. I was impressed with the rapport he created and care he took with the patient – a kind and caring doctor.

Driving back to the campus, I listened with increasing dismay to the students in the back seat discussing the consultation. They talked disparagingly of this doctor's paternalistic, doctor-centred approach. They noted that he failed to adequately elicit the patient's perspective on her medical condition or to engage her in discussion and decisions on the treatment options. They were concerned at his use of closed questions and apparent failure to provide opportunities for the patient to assert herself.

I wondered whether we had been watching the same consultation, and how we had arrived at such different interpretations of the doctor's behaviour.

In considering the above anecdote it would be easy to dismiss the student perceptions as just 'the arrogance of youth' or a reflection of their dependence on theoretical learning rather than clinical experience in interpreting the events. However, they highlight one of the key challenges for international and transnational medical education programmes – how to produce graduates with both the skills and sensibilities to operate effectively across different healthcare systems and contexts, with all that that entails. While the focus of this chapter is on models for delivery, we will come back at some point to this key requirement for students in a globalised world to acquire the multiple 'repertoires' they need for the diverse contexts in which they will find themselves in future practice.

The case studies in this chapter offer examples of transnational delivery in practice. They highlight the fact that for international and transnational medical education there is no blueprint, but rather many different permutations and combinations designed to meet the particular and often unique circumstances which characterise teaching and learning in any one location.

Whether consciously or unconsciously, we tend to use our own experience as a reference point in commencing new ventures. This is natural and not unexpected, but in the context of international ventures can be limiting. It can close our minds to new possibilities or ways of doing. On the other hand, innovation and change are approached with some caution in medical education, given the high stakes in ensuring quality and safety. The process of development of curricula within international medical education programmes therefore often involves a balance between these two imperatives – a need to be flexible enough to accommodate new and varied contexts, and a need to maintain a strong grounding in established and proven practice. This is the tension under which curriculum development often occurs, involving a conservative approach but willingness to explore alternatives and options as they arise or become necessary. This 'balancing act' is one reason why relationship building and the associated trust that it entails are key factors in the process by which collaborative curriculum negotiation and development occur within international medical education programmes, as illustrated in the case studies presented below.

As early as 1986, Hofstede was warning against the imposition of curricula from one country to another and questioning the viability of such a process, and his concerns remain relevant today. Whilst Bleakley et al. (2008) acknowledge the value of international partnerships and collaborations in medical education, however, they note that these tend to be driven by institutions of the 'modern, metropolitan West' and make assumptions about the universal applicability of particular learning methods currently in favour in Western medical education (e.g. problem-based learning). According to Bleakley et al., the Western medical curriculum is 'steeped in a particular set of cultural attitudes that are rarely questioned' (2008: 267). They advocate a more critical perspective in evaluating international medical education initiatives based on post-colonial theory. Although it is not within the scope of this chapter to address this issue in any depth, it is nevertheless important to acknowledge that the risks of neo-colonialism within transnational medical education programmes are real and require careful consideration.

So it is important to acknowledge that, when we talk of international or transnational medical education, we are *not* talking about the imposition or transferral of curricula – by definition, to be international or transnational implies some genuine collaborative curricular development and growth, genuinely reflecting elements of all parties involved in programme development and delivery. While transnational ventures often involve considerable relationship building in the early stages, respect cannot be something which ends at the dinner table – it has to translate into how programmes are organised, how collaboration is negotiated and the ways in which staff from different schools and countries are positioned in all communications. It must be real rather than tokenistic and enable all parties to have an equal voice in the curriculum as it moves forward. This is perhaps the greatest challenge facing transnational medical education programmes, and one which most involved would acknowledge has only partly been achieved in many such ventures to date.

This chapter is organised around four case studies, and seeks to draw from these specific examples some general observations. The first two case studies involved the establishment of full overseas branch campuses, with new medical schools being set up; the latter two have involved educational and institutional partnerships, with students completing different phases of their medical studies in different locations and institutions. Key issues raised in these case studies and requiring careful consideration in seeking best-practice approaches in transnational delivery include: legal and regulatory frameworks; relationships with government; curriculum equivalency in standards and content; staffing; coordination of clinical learning; contextualisation of teaching; learning and assessment materials; and accreditation processes. The challenge for achieving best practice in transnational delivery is not only *setting up* a programme which successfully navigates a course through these key issues and requirements, but establishment of processes which can grow and *be sustained* in the longer term, and withstand the pressures and constraints which inevitably arise in such ventures.

The Newcastle University Medicine Malaysia (NUMed) and Monash University Malaysia (MUM) case studies presented below illustrate a number of the key issues in the establishment of transnational delivery of medical education. As the first UK medical school to establish a branch campus overseas, both the University of Newcastle and the UK and Malaysian accreditation bodies were travelling through uncharted waters to an extent. Similarly, the Monash University venture outlined in the second case study presented both the Australian Medical Council (AMC) and Malaysian Medical Council (MMC) with particular challenges. This is why (as noted below) regular communication with the accreditation bodies as well as government departments can be so important, helping to circumvent issues before they arise as well as to find solutions to potential 'bureaucratic obstacles'.

Case study 20.1 Establishment of a branch campus medical school – Newcastle University Medicine Malaysia

Philip Bradley

In 2006 Newcastle University was invited by the Malaysian government to become part of the Educity development in Johor, Malaysia. The Educity concept is to provide an international student campus comprising a range of educational establishments from across the globe, each offering specific courses which together will be the equivalent of a conventional university. Newcastle University agreed to offer its MBBS degree and the NUMed campus opened in 2011.

NUMed was established as a Malaysian private company which is wholly owned by Newcastle University, UK. NUMed is registered as an independent private university and is subject to Malaysian law. As a UK organisation operating within an entirely different legal and regulatory framework, we have experienced inevitable frustrations with process. Processes that work well at home do not easily translate to another jurisdiction and having a good legal team negotiating the initial set-up was vital. It has been important to have governmental support for the project as NUMed has, on occasion, had to seek help from both Malaysian and UK governments to unlock bureaucratic obstacles. Establishing a branch campus from scratch has meant duplicating all those central university functions (e.g. human resources, finance) that many educators take for granted and which ensure smooth running of a campus. The value of the institutional memory shared amongst administrators is not recognised until it is absent.

(continued)

(continued)

The MBBS degree is awarded by Newcastle University and is a UK primary medical qualification. It is subject to accreditation by the MMC and the UK General Medical Council (GMC). This raised a number of issues, given that Newcastle was the first UK medical school to establish an overseas branch campus and there was no established mechanism for this process. We have had to work closely with the MMC and the GMC. The GMC's involvement with NUMed has led to proposals for amendment to the Medical Act and to changes in GMC regulations. Students are Malaysian and international. Home and European Union students are not allowed to enrol.

A requirement of GMC accreditation is that the programme of study in Malaysia must be of an equivalent standard to that in the UK. Students in Malaysia sit the same exams at the same time as the students in the UK. Ensuring that we can offer an educational experience that will allow our students to meet the requirements of *Tomorrow's Doctors* (GMC 2009) has been our top priority. Where possible, our teaching materials are contextualised to the Malaysia setting. A compare-and-contrast approach has been adopted, where UK practices are taught and then compared with current Malaysian practice. Fortunately, the Malaysian healthcare system is largely conducted in English and the MMC bases its policies largely on UK standards, so differences are minimised.

NUMed staff use IT to participate fully in all relevant UK curriculum management committees to ensure curricular harmonisation. Senior staff at NUMed are seconded from Newcastle, UK. Flying faculty help to maintain a UK feel to the course but are used sparingly. There are advantages of having a small local faculty largely focused on teaching as this ensures continuity for the students and faculty can innovate to improve the student learning experience. While the campus was under construction, the first two cohorts of students were taught in the UK and then transferred back to Malaysia. This meant that student numbers on the new campus rose rapidly, allowing the introduction of co-curricular activities to enhance the student experience.

Organisational differences in the approach to clinical education have required us to adopt a different teaching model to that used in the UK. Unlike in the UK, it is not the expectation in Malaysia that doctors within government hospitals have education as part of their remit. Thus it is not easy to use local practising clinicians as teachers. NUMed therefore employs its own clinical staff who accompany our students into the hospital and teach them at the bedside.

We have been able to deliver a UK medical degree within Malaysia at a branch campus in Johor. Maintenance of good relations with regulators and government has been vital to success. A solid legal framework is essential. Balance between UK content and local context is crucial. Equity of standards is maintained by having shared outcomes and shared assessment. Being able to teach within a healthcare system where English is widely spoken is important. Curriculum innovations in the branch campus can enhance teaching at home.

Case study 20.2 Establishment of Monash University's Jeffrey Cheah School of Medicine and Health Sciences, Malaysia

Shajahan Yasin

Monash University currently has three medical programmes, including a graduate-entry programme based in rural Victoria, Australia. The other two are undergraduate-entry 5-year programmes, one based in Melbourne, Australia and the other, the Jeffrey Cheah School of Medicine and Health Sciences (JCSMHS), in Kuala Lumpur, Malaysia.

MUM was established as a full branch campus of Monash University in 1998, upon the invitation of the Malaysian government. It is a joint venture between Monash University in Australia and the Sunway Group and is now co-owned by the non-profit Jeffrey Cheah Foundation. The medical school commenced operations in 2005 with the first two cohorts starting in Melbourne, while preparations for full operation in Malaysia were being completed. In 2007, three cohorts of students started Years 1, 2 and 3 in Malaysia. This medical school caters primarily to Malaysian students studying in their own country, and to date has produced four cohorts of medical graduates.

Years 1 and 2 are conducted at the main MUM campus in Kuala Lumpur. Years 3 to 5 are based at the clinical school in Johor Bahru, adjacent to the Sultanah Aminah Hospital, a large 989-bed tertiary care centre. Students complete most of their clinical learning in Malaysian hospitals and clinics, but also complete a minimum of 12 weeks on clinical placements in their final year at several hospitals in metropolitan Melbourne.

The hospitals and clinics where the students undergo their clinical experience are government facilities which prioritise services over teaching, and consultants in these centres are usually unavailable for the teaching of medical students except after hours. As a result, most of the teaching in the clinics and wards is done by full-time or part-time academic staff employed by the university. While Monash academic staff are encouraged to be involved in providing clinical services, this is sometimes difficult due to heavy teaching commitments and the need to conduct research. In addition the cost of all teaching has to be borne by the university and there is no government subsidy for teaching apart from the use of the health centres.

The course in Malaysia was accredited by the AMC in 2008 and by the MMC in 2010. AMC accreditation was given on the basis of a single accreditation across the three Monash medical programmes.

The medical programme in Malaysia has the same entry and exit criteria, same start and end dates and same learning objectives as the Australian programme. Students get the same Monash testamur on completion. Curriculum implementation is very similar, with close liaison between academic staff at the respective campuses. Where required, content is contextualised to take account of differences in healthcare systems, cultures and disease prevalence. In general, students get access to lecture and learning materials from both campuses and have equal access to online library resources, including e-books and databases.

Assessments, including written exams and Objective Structured Clinical Examinations (OSCEs), are identical and conducted at the same time (the time difference between Australia and Malaysia is 3 hours or less and this allows examinations to be conducted simultaneously). Examination processes, including blueprinting and standard setting, are jointly conducted, and examination items are jointly contributed. In general communication and collaboration between campuses are excellent, with large numbers of staff travelling both ways. Students from all three medical schools (undergraduate and graduate-entry) are considered as a single group in result review meetings and board of examiners' meetings. Students of JCSMHS have been performing on a par with the Australian-based students.

Although there are very few Australian academics on campus, there are active exchange visits by staff and a high degree of coordination and collaboration in teaching between the Australian- and Malaysian-based schools. Academic staff from both the Malaysian and Australian programmes liaise closely, have regular discussions and are members of the same curriculum and year-level committees.

(continued)

(continued)

As a single course implemented in several locations, governance of the programme has been a particular focus. Academic matters in the Malaysian programme are managed by a Director of Curriculum, with overview by a Deputy Dean (MBBS) who is based in Melbourne. Monash University educational policies and philosophies are reflected across all campuses, including MUM.

The governance structure has been designed to ensure that the quality and standards of the MBBS degree in Malaysia will be the same as that in Victoria. The committee structure, like the main course management committee and assessment committees as well as the year-level committees, serves all three medical programmes with active academic and student membership across all three programmes. Videoconferencing and teleconferencing are routinely used in all meetings.

Student exchange is a prominent feature and fairly large numbers of Australian campus-based students undertake units in Malaysia, especially in the later clinical years. Medical students are encouraged to be involved in staff research. Over the last 5 years research infrastructure and capacity have been added, with major research initiatives, including the Brain Research Institute of Monash Sunway (www.med.monash.edu.my/brims) and a community-based research platform (www.seaco.asia).

There have been a number of challenges over the years. Even though the AMC and MMC standards are similar, there are differences, and the need to satisfy both adds to the complexity of the programme. In addition there are governmental bureaucratic requirements that need to be satisfied.

The Monash medical programme in Malaysia has been very successful. Major reasons for this success have been the strong commitment of faculty; the decision to manage the Malaysian campus as a full branch campus with the same academic, quality and infrastructure standards; and the management of students as a single cohort. The need to satisfy local as well as Australian standards continues to pose challenges.

Staffing

The NUMed model employs a small local academic faculty to provide continuity while seconding senior staff from the University of Newcastle in the UK. Other academic teaching staff from the UK are flown in as required. Similar to the NUMed model, Monash University's JCSMHS has employed a significant number of local academic staff, many of whom have had opportunities to attend training in Australia to develop their teaching skills further. Like NUMed, it also has flown in academic staff from overseas as required, particularly in the formative years while building local capacity, and to deliver in curriculum areas where local recruitment proved difficult (e.g. medical ethics). However, the Monash University approach has also involved recruiting staff from within the region, for example, from Singapore, India, Bangladesh and Indonesia. Unlike the NUMed approach, senior management are all local, although all have significant international experience as both practitioners and educators. Most have worked for extended periods in either Australia or the UK, and bring a considerable degree of cross-cultural experience to their positions, as well as familiarity with both Malaysian and overseas healthcare and educational contexts.

Clearly, achieving the right balance of academic staffing is crucial, and while local and overseas staff typically have the same roles and responsibilities, there may be some differences in how they can contribute to the programme. For example, local teaching staff are familiar with local healthcare systems and contexts, and may be particularly well equipped to communicate and engage with local students in accessible ways. In addition, they can guide students in interacting with local patients and clinicians. Overseas academic staff, particularly those recruited or seconded from the university's main campus (in the UK and Australia in relation to the two case studies above) can help monitor and maintain curriculum equivalence, as well as provide an international perspective on teaching approaches and curriculum content.

While both the NUMed and MUM case studies highlight the importance of academic staff selection, undoubtedly transnational ventures place particular demands on administrative and support staff as well, and this should be acknowledged. Their capacity to operate effectively across cultures is crucial, as are the flexibility and versatility to cope with challenges as they arise.

Language and clinical learning

While in the Malaysian context English is relatively widely spoken, particularly within education circles, Malaysian society is highly diverse in terms of ethnicities, cultures and languages. Although English predominates within the healthcare system at the level of professional interactions, practitioner–patient interactions occur across a wide range of languages, and at government hospitals more often in the national language, Bahasa Malaysia. Therefore, as a learning space the clinical environment can present challenges that need to be considered. Interestingly, NUMed has found it necessary to employ its own clinical staff for bedside teaching, and these staff may have a role in mediating the language challenges for students in their interactions with patients.

In the case of MUM, a similar approach to managing clinical learning was adopted, involving both a dedicated clinical campus linked to a major public hospital in regional Malaysia and regular visits to a network of local clinics. Similar to NUMed, most clinical teaching at both hospitals and clinics is conducted by academic staff employed by the university, sometimes on a part-time basis, and staff are encouraged to maintain some involvement in provision of clinical care to patients.

In relation to patients' perceptions of doctors, Manderson and Allotey point out that 'ideas of professional competence are culturally informed' (2003: 83), and that behaviour viewed as appropriate and professional within one cultural context may be viewed quite differently in another. This may also apply to *clinicians'* perceptions and expectations of medical students, and highlights one of the challenges in addressing clinical learning within transnational programmes. That is, students are often learning within curricula derived primarily from one (usually Western) cultural context but doing much of their clinical learning within healthcare systems and cultural contexts sometimes quite different from that. As mentioned above, local teaching staff can play a key role in helping students navigate through this; to learn in ways which meet both curricula requirements and accommodate the expectations of patients and clinicians within the clinical environments in which most of their learning occurs.

Accreditation

While in theory the accreditation process for transnational medical education delivery is not markedly different from domestic accreditation processes, in fact the emphasis on ensuring quality and equivalence is often heightened. For this reason, accreditation represents not only a challenge, but an opportunity to ensure all aspects of a medical education programme meet best practice.

The MUM case study highlights the critical importance of accreditation from relevant medical councils in both the short- and longer-term viability of transnational medical education initiatives. This can significantly impact on recruitment of students, as well as on the capacity of the school to attract quality staff. It is an important 'measure' by which the credibility of the programme is gauged both locally and internationally.

The JCSMHS received accreditation from the AMC in 2008 and the MMC in 2010. It has been in negotiation with the governments of Singapore and Sri Lanka to initiate accreditation processes, due to regular intake of students from those two countries. In order to meet accreditation requirements for Australia and Malaysia, the medical school was required to demonstrate quality and equivalence across a wide range of elements, from the physical infrastructure of campuses, to the admissions processes, assessment, teaching content and provision of learning support for students. Quality and coverage of staffing to meet the breadth of the curriculum, not only in the commencing years but across the full 5 years of the degree, needed to be established and demonstrated, as did provision of processes for evaluation of programmes and staff development. The physical learning environment needed to be examined, as well as the electronic and virtual learning environments. Issues around adequate access to library and research support, as well as equivalent learning, language and pastoral support, needed to be addressed. In short, accreditation involved a comprehensive examination of the curriculum in the broadest sense, along with everything else that contributes to the total student experience of learning. This accreditation process is typically not a single event, but involves regular communication and meetings over an extended period, including visits to monitor sustainability and maintenance of standards.

Collaboration and 'positioning'

A fundamental principle underpinning the Monash University transnational venture was that, following a formative period where the Australia-based school took a leadership role, JCSMHS and the Australia-based Central Medical School would become equal partners in a shared, evolving curriculum. Importantly, an organisational structure was adopted which explicitly established the equal status of the two undergraduate medical schools in terms of governance, curriculum input and decisions on teaching and learning. As stated above, although initial communication tended to involve the Australia-based school 'mentoring' the new school in terms of teaching, learning and curriculum delivery, a gradual shift towards genuine two-way dialogue was required, and forms a fundamental requirement for sustainable transnational medical education delivery involving multiple schools and campuses in different countries.

Equivalence

Equivalence in curriculum, programmes, opportunities and support is an important concept in transnational ventures, and is often a key requirement of accreditation processes (as mentioned above). While achieving equivalence in terms of the physical learning environment is often relatively easy to demonstrate, equivalence in other areas is more complex. In particular, assessment is a crucial area where steps are required to achieve and maintain equivalence. These steps can include, for example, shared input into examination and assignment writing, shared marking, and shared involvement in blueprinting, moderation and other assessment-related processes, as outlined in the two case studies above. Other areas where equivalence is often necessary but sometimes overlooked is in the provision of pastoral and learning support tailored to meet the needs of both local and international students.

Contextualisation

In the selection and development of teaching, learning and assessment materials for use in transnational programmes contextualisation is often required. Put simply, this is because materials need to be appropriate and relevant for the location in which they are delivered, and should not disadvantage students due to factors such as assumed knowledge, unfamiliar cultural references, or contexts which are not authentic. Where teaching, learning and assessment materials (e.g. OSCE scenarios) are adapted, this may involve changing surface information such as names, locations, times and demographic information (e.g. regarding a simulated patient). However, contextualisation must also take into account differences in areas such as patient behaviour, the role of family members, healthcare resourcing, diet, gender roles, lifestyle factors, social and familial relationships, attitudes to (dis)ability, educational systems, language use, cultural norms and disease prevalence. In short, ensuring the appropriateness and relevance of teaching, learning and assessment materials through contextualisation is a complex area, often requiring rigorous trialling and a continuous cycle of improvement.

The two case studies examined above involved the establishment of full overseas branch campuses. Students complete the bulk of their studies at these, graduating with a qualification recognised as equivalent to that of students studying at the universities' main campuses located in the UK and Australia respectively. The intention is for students to graduate with a qualification that enables them to practise both in their country of study (in this case, Malaysia) and the country in which the core campus of their university is located. The two case studies that follow represent quite different models, in which students complete part of their degree in one country, and then relocate to a partner medical school (PMS) in another country for the second phase of their studies. Importantly, the curriculum delivered in Phase 1 has been developed to enable full credit transfer arrangements, and ensure an effective transition into the second phase. In the case of the International Medical University (IMU), this curriculum was developed deliberately to enable international collaboration, while in relation to the fourth case study, an existing curriculum from University of Queensland School of Medicine (UQSM) formed the basis for the institutional partnership developed with Ochsner Health System (OHS) in the USA.

Case study 20.3 The International Medical University, Kuala Lumpur, Malaysia

Victor Lim

The International Medical College (IMC) in Kuala Lumpur, Malaysia, was established in 1992. From its inception the college adopted an innovative approach to international collaboration in medical education. In this unique collaboration the IMC forged links with leading medical schools in the English-speaking world and developed a model of medical education where students spent an initial five semesters (Phase 1) in Kuala Lumpur. Upon successful completion of Phase 1 the student transfers to a partner medical school (PMS). The student would spend another 2–3 years in the PMS and graduate with the degree of the PMS. Students transferring to a graduate medical school would spend an additional intercalated year of primarily research work to qualify for the Bachelor of Medical Science (Hons).

The Phase 1 curriculum was a common curriculum developed by IMC with the assistance of leading medical educationists, including Ronald Harden and Ian Hart. This curriculum was a progressive, systems-based, integrated medical sciences course with early clinical exposure. The curriculum was not only innovative and unique in its learning–teaching methodologies; it had to be designed to a standard that is acceptable to some of the best medical schools in the world under the credit transfer arrangement. The original consortium of five schools had over the years increased to nearly 30, and these medical schools are located in the UK, Ireland, New Zealand, Canada, USA and Australia.

Early clinical exposure and the use of a skills laboratory were hallmarks of the Phase 1 curriculum at IMC. The Clinical Skills Unit established at IMC was the first of its kind in the Association of

(continued)

(continued)

Southeast Asian Nations region, and the design was based on the skills laboratories in Maastricht, the Netherlands and St Bartholomew's in London, the two major laboratories then in existence in Europe.

John S. Beck, an Emeritus Professor of Pathology from the University of Dundee, Scotland, was appointed the Foundation Dean of the IMC and Sir Patrick Forrest, Emeritus Professor of Surgery from the University of Edinburgh, Scotland, as the Associate Dean. In 1993, the IMC admitted its pioneer batch of 75 medical students.

In 1999, IMC was granted university status by the government of Malaysia and became the IMU. With this new status, the university was able to award its own degrees and the IMU Clinical School was established in Seremban to give students the option of completing the entire medical course in Malaysia. After Phase 1, the student transfers to the Clinical School and completes another five semesters to graduate with the MBBS (IMU). The IMU Clinical School admitted its first cohort of 46 students in 1999.

IMC, and later IMU, had the benefit of experienced and renowned educationists as members of its Board of Governors, an International Consultative Committee and a Professional Advisory Education Committee. An Academic Council (AC) was formed, comprising the Deans or their representatives from all the PMS. The AC functions as an external quality assurance body and meets at least once a year. This annual interaction is very useful to IMU, as during these discussions there is much exchange of new information and sharing of experience. IMU has been able to adopt many best practices as a result of this. The partnership with the many PMS enables the IMU to have access to a wide range of expertise in medical education and visiting experts from the PMS hold regular training sessions for IMU faculty in all aspects of medical and health professional education.

The IMU model for international collaboration and partnership in medical education has been highly successful. Between 1993 and 2011, a total of 2,519 students had transferred to PMS. Information was available on 1,445 students who transferred between 1993 until 2005. Of these, 1,251 (87 per cent) graduated from the PMS within the minimum possible time. Another 158 (11 per cent) completed their medical studies but required additional time. Only 36 (2 per cent) failed to graduate from the PMS. These results would indicate that there are sufficient commonalities in medical programmes worldwide for students to complete a portion of the course in one country and continue successfully with the programme in another (Chow et al. 2012).

The IMU has since launched other health programmes, including Dentistry, Pharmacy, Nursing, Nutrition and Dietetics, Medical Biotechnology, Chinese Medicine and Chiropractic. In all these programmes the university had adopted a model similar to that in medicine. Students have the option of completing the entire course in Malaysia or transferring to a partner university to complete their studies under credit transfer arrangements. In doing so, the university ensures that all its programmes are benchmarked to internationally acceptable standards.

Case study 20.4 Transnational medical education between Australia and the United States of America

David Wilkinson

In 2008 a partnership was established between the UQSM, Australia, and the OHS in New Orleans, USA, in order to establish a joint medical degree programme. The UQSM had set itself the vision to be 'Australia's Global Medical School' and in addition to a range of initiatives, including high levels of inbound and outbound student mobility, projects in developing-world settings, and a significant international medical student cohort studying in Australia, the school was keen to establish an offshore presence.

The OHS is an integrated academic health centre committed to high-quality clinical medicine, a range of teaching programmes and research. OHS was keen to develop its own medical degree, in a university partnership, building from its established affiliation agreements with local medical schools in Louisiana.

We enrolled our first students in January 2009, with a cohort of 16 students. Each cohort spends the first 2 years of the medical degree studying in Brisbane, Australia, alongside the onshore cohort of Australian and international students. The OSH cohort students then return to the USA for their clinical training. All students follow the same curriculum that is delivered in Australia, and all students sit identical exams, with quality assurance systems effective across all sites.

By 2013 the OHS cohort had grown to over 100 students entering each year, with a plan to increase the intake further to 120 each year. The first cohort has successfully graduated and all graduates have competed for, and taken up, residency programmes in the USA. These novel arrangements have been subjected to significant scrutiny by the AMC, and the arrangements are now accredited.

Students in the OHS cohort are all US citizens or permanent residents, and in addition to the normal examinations taken as part of their medical degree, they also take the United States Medical Licensing Examination (USMLE), in the same way that all US medical students do. This allows us to do some benchmarking, and to date we have seen that OHS students' scores on the USMLE match the US average for USMLE Step 1, while they exceed USMLE Step 2 average scores.

We have successfully established a novel programme of transnational medical education between the USA and Australia. The two partner organisations have invested significant time and effort into the partnership, which contributed to its initial success. Demand for places is high, and Medical College Admissions Test (MCAT) and grade point average (GPA) entry scores have been maintained. Student performance and progress within the degree programme has been positive, and success rates are as high as those experienced with the Australian and onshore international cohorts.

This arrangement is not typical, but it is innovative and has created much interest and commitment from within partner organisations. Starting with our existing curriculum it was relatively straightforward to expand the teaching programme to another site, even one very distant from the main sites. Significant effort was put into faculty development, with bilateral exchange visits occurring frequently. Deep institutional friendships have evolved and additional academic activities, focused around biomedical research opportunities, are now emerging.

Intercultural competence

Intercultural competence is now addressed within most medical education programmes; however its *broad* relevance comes into particular focus with the demands of transnational delivery. Heightened demands are placed on the intercultural awareness and competence of everyone involved, whether Deans, teaching staff, administrative staff or students. Transnational delivery highlights the absolute need for intercultural competency to be addressed (both in general and in relation to the medical context) within medical education programmes, for both staff and students, and for it to continue to be regarded as a key graduate attribute expected of all graduating medical students. It is of relevance not only in providing students with the knowledge, sensibilities and 'multiple repertoires' needed in clinical contexts, but also in facilitating engagement and learning in terms of student interactions with staff, fellow students and the curriculum itself.

Transnational education and the 'washback effect'

The process of curriculum development and renewal which accompanies transnational ventures can provide a measure of how effectively the internationalisation of curricula is occurring. The degree to which a curriculum is situated within a specific time, place and healthcare system, and the degree to which it embraces a broader global perspective, become clearer and more evident in the transnational development and delivery process. Transnational delivery has the capacity to provide students with the knowledge, skills, awareness and experience necessary for them to acquire the multiple 'repertoires' referred to at the start of this chapter. It also has the potential to impact positively on curriculum development and renewal in other ways.

The concept of 'washback' (Biggs 1996) has long been understood in medical education; it refers to the impact of assessment on what is taught and learnt (Cilliers et al. 2010). This impact can be positive or negative, influencing not only what is taught but also how it is taught. With transnational delivery a similar effect can occur in relation to the curriculum. Where genuine collaboration on curriculum development and renewal is occurring across schools and countries, the possibility becomes real of a positive washback effect, with innovative content and approaches developed as part of delivery within one medical school or at one campus informing curriculum development and delivery at the other. Such positive processes, akin to a 'washback' effect, are alluded to in both the MUM and NUMed case studies. Effectively, curriculum development and renewal at the overseas school or branch campus can positively impact on the way the curriculum is understood and delivered at other schools or campuses. Where meaningful collaborative processes have developed, this effect could be expected to occur both forward and backward. In this way transnational initiatives have the potential over time to produce richer, less static curricula, creating not only best practice, but a platform for 'next practice' (Hanlon 2007).

Conclusion

The four case studies presented in this chapter remind us that transnational medical education can take many different forms. However, what the ventures described in each case study have in common is a shared commitment to curriculum internationalisation and a belief in the value of transnational collaborations for both institutions and individuals. The anecdote which opens this chapter can serve one more purpose – to remind us that at the end of all the planning, implementation, contextualisation, accreditation and evaluation required in transnational delivery lies the fundamental imperative to equip graduates to meet the needs of an individual, often vulnerable, patient. Within an increasingly globalised world and increasingly diverse healthcare contexts, transnational delivery offers much potential to produce graduates with the necessary flexibility and versatility to manage the complex and varied needs of patients within and across healthcare systems, now and into the future.

Take-home message

- International or transnational curricula imply genuine collaborative curricular development and growth, reflecting elements from all parties involved.
- There is no blueprint, and curricula need to be designed to meet the particular needs and circumstances of teaching and learning in the local context.
- Particular attention needs to be paid to issues of staffing, language and clinical learning, accreditation, equivalence and contextualisation between the partner organisations.

- Transnational delivery requires intercultural competency and sensitivity at all levels for staff and students to work in a multitude of environments.
- Genuine collaboration and curriculum renewal offers the potential for positive 'washback' for all partner institutions in the way curricula are understood, designed and delivered.

Bibliography

Biggs, J.B. (1996) 'Assessing learning quality: Reconciling institutional, staff and educational demands', *Assessment and Evaluation in Higher Education*, 21: 5–16.

Bleakley, A., Brice, J. and Browne, J. (2008) 'Thinking the post-colonial in medical education', *Medical Education*, 42: 266–70.

Chow, J., Boohan, M., Carmichael, A., Lim, V. and Peters, S. (2012) 'The International Medical University partnership: Lessons from a 20 year programme of international medical education and workforce development', unpublished conference paper, Ottawa Conference, 9–13 March, Kuala Lumpur.

Cilliers, F.J., Schuwirth, L.W., Adendorff, H.J., Herman, N. and Van der Vleuten, C.P. (2010) 'The mechanism of impact of summative assessment on medical students' learning', *Advances in Health Sciences Education*, 15: 695–715.

General Medical Council (GMC) (2009) *Tomorrow's doctors: Outcomes and standards for undergraduate medical education*, London: GMC. Online. Available HTTP: www.gmc-uk.org/New_Doctor09_FINAL.pdf_27493417.pdf_39279971.pdf (accessed 10 June 2014).

Hanlon, V. (2007) *'Next practice' in education: A disciplined approach to innovation*, London: Innovation Unit. Online. Available HTTP: http://www.innovationunit.org/sites/default/files/Next%20Practice%20in%20Education.pdf (accessed 23 March 2015).

Hofstede, G. (1986) 'Cultural differences in teaching and learning', *International Journal of Intercultural Relations*, 10: 301–20.

Manderson, L. and Allotey, P. (2003) 'Cultural politics and clinical competence in Australian health services', *Anthropology in Medicine*, 10(1): 71–85.

21
CREATING AND SUSTAINING MEDICAL SCHOOLS FOR THE 21ST CENTURY

David Wilkinson

Medical schools must respond to a multitude of challenges if they are to remain vibrant in the 21st century.

While all medical schools have a common goal – the graduation of doctors – the settings within which this noble work occurs are highly variable, as are the needs of the communities that medical schools serve. The critical challenge for the 21st century is surely for medical schools to understand and address this apparent paradox: all schools have to do fundamentally the same thing, but often for very different reasons and hence often in very different ways.

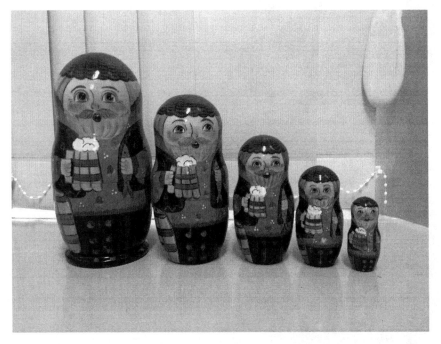

Figure 21.1 The Russian doll. (Courtesy of Cary Dick.)

A doctor is a doctor is a doctor. In other words, all doctors should graduate with a common core defined set of attributes. This does not mean that all doctors are or should be the same – far from it. Think of the *matryoshka* (Russian) doll (Figure 21.1). All doctors should look the same in terms of the smaller (inner) dolls. We might call the smallest doll the core knowledge that *all* doctors need, the second doll might be the core clinical skills that *all* doctors need, and we might call the third doll the core professional attitudes that *all* doctors need. Beyond that we might have four, five or six dolls that enhance or add to the core, and different medical schools will choose different additional dolls. One school might focus on biomedical research and focus on graduating doctors who are ready to take on further training and to become clinician scientists, while another school might have a focus on rural medicine and the development of primary care physicians, and yet another may have a preventive health and public health medicine perspective.

The key to getting this right in the 21st century is for medical schools to understand and embrace the apparent paradox, clearly define their individual mission, understand the vital importance of their social accountability and then to be able to demonstrate both the attainment of the core attributes needed by any doctor as well as the additional attributes that defines their graduates and their medical school. The case study from Southern Illinois University School of Medicine (SIUSOM) discusses the way in which they identified a set of critical clinical competencies (CCCs) that are guaranteed attributes of their graduating doctors.

**Case study 21.1   Mandatory versus curricular objective.
Do we mean it when we say it? Southern Illinois University
School of Medicine**

Debra L. Klamen

SIUSOM is a 4-year, public school of relatively small size (72 students per year) in the middle of Illinois. It has since its creation been built on a culture and expectation of innovation in medical education. The school has noted that the frequency with which major stakeholder groups call for educational reform for medical students highlights the fact that there are problems in the current system. To that end, we have begun to develop a new curriculum to address some of the problems that we see.

We believe that students need to graduate with a consistent set of clinical decision-making skills that enable them to function in residency and beyond. We are working on a new CCC curriculum. Students will have, upon graduation, the ability to diagnose and provide the initial management for 12 defined CCCs, for example abdominal pain and headache (these 12 will encompass 90 per cent of diagnoses seen in ambulatory and acute care settings). This will be achieved through longitudinal exposure to the CCCs, with active engagement in deliberate practice. Immediate feedback will be provided and there will be multiple opportunities to refine performance through repetition.

A combination of standardised patients (SPs), online interactive computer-based scenarios, demonstrations of expert clinical reasoning and direct observation will contribute to this curriculum. Every year for the first 3 years, students will learn some of the diagnoses related to the 12 CCCs, resulting in practice on all 12 of them every year. There will be annual uncued SP assessments of these clinical reasoning skills using SPs as well as clinical reasoning tools developed at SIUSOM. A senior clinical competency standardised patient examination will be given at the end of the third year. Passing levels will be pre-set at 85 per cent initially for each case (notably, most passing levels for uncued SP exams must be set at the 60–65 per cent level to avoid high levels of failure in the usual

(continued)

(continued)

curriculum). While it may seem unimpressive to guarantee 12 CCCs by graduation, since many schools have upwards of 700 graduation objectives or more (the 1976 publication by SIUSOM of graduation objectives ran to 800+ pages!), these 12 competencies are *mandatory* for all and must be achieved before graduation is permitted.

While the words 'graduation objectives' imply that all are mandatory, they are in fact, not. Indeed, the author asked seven clerkship directors at SIUSOM the following questions about their clerkship objectives:

1   Can you guarantee all students can do them all (by the end of the clerkship)?
2   Can you guarantee that *any* student can do them all?
3   Can you guarantee that 50 per cent of the objectives are done by all? (And if so, which 50 per cent?)
4   Can you guarantee that even *one* competency on the list is done by *every* student?

This led to some interesting conversations, but the consensus among all the clerkship directors was that the answer to all four of the above questions was 'No'. The guarantee that our graduates can do 12 CCCs goes from unimpressive to bold when seen in this light.

While SIUSOM is only at the very beginning of the new CCC curriculum, problems have already arisen. Breaking out of the usual two-by-two format of medical school causes those in the first 2 years to lament the loss of time for basic science, and those in the third year to resist any attempt to encroach upon 'their' siloed curricular weeks. The whole notion of guaranteeing 12 CCCs upon graduation throws up alarms in both directions: (1) Will we actually stop students from graduating? We can't do that! (2) Why are we guaranteeing only 12 CCCs? What about the other 688? Despite this, an active, and growing, number of converts to this new way of thinking is swelling the ranks of case developers. A whole host of assessment tools are being developed to enable this new curriculum (and its students) to be evaluated, and the school finds itself to be invigorated as we attempt to meet the needs of the students and patients of the 21st century.

Paradoxical medical education: medical school, medical degree, medical graduate

One definition of paradox is 'a seemingly absurd or self-contradictory statement or proposition which when investigated or explained may prove to be well founded or true' (www.oxford-dictionaries.com).

One of the great pleasures and privileges that medical deans have is to visit medical schools and medical programmes around the world. Consistently, when I do this, I hear the refrain that the school that I am visiting is 'different' from others, or at least seeks to be different. The claim of difference may apply against other schools in that region, that country or even the world. 'Our graduates are different because . . . ' or 'Our graduates are better because . . . '. And then, during the same visit I usually hear about and am shown evidence for how medical schools and medical programmes are all so very similar, and indeed, how leaders feel compelled to ensure that their school matches other schools. What is going on here?

I suggest that this apparent paradox – the urge to differentiate while also producing the same 'thing' (a doctor), and also needing to show how similar our schools are (so that we can be accredited, accepted within the medical education community and achieve some level of credibility), is a useful framework for considering the core challenge for sustainable and relevant medical education in this century. The second case study from Australia discusses some of the issues raised in trying to develop new medical schools to meet the needs of communities, one a lower-socio-economic area, and the other rural and remote.

Case study 21.2   A tale of two medical schools in Australia

Ian Wilson

Coming from a medical school that had existed for almost 125 years to a greenfield site as the second academic appointment of a new School of Medicine was exciting.

I was appointed as the Head of Medical Education and my role was to develop and implement the medical curriculum. A number of decisions had been made before I arrived. The school was to be situated in a lower-socio-economic area and was to produce doctors capable of working in such areas. In order to maximise the intake of students from the local region it was to be a school-leaver programme and there would not be any subject prerequisites. Combined with a small reduction in the required matriculation ranking, these decisions were designed to overcome the academic under-performance seen in lower-socio-economic areas. It had also been decided that we would purchase an existing curriculum that covered the first 2 years of our programme.

This left a number of large undertakings:

1. rewriting the curriculum for the first 2 years, based on a curriculum that covered 30 months. The problem-based learning (PBL) tutorials needed rewriting in the context of a different setting;
2. developing a selection process that reflected the aims of the programme;
3. hiring and training staff to work in a PBL environment;
4. keeping the accrediting body appraised of and happy with our developments;
5. developing and implementing our assessment processes and policies;
6. developing the clinical attachments and undertaking difficult negotiations with other medical schools that saw the new school as an interloper;
7. developing a strong relationship with the central university to ensure the medical school was developed as a modern school, meeting accreditation requirements.

None of these was particularly easy and each required developing a project team to have a clear picture of what we needed and give attention to detail. The leadership group had to maintain a detailed knowledge of the developments so that the programme had some level of integration. The highlights for me were developing a selection process that meant we took 55–60 per cent of our intake from the local region; a programme of recruitment and support for Indigenous medical students; developing a programme so that each of our students would undertake a 5-week attachment in an Indigenous health facility; and receiving very positive feedback about the quality of our graduates.

After the first graduation I took up a position in another new medical school. This had started at the same time as the school mentioned above. However it was quite different, with graduate entry to a programme with a regional, rural and remote focus. It had a number of exciting innovations, including a 12-month longitudinal integrated curriculum based in rural and regional communities.

With good reports as to the quality of the graduates and with an intake of around 70 per cent of students with a rural and regional origin, and with over 50 per cent of graduates undertaking

(continued)

> *(continued)*
>
> their internship in rural or regional settings, the programme was running well. This programme, like most, if not all, new schools, suffered from problems of integration. Each of the years or phases was developed by a different team. While there were common team members, particularly among the senior staff, the pragmatic decisions required to get the programme up and running on short deadlines meant that the transitions are not always as smooth as they could be. This integration of the programme is now well under way. The second issue that affects most new schools is that as the initial excitement dies down more attention needs to be paid to the retention of the non-salaried teaching staff and the maintenance of effective relationships.
>
> This case study has concentrated on the educational aspects of starting a new school. It is obvious from the above that a new medical school needs a strong medical education team to develop and implement the programme. A school also needs a strong leadership team with a common, well-articulated vision of what the school will achieve. The leadership team requires the support of the central university. This leadership requires an integrated vision of the programme, the graduates, the research and the administration.

Clarity of language

In considering this issue we need to be clear about the language that we use. We risk confusion and uncertainty otherwise. The one consistent term that we can all use is a 'medical degree'; the period of study that leads to graduation as a doctor. Many universities and medical schools use the term 'medical course' to describe the entire period of study, while others use the term 'medical programme' for the same purpose. And, often times we will substitute 'medical school' for 'medical course' or 'medical programme'. Most medical schools, but not all, are part of larger universities, and the organisational structures of medical schools within the parent universities are highly variable. Some schools are part of health science faculties, some are more stand-alone or independent, and others are more closely affiliated with a hospital or health system than a university. Some medical programmes or courses are delivered without a medical school *per se*, and are part of (for example) a health sciences faculty.

This organisational context is very important because there are very different structures and processes that lead to an (apparently) consistent output – the doctor. Furthermore, these organisational realities can help frame and define a school's mission. For example, schools located within very highly ranked research-intensive universities need to think very clearly about what their mission really is. These schools have the opportunity to consider making explicit use of this research-intensive environment. New medical schools have an exciting opportunity: they can define their mission from the outset, and indeed, often their establishment will be explicitly mission-driven, and in a highly specific way. The Australian case study highlights some of the advantages and disadvantages of developing programmes in new medical schools. Long-established schools may find it more difficult to review, revise and refine their mission, but accreditors are increasingly interested in these matters.

These issues matter in the 21st century, for both new and established schools.

What the 21st century demands of doctors

There are three major themes around which the debate about what we need from medical graduates today can occur:

- theme 1: 'the same as we have always needed';
- theme 2: 'new-technology doctors';
- theme 3: 'it depends where you are'.

Irrespective of which century, or which part of the world, we are in, the core attributes that we need of our graduates are timeless. These include the ability to take a history, perform a physical examination, communicate effectively with patients and colleagues, establish a differential diagnosis and develop a management plan. In addition doctors have always enjoyed a key leadership role within the delivery of healthcare, and while this has evolved recently, with an appropriately greater emphasis on team-based care, doctors still hold positions of authority and leadership, and this will continue.

However, especially in the developed world, medicine is changing very rapidly indeed. The explosion in medical knowledge, the remarkable developments in biology, biotechnology, genetics and biomedical sciences more generally, together with extraordinary developments in medical imaging technologies, mean that for many doctors, especially in the more developed parts of the world, deep understanding of the science that underpins medicine is increasingly important. These 'new-technology doctors' will also be more adept at using computers, interrogating and using big datasets, and many will be key developers of new technologies and their applications, often working in partnerships with engineers and IT specialists, for example.

But, the new-technology doctors are not necessarily relevant to the millions of people in the still developing parts of the world where clean water, sanitation, immunisation, primary healthcare and access to a suite of hospital services are the factors that drive human health. Context therefore is critical, and, I argue, this is why now (more than ever, perhaps) each medical school needs to decide what its mission is. The third case study from Canada highlights the ways in which local contextual issues of a regional maldistribution of doctors led to universities investigating ways to improve provision in underserved areas.

Case study 21.3   Developing a distributed model of medical education to help meet the healthcare needs of the population of British Columbia, Canada

David Snadden

Faced with a projected shortage of physicians and a poor distribution of physicians outside of main urban centres in British Columbia (BC), Canada, the Faculty of Medicine at the University of British Columbia (UBC), the provincial government and partner universities worked together not only to double the number of medical school places each year, but to find ways of distributing medical education to underserved areas. While there are examples in the literature of medical schools that had set up regional campuses, these were often for 1 or 2 years of the curriculum. In BC, the model developed was to distribute all 4 years of the medical curriculum in partnership with regional universities and to connect students and postgraduate residents by audiovisual technology (Snadden and Bates 2005).

Two campuses were created, one in partnership with the University of Northern British Columbia, 800 km north of Vancouver, and one in partnership with the University of Victoria on Vancouver Island.

(continued)

(continued)
New facilities were built at the partner universities to accommodate the needs of pre-clinical education, and clinical education facilities were created at the local hospitals in partnership with the health authorities. The annual class intake was planned to increase from 128 to 256, with the distributed campuses initially taking 24 students and increasing this to 32 after 3 years. The same admissions processes and criteria were used for all sites, but the northern site used an additional rural suitability score to identify students most likely to succeed in a northern Canadian environment.

At the time of admission students rank their site preferences. All students spend their first semester in Vancouver and then move to their distributed site for the rest of their education. All students follow the same curriculum and sit the same exams. The curriculum is centred on small-group learning, with some didactic lectures. All lectures and labs are connected by audiovisual technology and for lectures one instructor is generally used for the whole class. A lot of material is available through the Faculty of Medicine online learning system and all histology is delivered through digitised images. Clinical education is widely distributed throughout BC using major teaching hospitals, regional and community hospitals and family practice settings. There are several integrated clerkship sites in small communities (Worley et al. 2000) that students compete to go to. Postgraduate residency training places were also increased, and distributed within the limits of residency rotation requirements.

All sites have recruited local physicians to become teachers, developed research programmes and worked with hospitals and health authorities to create academic environments. The degree of cultural change in 10 years has been significant.

In 2010 a third distributed campus in the interior of BC, the Southern Medical Program, was established at the University of British Columbia Okanagan Campus, adding a further 32 places to the medical school intake. A planned increase of residency position, primarily in family practice, has been established to ensure the number of available residency positions matches the numbers of graduating students.

Building distributed campuses takes considerable planning, effort and commitment from many partners, including university faculty, government, health authorities and communities (Snadden et al. 2011). A major initial concern was whether a rapid distribution would maintain the quality of the graduates. Student performance, therefore, across all sites was evaluated rigorously and there was found to be no difference in academic performance, or in success rates in the Canadian National Residency Match, and while each campus has its own unique culture and 'flavour', the educational outcomes are comparable. There is a difference in the types of residency positions chosen by students from different sites, and more students from the distributed sites choose family practice as their first-choice career. The early outcomes of the programme show that students are entering practice in rural areas of BC more frequently than prior to the expansion of the medical school. In addition physician numbers increased significantly at the underserved northern site in advance of students graduating from the programme as the opportunity to engage with medical education and research has been attracting physicians to the area.

Governance throughout the system is a collaborative endeavour with all sites working together, and with leadership distributed around the province. We found it important to continue to maintain and build relationships across the programmes by ensuring face-to-face as well as remotely connected meetings, and by ensuring participation in major governance meetings by all of our sites. We also found we had to revisit and reinforce the reasons for distribution and the values surrounding it as new people came into the system, both internal to the Faculty of Medicine and externally in our partner organisations, who did not have institutional memory.

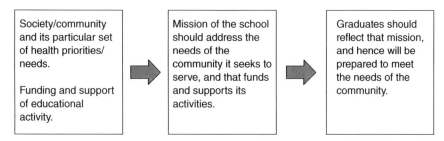

Figure 21.2 A simple model linking societal needs to medical school outcomes.

Medical schools, medical graduates and a mission for the 21st century

Each school needs to appreciate that its graduates must all look the same at the core: that is, all doctors must be able to demonstrate that they have the core attributes that are expected of them by society. However, all schools also need to be clear about what it is, in their mission, that makes them different. Not different simply for the sake of being different but different for the sake of being socially accountable (see the Australian and Canadian case studies).

Some medical schools have a very focused mission, seeking to train doctors for a clearly defined geography or social need. Geographical need is perhaps the easiest to see and appreciate, and so schools in parts of sub-Saharan Africa, for example, will typically have a mission that is focused on producing doctors ready to work in that setting, and hence graduates will be especially knowledgeable about the diseases in their area, and the technologies available to them. Some of the attributes needed of graduates from these schools are identical to, while other attributes are different from, graduates of schools in (for example) highly developed societies.

There is no suggestion here of difference in quality, value or importance; on the contrary this is all about difference in need.

A simple framework is shown in Figure 21.2.

Linking mission with social accountability, with curriculum

There has recently been a renewed and enhanced interest in the issue of social accountability of medical schools and medical education. One critically important focus operating at the global level has been the Global Consensus for Social Accountability of Medical Schools (GCSAMS), supported by the World Health Organization, and the World Federation for Medical Education, amongst others, and with input from 130 individuals and organisations (GCSAMS 2010: 1).

Twenty-first-century medical schools, whether they be new or established, should not see the Global Consensus statement as being restrictive or threatening. Rather it is a guide, and should be used within context, as a catalyst, a reframing of priorities. The statement provides an opportunity for schools to rethink their purpose, and to articulate this clearly and formally within their mission. Then, once the mission has been determined, work can begin on becoming clear on how the curriculum delivers upon the mission.

So, the challenge we all face is the clarity and specificity around the linkage between mission, social accountability and curriculum or programme/course structure. For example, in Australia over the last 10–15 years there has been a major investment in infrastructure to support distributed, rural medical education. About one-third of the Australian population lives in rural and remote settings, with many of these (often very small) communities facing severe medical workforce shortages. As part of the response to this workforce shortage, governments have invested heavily in developing an academic network of rurally based University Departments of Rural Health and Rural Clinical Schools, with large numbers of Australian medical students spending at least 1 year studying medicine in these settings. Thus, the issue of social accountability with a rural perspective has become embedded in the mission of many Australian medical schools. Curriculum has changed so that rural health issues are addressed in a deliberate and systematic manner, and course or programme structure has been changed to accommodate this. Common across Australia, 25 per cent of all Australian students in our cohort are required to spend at least half of their clinical training time (one of the two clinical training years in our case) in a rural or remote setting; and all Australian students do at least one 8-week term in a rural setting.

Similarly, at a sectoral level, all medical deans in Australia and New Zealand commit to a range of initiatives that focus on the enhancement of the health of Indigenous peoples in our two countries. These initiatives include recruitment of Indigenous students through special access schemes, a focused Indigenous health curriculum and placements in Indigenous health services. These expectations have even become enshrined in our accreditation standards. Some schools choose to develop a deep focus in this area, making their mission even more focused on this key aspect of social accountability, and they then make further adjustments to curriculum to accommodate this. A diversity of focus, interest and expertise is thereby developed, while at the same time all schools meet an agreed standard.

Social accountability need not always relate to areas of absolute or of relative disadvantage. Some schools make a deliberate choice to focus on, for example, medical research and the development of future doctors who will work in academic health centres, and as part of research teams. This is equally legitimate. Other schools have been established to meet the needs of a specific geographic location, even within a rich country such as the USA.

The point to be made though is that the challenge for all of us still relates to understanding our social accountability (whatever form it takes), linking it to our school's mission and then designing our curriculum to deliver on the mission.

Defining and documenting outcomes and attributes

I argue that in the 21st century medical schools have an absolute, non-negotiable responsibility to demonstrate to society that our graduates have met a defined standard. Not all of us do this currently; indeed, practice around the world is highly variable.

In Australia, for example, all medical schools design and deliver their own exams and students graduate based upon their performance on these exams. We have a very rigorous accreditation system, but we do not have a national licensing exam, and there is limited collaboration between schools in terms of assessment. There is no systematic programme of external examiners as part of internal assessment. Hence there is no opportunity for schools or students to confirm attainment of a specific standard. In the USA there is a medical licensing exam that all doctors must take (and pass) if they wish to practise medicine in the USA; this suite of assessments occurs through medical school and into medical practice training. Medical schools in the UK are well down a track of formal collaboration where they are all sharing exam questions and using common questions as part of their internal exams. Other countries are also using, or planning, similar approaches.

Schools need to consider how best to demonstrate and document, to their various constituencies, that their graduates do meet a defined standard. There are many ways to do this, but simply asserting that their own internal exams are proof is no longer acceptable.

Demonstrating the non-core attributes that may be more explicitly linked to social accountability and mission may be harder to do. Quantitative assessment and documentation (exams) may work for some schools and some attributes. In other cases, a more qualitative evaluation may be more appropriate. A new initiative led by the Association for Medical Education in Europe (AMEE), called ASPIRE (www.aspire-to-excellence.org), has been established in order to identify and recognise excellence in medical education. Prior to ASPIRE, there was no mechanism for this to occur. One of the three areas of focus that ASPIRE chose to be part of its launch is 'social accountability'. Effectively, ASPIRE has set the standards expected of medical schools who wish to demonstrate excellence in their practice of social accountability. Hence, schools that are successful in achieving recognition through ASPIRE can legitimately demonstrate (and not simply assert) achievement.

Medical schools are important. They are highly visible, and their many constituents (funders, owners, staff, students, alumni and the communities that they serve) often feel a deep sense of connection. The fundamental challenge for new and established medical schools now is to rethink and refine their mission, having thought about their responsibility in terms of social accountability, and then to go on and design their curricula appropriately and to demonstrate how their graduates have met the desired attributes.

This is not a call for wholesale change. As articulated by the Global Consensus, this is an opportunity for the 21st century and it is a responsibility. If we focus on what our noble purpose really is – the graduation of doctors fit to serve society – the rest will follow.

Take-home messages

- There is a set of core knowledge, skills and attitudes that all doctors should graduate with. Beyond this, knowledge and skills should vary according to a range of differing priorities and issues.
- Differing priorities and issues will reflect the local circumstances of the medical school and its social, economic and geographic context.
- The social accountability of medical schools is of vital importance, and should be considered in the framing of their mission and curriculum.
- In the 21st century, technology has had a major impact on medical knowledge and practice in the developed world, but is of less relevance where fundamental health needs are not yet met.
- Outwith contextual differences, all 21st-century medical schools have a responsibility to demonstrate that graduates meet a defined, universal standard.

Bibliography

Global Consensus for Social Accountability of Medical Schools (2010) *The consensus document*. Online. Available HTTP: www.healthsocialaccountability.org (accessed 30 June 2014).

Snadden, D. and Bates, J. (2005) 'Expanding undergraduate medical education in British Columbia: A distributed campus model', *Canadian Medical Association Journal*, 173(6): 589–90.

Snadden, D., Bates, J., Burns, P., Casiro, O., Hays, R., Hunt, D. and Towle, A. (2011) 'Developing a medical school: Expansion of medical student capacity in new locations: AMEE guide no. 55', *Medical Teacher*, 33(7): 518–29.

Worley, P., Silagy, C., Prideaux, D., Newble, D. and Jones, A. (2000) 'The parallel rural community curriculum: An integrated clinical curriculum based in rural general practice', *Medical Education*, 34(7): 558–65.

22
RECOGNISING LEADERSHIP AND MANAGEMENT WITHIN THE MEDICAL SCHOOL

Khalid A. Bin Abdulrahman and Trevor Gibbs

Over the past two decades there have been significant changes in the organisational structure within medical schools around the globe.

Effective leadership and management are considered essential for the development and sustainability of an effective organisation (Long 2011). Today's medical schools are complex, adaptive organisations (Glouberman and Zimmerman 2002) that are measured on their effectiveness at fulfilling multiple functions: creating world-class healthcare practitioners; employing and developing world-class faculty; demonstrating expertise in research, teaching and service; maintaining a national and international perspective; and having to succeed in creating a financially stable and increasingly unique and recognised institution.

A successful school fulfils its mission through leadership and management, together. Without leadership, medical schools fail to keep pace with changing circumstances, and fail to produce graduates with the capacity to provide high-standard healthcare for the 21st century (Boelen et al. 2013). Large amounts of money are spent developing world-class medical schools that aspire to produce world-class health practitioners. The responsibility for this is placed firmly in the hands of the leaders of the school, who through leadership seek to satisfy this aspiration. However, the path to success is not an easy one and the concept and development of leadership are fraught with difficult challenges. For too many years there has been a barrier between 'the clinicians' and the organisational leadership. A lack of leadership training, a disjointed career structure and a wide differential in financial remuneration created barriers for clinicians and academics seeking to become involved with, and to assume responsibility for, leadership within the institution. The emergence of health managers, particularly in the UK, Europe and the USA, has disincentivised clinicians from becoming managers (Hamilton et al. 2008), while some of the 'blame catastrophes' occurring in certain hospitals have driven clinicians away from taking leadership roles (Department of Health 2002). Given the symbiotic relationship between clinicians, health services and medical schools, it is inevitable that reluctance to take on a leadership role has also pervaded the medical school. For many, leadership still remains a rather nebulous and ill-structured concept, probably related, in part, to its variability in definition, its overlap with the concepts of leader and management, and its necessary dynamic quality, suggesting that leadership continuously needs to be adaptive to changing and variable circumstances. If medical schools are to move forward, this confused state around the subject of leadership and management needs clarification, while at the same time recognising that there are specific roles for those with responsibility to support this move. The emergence of 'adaptive leadership' addresses many of these concerns (Heifetz et al. 2009; Thygeson et al. 2010).

This first part of the present chapter will use three commonly heard statements to distinguish between the terms leadership, management and leaders, while the second half will use three cases drawn from specific medical schools to illustrate how the qualities of each can effectively promote conditions that can deliver a quality product.

The what and why of leadership

The following quotations, taken from years of experience in medical education, go some way to support the lack of clarity between the three terms.

- 'I was appointed as a leader and therefore I already must have leadership skills.'
- 'Leaders are born leaders and therefore leadership cannot be taught.'
- 'I only manage programmes and therefore I do not need leadership skills.'

Leadership is frequently quoted as an essential skill required of anyone who takes responsibility for developing an educational institution, and in relation to this chapter, a medical school. However, it is difficult to argue against the similar presence of effective management and leaders in the development of that same institution. If we are to agree with Jonas and colleagues (2011) in their paper describing the importance of clinical leadership within the UK National Health Service (NHS), leadership is vital to the success of healthcare organisations, bringing quality, cost-effectiveness, change management and direction, and it is a quality that should pervade the whole organisation. They consider that these markers of effective leadership translate to all organisations that desire to succeed in a competitive world. Medical schools are employers and as such the effective management of their workforce is essential. We also attest to the importance of medical school leaders in their specific fields; indeed, most medical schools rely on specific specialty leaders to generate research income and to bring national and international status to the school.

Hence, it appears that we have three interchangeable terms, frequently used incorrectly due to a lack of clarity in their definitions and applications.

According to Kotter (1990), management is a relatively recent concept. He suggests that it has risen to prominence only within the last 100 years in response to the development of large complex organisations such as the railroad systems and the automotive industries. Management involves a series of processes, categorised into three groups: planning and budgeting; organising and staffing; and controlling and problem solving. Kotter states that leadership is different, it 'does not produce consistency and order . . . it produces movement' (1990: 4).

> Strong managers produce predictability and order, but leadership involves creation, communication and implements visions of the future which enable companies to change themselves in a changing competitive marketplace.
>
> *(Kotter 1990: 4)*

In describing the ten roles of an effective manager, Mintzberg (1990) gave importance to the role of being a leader, by which he meant the setting of goals and assessing employee performance as well as mentoring, training and motivating employees.

More recently, the work of Heifetz (1994) has been influential in clarifying our understanding between management and leadership and has introduced an educational element into our definitions. Heifetz redefines leadership as 'an activity rather than a position of influence or a set of personal characteristics' (1994: 20). He proposes that we discard our ideas that 'leaders are born and not made' and that leadership becomes a learned quality, the teaching of which relates to learning how to help others to close the gap between solving technical problems (managerial skills) and problems arising in a complex, changing world in which the interdependence of environmental, societal and cultural factors is both part of the problem and the solution. Heifetz describes these latter factors as 'adaptive' and effective leadership as involving learning how to recognise the conditions that promote their emergence and how to help people address the challenges they face as they seek to resolve problems. Heifetz considered leadership as the capacity to adapt, to learn, to change, to narrow the gap between the past and the developing present, by creating energy, resources and ingenuity to change the circumstances.

'I was appointed as a leader and therefore I already must have leadership skills'

From the seminal discussions of Kotter, Mintzberg and Heifetz, we can deduce that there are plenty of leaders who hold assigned positions yet lack leadership skills and there are plenty of people who are not formal leaders that show leadership skills. It is possible to be a leader yet fail to demonstrate leadership skills and at the same time possible to demonstrate leadership skills without a formal (structural) leadership position; leaders and leadership are not the same thing. The *Oxford English Dictionary* (2012) defines a leader as 'a person who leads or commands a group, an organisation or a country'; taking that further, a person who takes the lead, an expert within his field or someone who is at the top of her profession. Leaders usually lead by example, from the front or the top of the hierarchy, and expect others to follow, frequently without discussion or group agreement.

Taylor and colleagues (2008) characterise effective leaders in academia as those who can identify with specific areas of academic or health professionals practice and 'take the lead' in developing themselves and taking others with them. Counter to that, leadership is a much more complicated concept and, for some, considered to be a collection of attributes. Bland and colleagues (1999) were some of the first to describe leadership as a collection of qualities when they presented a study of the leadership skills related to a successful university–community partnership. Their description of leadership included envisioning, collaboration, cooperation, communication, valuing systems and being able to set achievable goals. However, we have to understand in their study that they were looking at the subject through a more static or normative process, similar to the description of leadership provided by Lieff and Albert (2010, 2012). In their studies they divided best leadership practice into four domains of skill:

1 intrapersonal (role modelling, communication, envisioning);
2 interpersonal (valuing relationships, supportive, cooperative, collaborative);
3 organisational (facilitating change, having both a personal and shared vision, management of people and time);
4 systematic (organisational understanding, political awareness, societal need).

McKimm (2004), in her study of educational leaders, added other important qualities in the form of strategic and analytical thinking skills, personal development, self-awareness, risk taking, tolerance to uncertainty, and professional and contextual awareness.

It was Heifetz, though, who felt that these qualities were more qualities of a leader and leadership was something very different – 'adaptive work' (Heifetz 1994; Heifetz et al. 2009):

Adaptive work consists of the learning required to address conflicts in the values people hold, or to diminish the gap between the values people stand for and the reality they face. Adaptive work requires a change in values, beliefs or behaviour.

(Heifetz 1994: 22)

Adaptive work requires learning. The tasks of leadership consist of choreographing and directing the learning process in the organisation, institution or group. Leadership with or without authority requires an educative strategy.

'Leaders are born leaders and therefore leadership cannot be taught'

Leadership is about knowing yourself and understanding others (Held and McKimm 2011) and in a complex environment the skills required for effective leadership are not inherent within the individual, nor do they come naturally. They need to be learned, understood and supported by theory; they need to be developed and evaluated. Those showing effective leadership also need to adapt to the ever-changing world of education and healthcare – i.e., show adaptive leadership (Heifetz and Linsky 2004). Medical and healthcare education in medical schools is complex (Sweeney and Griffiths 2002; Mennin 2013). Leadership within this complex environment requires careful and iterative navigation to learn about new policies, new strategies, financial and political systems and professional regulations. These are certainly not inherent in an individual – effective leadership has to be learned and practised.

Readers taking an interest in leadership will learn that there are many theories and models that underpin leadership. Describing all of these is beyond the scope of this chapter, but for more information, readers are directed to the relevant chapter by McKimm and Lieff in the 2013 book *A Practical Guide for Medical Teachers*.

'I only manage programmes and therefore I do not need leadership skills'

The managers in medical schools are those individuals who are usually tasked to specific activities; to lead because of their academic or clinical experience or expertise. This has held true for many years. However, as medical education develops and medical curricula become more complex with competency-based education, integrated, community-based and interprofessional learning, electronic learning platforms and new methods of assessment, the managerial tasks themselves also become more complex. Northouse (2004) in describing leadership considered that managers produce order and consistency, while leadership is about producing change, direction and movement. John Kotter (1999) identified the need for two distinct and complementary systems to deal with the complexity of institutions; he called for both management and leadership, with leadership being a learned skill that complements management. He based this upon his observation that many institutions were indeed over-managed – too many people making decisions but not in a coherent or purposeful direction, eventually leading to fragmentation and ineffective learning. Leadership provides the vision for change that leads the institution in a coherent direction for learning and working together. However, in reality, it is more appropriate that they both blend into one another – the manager assuming more leadership skills, whilst leadership *per se* envelops being a manager, depending on the situation. Charles Handy (1993) draws a relevant analogy in his work describing organisations. He likens a manager to a general practitioner (GP) dealing with a patient – the first point of call for a problem that requires an answer. In doing that the GP uses four basic actions:

1   symptom identification;
2   diagnosis;
3   decision regarding appropriate management;
4   management of the patient.

Leadership at a college or regulating body level provides direction and vision. Much has changed from the date of this analogy. The workings within a 21st-century healthcare system often place more responsibility on the manager, in terms of responsibility and accountability, and they tend towards a manager also requiring leadership skills.

From theory to practice

So far this chapter has discussed the concept of leadership, management and leaders as individual concepts that in the complex worlds of healthcare and medical schools frequently overlap in definition and roles. Theory is of limited relevance without practice. Now we turn to examples of some of those definitions and theories in practice through three different models of leadership and management from three medical schools.

Case study 22.1   Recognising leadership, management and other responsibilities within the medical school – an example from Pakistan

Rukhsana W. Zuberi and Farhat Abbas

Aga Khan University (AKU), Pakistan, is a renowned, internationally recognised private academic institution. The Medical College admits 100 students per year in a 5-year curriculum. The Curriculum Committee (CC), the responsible academic body for undergraduate medical education (UGME), reports directly to the Dean. The curriculum has been systems-based from its inception, with department heads and students as UGME-CC members.

Organisational structure within AKU Medical College

A curriculum review by the Department for Educational Development (DED) in 1999 recommended an integrated, outcome-based curriculum. As the curricular framework developed, the curriculum management structures were aligned to it in order to sustain the change. In 2002, the Mintzberg strategy for planning and management was instituted with the renewed curriculum (Mintzberg 1992, 2009). Decision-making power became centralised in the UGME-CC. Through its subcommittees for the different phases and elements of the curriculum, authority was devolved to those responsible for curricular planning, delivering and monitoring.

Curriculum committee

The UGME-CC chair held a Masters in Health Professions Education (MHPE – Maastricht University) qualification. The two co-chairs represented basic and clinical sciences. Multidisciplinary teams were organised to plan, coordinate, implement and evaluate the longitudinal themes, which cut across all 5 years of the curriculum. These coordinators had access to all Year Committees and were members of the

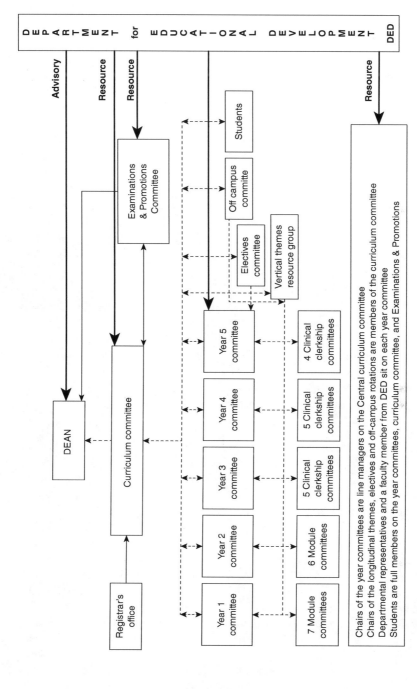

Figure 22.1 Leadership and management of the undergraduate medical curriculum, Aga Khan University Medical College.

(continued)

> *(continued)*
>
> CC. There were two student members on UGME-CC: one from Year 1 or 2 and one from Year 5. There was a student member on each Year Committee. A curriculum office with its own budget was created.
>
> ### *Examinations and Promotions Committee*
>
> AKU is accountable to society and its community for the quality of its medical graduates. The Examinations and Promotions (E&P) Committee is chaired by a faculty member with demonstrated interest in medical education. Membership includes four faculty members, with no responsibility towards any phase of the curriculum, and two Year-5 students. All student members on all educational committees are full members and are elected by the students.
>
> ### *Cross-representation*
>
> To ensure cross-representation, the chair of the UGME-CC is a member of the E&P Committee and vice versa. The Associate Dean of Education (also chair of the DED) and the Senior Associate Registrar are members of both the UGME-CC and the E&P Committee.
>
> The DED is responsible for the philosophical underpinnings of educational programmes and for all examinations. It focuses on improving curricula, pedagogy, use of e-learning, web-based resources and assessments. The DED leads self-studies for programme evaluations. All DED faculty members have or are in the process of acquiring a Masters or PhD in Health Professions Education (HPE). The DED has membership on all Year Committees, the UGME-CC and the E&P Committee (Figure 22.1).
>
> Faculty members aspiring towards careers in medical education were recruited for joint appointments between the DED and other clinical/basic science departments as educational coordinators. They facilitate the implementation of educational principles, philosophies and policies in the other departments and assure quality.
>
> The DED offers a 5-day Introductory Short Course in Health Professions Education mandatory for all new, incoming faculty members. It offers retreats, workshops and courses and has recently initiated a Master's degree in HPE for developing researchers and leaders. It is a resource in medical education for other national institutions as needed.
>
> (Acknowledgements to Dr Zoon Naqvi, Dr Rashida Ahmed and the late Dr Robert Maudsley.)

What can be learned from the Aga Kahn case study?

- Initially, the curricular review by the DED recommended an integrated outcome-based curriculum. Before work began they decided upon a recognised theory of organisational management; they demonstrated leadership through vision and organisational skills by adopting a valid and well-tested approach to organisation management – the Mintzberg matrix of organisational management.
- Although major decision-making power became centralised in the UGME-CC, there was a planned devolution of tasks to appointed subcommittees and named individuals – collaboration and cooperation.
- New skills required in modern medical education were agreed – the UGME-CC chair already had a recognisable higher qualification and there was support for others to follow, supporting the workforce.

- A multidisciplinary team approach was instituted, creating equity, cooperation and coordination.
- There appeared to be a shared understanding of the curriculum, achieved through a defined organisational structure, enhanced through integration and equal access to all elements of the curriculum – effective communication skills.
- Student engagement in the process and social awareness ensured a cooperative and shared process.
- There was a willingness to share educational skills within society through educational courses.
- Creating a separate budget for the curriculum office allowed financial flexibility, but also delegated responsibility.
- The level playing field that appears to exist in the managerial structure supports both a top-down and a bottom-up approach, where all involved are allowed a say and shared vision within the curriculum.
- The DED is positioned to recognise and respond to the need for change – an important issue in the changing world of medical education.
- The whole process was structured around need: the need in 1999 for curricula renewal in the medical school, set within a specific environment using modern methods of medical education.

Case study 22.2   Starting a new medical school in Southern Africa – University of Namibia Medical School

Jonas Nordquist

Namibia and the lack of health professionals

The World Health Organization (WHO) demonstrated, in its 2006 *World Health Report*, the urgent need to train health professionals in all parts of the world, and this was specifically critical in Africa (WHO 2006). This case addresses the leadership challenges when starting a new medical school in Namibia, a country previously dependent upon graduates from other countries and whose indigenous students frequently failed to return to their mother country.

Namibia is a middle-income country in Southern Africa with a population of approximately 2.3 million. Human immunodeficiency virus (HIV)/acquired immunodeficiency syndrome (AIDS), tuberculosis and other infectious diseases threaten the population, as well as its economic development.

In a national comprehensive vision from 2004 (*Namibia Vision 2030*: Republic of Namibia 2004), a number of actions were identified to improve the health system and health education. Focus was needed on training medical and paramedical personnel, with a focus on rural and community health and the prevention of HIV/AIDS. Primary care was highlighted as a priority area.

The birth of the first Namibian School of Medicine

In 2009, a five-person taskforce of national and international members was appointed with the mission of designing a new medical school in only 5 months, with content, curricula, admission, recruitment of staff, and the design of the new infrastructure all being addressed. In parallel, the recruitment of faculty and students was organised at a central level within the University of Namibia – in effect, three parallel processes conducted by two separate groups.

(continued)

(continued)

One of the central challenges was to select an appropriate curriculum model. Due to the short time span, familiarity with the systems and similar pattern of diseases, the taskforce looked into curricular models in the region. A 5-year undergraduate curriculum, mainly based on the classical pre-clinical and clinical Flexnerian model, was chosen, but with a strong emphasis on active learning.

The school officially opened in August 2010, admitting 59 out of 750 applicants. Even though the infrastructure was not yet completed at that time, a lot of emphasis was placed on designing a new medical school where the physical infrastructure would align with the curriculum and also reflect the underlying values of the new school (Nordquist and Sundberg 2013): a vibrant, inviting and dynamic place, where colours and materials should be Namibian and mirror the needs of Namibia. The buildings had also to be designed for hybrid curricula, with small tutorial rooms, labs, lecture theatres, IT suites and seminar rooms. Health professionals in fields other than medicine (pharmacy, dentistry and physiotherapy) will in the future also be graduating from new schools developed and developing within the university.

Planning is crucial and must be given more time than just a few months, but, in this case, the political urgency to start a new medical school made this impossible. The relationship with and expectations of the Ministries of Health and Ministries of Education concerning universities is an interesting and sometimes delicate political issue. There is also a need to create alignment between different planning processes, and taskforce members should ideally represent different disciplines and stakeholder interests; in particular, it is of great importance to include clinicians and the potential providers of clinical rotations into this process at a very early stage. Another important lesson is to develop a local vision of the enterprise of a new medical school that can guide all the different taskforces and groups involved in setting up the new medical school. There is an obvious risk that many decisions otherwise will be based on different mental models that have not been made explicit. If there are different groups involved (as in this case), one might run into a situation where different groups have different mental models or ideas about the new medical school. This is not productive and leads to miscommunication. Mistakes and such miscommunication can be avoided if local visions are created and expressed by groups involved. Many decisions might also be made on technical grounds, with no alignment with the overall vision of the new medical school. If possible, local visions (if they are properly developed) should strive for alignment with other national and international strategies.

The curricula developed have to honour the local needs, both in terms of content and its implementation. Everything has to be localised – a simple copy-and-paste strategy doesn't work. Also, the physical design of a new medical school is a strategic decision and has to align with the ideas behind the curricula. The development of the new medical school in Namibia demonstrates this.

What important features can be learned from the University of Namibia case study?

- This case study differentiates the roles and responsibilities of leader, leadership and management.
- The political leaders decided on the development of an urgently needed medical school – a poorly thought-out but socially necessary activity.
- Leadership was sought by the selection of national and international experts within their field.
- Leadership skills in planning, discussion and communication with the political leaders overcame the initial barriers.

- Compromise was made in adopting a more traditional yet achievable curriculum, rather than reaching for unobtainable heights in curriculum design.
- Inclusivity was a feature of early discussions, with early involvement of all those connected with the curriculum.
- Parallel processing of essential activities, associated with delegation and responsibility of tasks, reduced the time factor to completion, appointing managers with designated roles and delegated responsibilities.
- The leadership had a particular vision of the medical school which encapsulated the needs of the students, faculty and society in planning the school.
- Expertise in design matched the curriculum style, the students and national and local needs, even to the level of using the national Namibian colours, all achieved through vision, expertise and effective communication.
- Cohesion of thought and activity pervades the planning, development and delivery of the medical school.
- Despite the political pressures and the problems created, adaptive leadership brought about change.

Case study 22.3   Steps towards establishing a new medical college in Saudi Arabia – an insight into medical education in the Kingdom

Khalid A. Bin Abdulrahman and Farid Saleh

Medical education in Saudi Arabia has evolved since the late 1960s when the first medical college was established and named after the late King Saud Bin Abdulaziz. Four other medical colleges were later developed and these five remained the only colleges graduating doctors for the next 30 years.

In 2006, the country's statistics showed that the percentage of Saudi nationals holding a medical degree and practising in the public health sector was less than 20 per cent. This alarming figure necessitated the issuing of a royal decree by King Abdullah bin Abdulaziz Al-Saud, the Custodian of the Two Holy Mosques, and the Chairman of the Council of Ministers and Higher Education Board to develop and expand medical education in the Kingdom. It resulted in the establishment of many new medical colleges and expansion of some of the existing ones. There are currently 28 public and six private medical colleges in the Kingdom, with five more public colleges on the verge of being established in the near future.

The College of Medicine at Al-Imam Mohammad Bin Saud Islamic University was founded in 2007 and became operational during the academic year of 2008–9. The vision was to help in revolutionising medical education in the Kingdom and graduate medical doctors who demonstrate those skills required of a doctor equipped for the 21st century. To achieve this goal, careful and lengthy planning, testing and retesting followed. Despite the urgent need to establish new medical colleges in the Kingdom, careful considerations were made in order not to compromise the time that should be allocated to each of the developmental steps while planning the establishment of the College of Medicine at Al-Imam University. The main goal that was kept in mind, and subsequently integrated in all these steps, was innovation in medical education. Soon after the appointment of a founding dean, a subcommittee derived from the Saudi Medical Colleges Deans' Committee was created and chaired by the founding dean. It included the deans of three

(continued)

(continued)

new medical colleges. The main goal of the subcommittee was to review the status of medical education in the Kingdom and to produce a list of fundamental steps to be followed by any new medical college to be established in the country.

An important cornerstone in establishing a new medical college is the appointment of a founding dean, who should have an excellent background in medical education and leadership, management and communication skills. These skills are essential for surveying medical education nationwide; communicating a unique vision, missions, goals and objectives pertaining to the new medical college; providing leadership in the implementation of these missions, goals and objectives; and acting as a catalyst for securing the resources needed for the proper accomplishment of the various tasks. In addition, the founding dean should have the expertise in planning, developing, evaluating and implementing medical and allied health curricula.

The recommendations made by the subcommittee included the need for the medical college to take into consideration, right from the beginning, both institutional and programme accreditation, based on international and national standards and requirements. To achieve this goal, five main pillars of a medical college were planned by the six main taskforces, headed by the founding dean. These five pillars were: the setting of the institution; the medical programme; the student division; the faculty division; and the resources needed. The sixth taskforce was a liaison committee, whose role was to accumulate and share information and activities derived from the other five main task forces. Embedded among the five pillars are 21 domains, which include administration and governance, the academic environment and the programme's essential elements, namely curriculum management, objectives, design, content, teaching, evaluation and the learning environment.

Other domains embedded in the five pillars pertaining to students are their admission and selection criteria, premedical requirements, counselling, and ethical and professional conduct. Still other domains embedded in the five pillars and pertaining to the teaching staff (both faculty and teaching assistants) include their number, experience and qualifications. The last domain pertains to the finance, space, clinical affiliations, information technology, support staff, library and other educational resources. Planning for the domains listed above was allocated to the six main taskforces described earlier, based on the pillars to which these domains belong. The recommended action plan towards establishing a new medical college in the Kingdom, along with the suggested timeframe, is summarised in Table 22.1. Moreover, the new medical college was designed with the healthcare needs of the community and region in mind, and to increase the supply of well-qualified physicians who are compassionate and who will be inclined to practise in the community and region, and enhance the academic standing of the university to which it belongs. The latter should facilitate the new establishment process by bypassing bureaucracy and by considering the new college as a 'newborn baby' that requires special attention and care for 5 years following its birth.

Table 22.1 Development action plan: the College of Medicine at Al-Imam Mohammad Bin Saud Islamic University

Administrative affairs

- Founding dean and job description – first 6 months
- Vice-deans – first 6 months
- Executive secretary – first month
- Director of staff affairs – first month
- Supervisor of student affairs – first month

- Calculation of costs – first 3 months
- Formal delineation of the relationship between the medical college and the parent university
- Director of finance – first 3 months

Admission and enrolment of students, and other student affairs

- Conditions and regulations for student admission – first month
- Maximum and minimum number of students – first month
- Written procedures and standards for the evaluation, progress, counselling and graduation of students and disciplinary actions

Faculty affairs

- Number, qualifications, experience and specialties of faculty members – first 6 months
- Medical education specialist – first 2 years
- Faculty development program – first year
- Teaching assistants – first year

Curriculum

- Mission statements – first 3 months
- Objectives and outcomes – first 3 months
- Competencies – first 3 months
- Preparatory year – first 3 months
- Pre-clinical and clinical years – first year
- Internship year – first 2 years
- Delivery methods
- Assessment methods

Educational environment and infrastructure

- Temporary college administration building – first month
- Space needs for the preparatory, and pre-clinical and clinical years – first 2 and 6 months, respectively
- Design of the university hospital – first year
- Cooperation agreements with regional health sectors – first 2 years
- Learning resources within and outside the college, including the library and information technology – first 6 months

Temporary college board

- Nominating the members – first 2 months
- Nominating the secretary – first 2 months

What important features can be learned from the Saudi Arabian case study?

- The decision to establish a new medical school was based on societal and national needs, and supported by a forward-thinking political ideal.
- A structured approach to planning and development, although it may take time and resources, led to a successful outcome.

- The appointment of a founding dean with specific qualifications in medical education and with leadership skills was one of the first priorities in the schools development.
- Early communication with other medical schools, enhancing collaboration and cooperation, was essential to develop a series of schools that all had the same important vision – the development of high-quality institutions tailored to the needs of the Kingdom of Saudi Arabia.
- A clear definition of the mission of the school and a very clear plan of its organisational structure enabled a shared understanding of what the school was aiming to be and to achieve.
- The school used the accreditation process, through which it would pass in the future, as a template for curricular construction.
- The detailed plan allowed a clear vision and definition of the roles and responsibilities of all those involved in the medical school, supporting effective management and responsibility.
- A realistic timeframe underpinned the development plan.

The role of the medical school and medical education is paramount in today's complex world. They are at the heart of producing doctors equipped to deliver high-quality healthcare for the 21st century and beyond. Whereas history has supported the top-down 'leader' model of management, contemporary challenges have necessitated the development of a new approach to institution leadership and management. Those tasked with taking charge of medical schools are required to develop diverse and essential skills, most of which have to be learned, developed and adapted over time and adapted to changing circumstances. These skills, under the broad umbrella of leadership, should now take priority over the previous political and academic qualities expressed by past leaders of medical schools, and used as a basis for appointment.

Medical education is rapidly evolving; new styles and forms of medical schools are fast developing; societal pressures demand a new style of healthcare; effective leadership is at the fore.

Take-home messages

- Medical schools are complex environments requiring effective leadership and management.
- Confusion occurs between the terms leadership, management and leader; clarity of these terms is important.
- Previous definitions of leadership do not accommodate the complex world of institutional organisations.
- Adaptive leadership is a more appropriate style, requires a change in values, beliefs or behaviour and is an educative process.

Bibliography

Bland, C.J., Starnaman, S., Hembroff, L., Perlstadt, H., Henry, R. and Richards R. (1999) 'Leadership behaviours for successful leadership–community collaborations to change curricula', *Academic Medicine*, 74(11): 1227–37.

Boelen, C., Gibbs, T. and Dharamsi, S. (2013) 'The social accountability of medical schools and its indicators', *Education for Health*, 25(3): 180–94.

Department of Health (2002) *Learning from Bristol: the Department of Health's response to the report of the Public Inquiry into children's heart surgery at the Bristol Royal Infirmary 1984–1995*, London: The Stationery Office. Online. Available HTTP: https://www.gov.uk/government/uploads/system/uploads/attachment_data/file/273320/5363.pdf (accessed 24 March 2015).

Glouberman, S. and Zimmerman, B. (2002) *Complicated and complex systems: What would successful reform of Medicare look like?*, Canada: Commission on the Future of Health Care in Canada.

Hamilton, P., Spurgeon, P., Clark, J., Dent, J. and Armit, K. (2008) *Engaging doctors: Can doctors influence organisational performance?* London: NHS Institute for Innovation and Improvement and Academy of Medical Royal Colleges.

Handy, C.B. (1993) *Understanding organisations*, London: Penguin.
Heiffetz, R.A. (1994) *Leadership without easy answers*, Cambridge, MA: Belknap Press of Harvard University Press.
Heifetz, R. and Linsky, M. (2004) 'When leadership spells danger', *Educational Leadership*, 61(7): 33–7.
Heifetz, R., Grashow, A. and Linsky, M. (2009) *The practice of adaptive leadership: Tools and tactics for changing your organization and the world*, Boston, MA: Harvard Business Press.
Held, S. and McKimm, J. (2011) Emotional intelligence, emotional labour and effective leadership. In M. Preedy, N. Bennett and C. Wise (eds) *Educational leadership, context, strategy and collaboration*, Milton Keynes: The Open University.
Jonas, S., McCay, L. and Keogh, B. (2011) The importance of clinical leadership. In T. Swanick and J. McKimm (eds) *ABC of clinical leadership*, Oxford: BMJ Books/Wiley-Blackwell.
Kotter, J.P. (1990) *A force for change: How leadership differs from management*, New York, NY: The Free Press.
Kotter, J.P. (1999) *What leaders really do*, Boston, MA: Harvard Business School Press.
Lieff, S. and Albert, M. (2010) 'The mindsets of medical education leaders: How do they conceive of their work?', *Academic Medicine*, 85(1): 57–62.
Lieff, S.J. and Albert, M. (2012) 'What do I do? Practice and learning strategies of medical education leaders'. *Medical Teacher*, 34(4): 312–19.
Long, A. (2011) Leadership and management. In T. Swanick and J. McKimm (eds) *The ABC of clinical leadership*, Oxford: BMJ Boooks/Wiley-Blackwell.
McKimm, J. (2004) *Special report 5: Case studies in leadership in medical and health care education*. York, UK: The Higher Education Academy.
McKimm, J. and Lieff, S.J. (2013) Medical education leadership. In J. Dent and R.M. Harden (eds) *A practical guide for medical teachers*, Chapter 42, London: Churchill Livingstone–Elsevier.
Mennin, S. (2013) Health professions education: Complexity, teaching and learning. In J.P. Sturmberg and C. Martin (eds.) *Handbook of systems and complexity in health* (pp. 755–66). Heidelberg: Springer.
Mintzberg, H. (1973) *McGill University School of Management, The nature of managerial work*, Canada: Harper and Row.
Mintzberg, H. (1990) *Mintzberg on management*, New York, NY: The Free Press.
Mintzberg, H. (1992). *Structure in fives: Designing effective organizations*, Upper Saddle River, NJ: Prentice Hall.
Mintzberg, H. (2009) *Tracking strategies: Toward a general theory of strategy formation*, New York, NY: Oxford University Press.
Nordquist, J. and Sundberg, K. (2013) 'An educational leadership responsibility in primary care: Ensuring the physical space for learning aligns with the educational mission', *Education for Primary Care*, 24(1): 45–9.
Northouse, P. (2004) *Leadership: Theory and practice* (3rd edn), London: Sage Publishing.
Oxford English Dictionary (2012) Online. Available HTTP: www.oed.com (accessed 28 December 2014).
Republic of Namibia (2004) *Namibia Vision 2030 policy framework for long-term national development*. Windhoek: Office of the President.
Sweeney, K. and Griffiths, F. (2002) *Complexity and health care: An introduction*. Abingdon: Radcliffe Medical Press.
Taylor, C.A., Taylor, J.C. and Stoller, J.K. (2008) Exploring leadership competencies in established and aspiring physician leaders: An interview based study, *Journal of General Internal Medicine*, 23(6): 748–54.
Thygeson, M., Morrissey, L. and Ulstad, V. (2010) 'Adaptive leadership and the practice of medicine: A complexity-based approach to reframing the doctor–patient relationship', *Journal of Evaluation in Clinical Practice*, 16(5): 1009–15.
World Health Organization (2006) *World health report*. Geneva: WHO. Online. Available HTTP: http://www.who.int/whr/2006/en/ (accessed 28 December 2014).

23
HOW TEACHING EXPERTISE AND SCHOLARSHIP CAN BE DEVELOPED, RECOGNISED AND REWARDED

Deborah Simpson, Maryellen E. Gusic and M. Brownell Anderson

> The teacher is one of the most powerful assets of a medical school. Content expertise is not the same as teaching experience.

Every day, in every part of the world, medical students and postgraduate trainees are engaged in learning to be physicians. Educators have been teaching the sciences fundamental to the understanding of health and disease (e.g. anatomy, physiology) since antiquity, when clinical educators/physicians like Hippocrates travelled around Greece to train medical students (Grammaticos and Diamantis 2008). Indeed as Aristotle said, 'Teaching is the highest form of understanding', and begins with what the teacher knows – the subject matter of the teacher's field (Boyer 1990). Yet teaching is more than transmitting knowledge from one's discipline; it requires a dynamic synergy between one's knowledge of subject matter and skills as a teacher. The latter requires a knowledge of the principles of learning, educational methods, instructional resources and knowledge of learners (Irby 1994).

On a daily basis, teachers systematically approach their task by:

1. identifying clear goals for their teaching interactions;
2. assuring that they are adequately prepared (current in their subject and as teachers);
3. selecting the appropriate methods for teaching and assessment with attention to delivery platforms (e.g. classroom, clinical rotations, community, web/online), and possible approaches to meet their goals within the time/resources available (e.g. lectures, podcasts, small-group discussions, simulations, multiple-choice assessments);
4. analysing the results to determine the extent to which learning occurred;
5. sharing those findings with colleagues (e.g. course leaders, curriculum committees, other educators); and then
6. critically reflecting on their efforts in order to revise and improve, in preparation for the next educational event (Glassick et al. 1997).

This stepwise, systematic approach to how educators approach their work is synonymous with what it means to be a 'scholar'. Scholars in all fields – be it scientists seeking discoveries, community health officials seeking the root cause(s) for a disease outbreak or teachers seeking to prepare and certify our next generation of healthcare professionals – approach their tasks by beginning with clear goals and adequate preparation and conclude with reflective critique.

The work of educators goes beyond the 'act' of teaching. Educators are involved in at least four additional domains of activities, each requiring a scholar's approach: curriculum development; advising/mentoring; learner assessment; and/or educational leadership/administration (Simpson et al. 2007). While educators typically approach their work using elements associated with a scholar's approach (e.g. clear goals = defined objectives linked to competencies), the rigor and value of this work often go unrecognised and undervalued. The criteria associated with a scholar's approach in each of these five educator activities have been elucidated through a systematic, evidence- and stakeholder-based process and can be used to frame educator development initiatives and processes for educator recognition/reward decisions (Gusic et al. 2013, 2014). Explicitly framing our educational work as the work of educational scholars allows us to identify and address gaps in our scholarly approach and stand as equals with our research colleagues.

How do we begin?

First we present the educator-as-scholar framework (Gusic et al. 2013) and then we illustrate its application for individual and programmatic faculty development and for recognition and reward of educators through several case studies. The scholar framework uses a common structure to ascertain the degree to which we engage in, and can demonstrate, the value of our work as educators (Table 23.1): the first column presents the stepwise approach used by scholars in any field, and the second column provides both broad and specific quality indicators that can be used for assessment of one's work as an educator. Independent of the domain of educational scholar activity (e.g. teaching, curriculum, learner assessment), the framework is consistent: the necessary steps are listed in the first column. Indicators related to *significant results* are adapted from Kirkpatrick and Kirkpatrick's (2006) four-level model for measuring the outcomes of training programmes (satisfaction/reaction, learning, application of learning, impact). The *effective presentation* indicators are outlined using accepted standards for scholarship across all fields, as outlined by Hutchings and Shulman (1999): scholarly work must be reviewed by peers and shared with others/disseminated in a format that others can use or adapt. To see the broad and detailed indicators for each of the other educator activities (e.g. curriculum, advising/mentoring, learning assessment, administration/leadership), access is available through MedEdPORTAL, a peer-reviewed repository of educational materials (Gusic et al. 2013).

Illustration of scholar approach in four case studies

To demonstrate how the scholar approach works to transcend differences in our institutions and organisations, we apply the approach to several case studies with four objectives; that is, to demonstrate how this framework can be used to:

1 provide guidance to medical educators who are teaching multiple learners, in a variety of settings (e.g. classroom, community, health system);
2 identify needs and inform the design of faculty development efforts;
3 assess the quality of our work as educators;
4 return educators to be amongst those who, like Hippocrates, are recognised and esteemed.

While each of the six scholar elements outlined in Table 23.1 can be identified in each case, we will highlight several elements within each of the first two cases, allowing a richer illustration of the approach, and then offer a combined analysis for the last two cases, to provide an integrated perspective.

Table 23.1 Scholar framework – broad and specific indicators for teaching activities

Scholar approach	Indicators of scholar approach in teaching (used to judge work)
Clear goals	Learning objectives for the teaching session(s) are: • Based on documented needs of learners • In multiple domains (e.g. knowledge, skills, attitudes, behaviours) • Stated clearly: specific, measurable, achievable, realistic and timely (SMART) • At appropriate level for targeted learners

Adequate preparation	• Congruence with institutional/programme goals and integration with other components of curriculum:
	  ○ Material is comprehensive and is integrated logically with other curricular components
	  ○ Subject matter is at depth and breadth matched to learners' needs and time available
	• Use of best practices and the literature, professional development activities and personal experience
	  ○ Material is up to date and evidence-based
	• Resource planning:
	  ○ Resources needed for teaching are specified and available
	  ○ Adequate preparation for use of technology

Appropriate methods	• Teaching methods aligned with learning objectives and are feasible, practical and ethical
	• Employs suitable range and variety of teaching strategies supported by learning theory, best practices, literature review:
	  ○ Uses interactive approaches and promotes self-directed and collaborative learning
	  ○ Uses methods that promote critical thinking and reasoning skills
	• Innovative teaching methods used to achieve objectives:
	  ○ Provides evidence of innovation (e.g. novel strategies to promote learning)
	• Teaching methods include ways to monitor learners' progress
	
	If technology is used, it:
	• Aids achievement of the objectives
	• Is interactive (e.g. teacher to learner, peer to peer, learner to teacher and content, learner to technology)
	• Is easy to navigate

Significant results	**Satisfaction/reaction** • Rating of teaching by learners, peers, experts • Comparison of learner ratings to ratings of other teachers (internal, external) **Learning** • Evidence of learning based on measurable changes in knowledge, skills, attitudes and behaviours • Comparison of learner performance to established benchmarks and/or to other learners' performance in previous years

Scholar approach	Indicators of scholar approach in teaching (used to judge work)
	Application
	• Demonstration of skills/behaviours learned from teaching activity in subsequent settings, curricular components
	Impact
	• On educational programmes and processes within and/or outside institution
	• Positive evaluation by knowledgeable peers, educational leaders, curriculum committees
	• Recognition via awards, incentives, promotion
Effective presentation	Recognised as valuable by others (internally or externally) through:
	• Peer review + Dissemination (1 and/or 2 below):
	1 Dissemination (presentations/publications)
	○ Peer-reviewed publications/presentations of teaching strategies and/or instructional materials
	○ Invitations to provide faculty development, conduct workshops or do presentations about teaching locally, at other institutions, in other regional, national, international venues
	○ Invitation to peer review other teachers locally or at other institutions
	2 Adopted/adapted by others:
	○ Breadth of dissemination and adoption of teaching methods/materials: local, regional, national, international
Reflective critique	• Reflection and results of evaluations used for ongoing improvement:
	○ Critical analysis of teaching activity using all information from others and from self-assessment
	○ Evidence of ongoing improvement of teaching activity based on critical analysis and reflection

Source: Adapted from Gusic, M.E., Baldwin, C.D., Chandran, L., Rose, S., Simpson, D., Strobel, H.W., Timm, C. and Fincher, R.M. *Academic Medicine* 2014, 89(7):1006–11; and Gusic, M.E., Amiel, J., Baldwin, C., Chandran, L., Fincher, R., Mavis, B., O'Sullivan, P., Padmore, J., Rose, S., Simpson, D., Strobel, H., Timm, C. and Viggiano, T. (2013) *Using the AAMC toolbox for evaluating educators: You be the judge!,* MedEdPORTAL. Online. Available HTTP: www.mededportal.org/publication/9313 (accessed 6 August 2014).

Case study 23.1   Dr Lasz Lo – clinician teacher (teaching activity category)

Deborah Simpson, Hina Mahboob, Richard J. Battiola and John R. Brill

A practising physician employed by a large non-profit healthcare system in the USA, Dr Lasz Lo regularly has students and residents rotating with him on his hospital rounds and in clinic. He enjoys the opportunity to teach and feels it is his duty to give back because of his respect for those who trained him. Dr Lo often spends extra time to learn about trainees as people and provide guidance to them as future physicians.

'Medicine', Dr Lo often tells his learners, 'is the highest calling one can have… Our patients trust us to help them stay well, to care for them in time of need, and to treat them as our equals. We must

(continued)

(continued)

never violate that trust.' Dr Lo has high expectations for himself and for his learners specifically because he often cares for the neediest of patients. Many of Dr Lo's patients are poor (choosing to spend their limited funds on housing and food for their families rather than medications) and suffer from multiple chronic conditions, even those at a young age. Patients often struggle to get to his clinic because transportation options are limited. Time for teaching, given this complex patient population, is limited, as he is often running 'behind'. The healthcare system encourages teaching, but its first priority is patient care, providing regular reports to Dr Lo about his performance on various quality and safety measures.

Recently, Dr Lo was contacted by the physician who supervises the healthcare system's student education. According to the supervisor, students have been reporting for the last year that Dr Lo is disorganised (e.g. their start time with him is unpredictable, their roles are unclear); interrupts students as they present cases; has unrealistic expectations for what they can do at their stage of training; and doesn't tell students what they are supposed to learn. Dr Lo is shocked! He had always been told that he was a good teacher. Dr Lo is angry and frustrated that his students never talked to him about their concerns and that this was the first time he had learned that this was a problem. Demoralised, Dr Lo wonders if he should continue to teach as he doesn't have time to spend 'reading'. His teaching already takes time away from his patients and his family. The supervisor, who doesn't want to lose Dr Lo as a clinical preceptor, sits down with Dr Lo to share strategies about how he might enhance his work with learners.

Providing guidance to educators

Clinical teachers like Dr Lasz Lo have an extraordinarily difficult task: to assure the highest quality of care for their patients and to teach learners who expect high-quality education in a dynamic, fast-paced setting. Applying the teacher–scholar framework can provide Dr Lo and his supervisor with specific guidance to improve teaching. The analysis below represents the approach the supervisor can use in working with his colleague, Dr Lasz Lo.

Clear goals

Students, teachers and supervisors at clinical sites must have an agreed-upon set of SMART learning objectives for the experience. These objectives must be explicit and shared with both the teacher and the learner so that each has the same expectations for the experience.

Adequate preparation

Annually, supervisors should ensure that the unit and the teachers are ready to teach by working with teachers to:

1. confirm that teachers and learners have shared these goals and agree that they are attainable within the time available;
2. delineate specific roles and responsibilities for all students rotating through the department that are aligned with expectations for their stage of training;
3. match any assignments for students to the goals for the rotation, roles and responsibilities;
4. provide teachers with a brief (3–5 minute) 'teaching script' to use in orienting learners to their teams and to their roles/expectations. The supervisor can use existing resources and templates widely accessible on the web to adapt to the system/setting as resources for teachers.

Appropriate methods

Healthcare teams and their members function most effectively and efficiently when: they have shared values (to provide the safest and highest quality of care possible); they have clear roles and responsibilities (e.g. students are responsible for . . .); and members accept accountability and perceive that the team leader will create a safe and respectful environment in which any team member (even a student who feels at the lowest rung on the ladder) can raise a concern or question. The supervisor can help Dr Lo and other teachers create an environment that promotes learning, by sharing strategies to meet teaching goals. Examples include:

1. a 10–15-minute orientation when the 'team is formed' (e.g. when a medical student begins the rotation) that reaffirms the team's shared values, members' roles and responsibilities and accountabilities;
2. 'activity of daily living' schedules and templates for students to provide clear structure (e.g. start at 7:00 a.m.; case presentation for inpatient versus outpatient; map of facility; and team call numbers). Start simply, adding an element or two for each rotation so that students do not become overwhelmed with these tasks.

Case study 23.2   Supporting the continuum of faculty development through the Department for Educational Development, Aga Khan University, Pakistan

Rukhsana W. Zuberi, Syeda K. Ali, Sheilla K. Pinjani, Shazia Sadaf and Naveed Yousuf

Aga Khan University (AKU) is a not-for-profit private university with campuses in Asia, East Africa and the UK. A School of Nursing was established in 1982, followed by establishment of the Medical College in 1983. Faculty members are recruited for their specialty-based expertise, but generally need support to enhance their teaching expertise. In response to this need, the Department for Educational Development (DED) was created to support faculty as teachers and scholars through programmatic interventions ranging from individual consultations, to serving as educational experts on academic committees, conducting workshops and annual retreats, and administering certificate and graduate degrees in health professional education (HPE). DED faculty have Masters or doctoral-level qualifications in Medical Education/HPE from the University of Illinois at Chicago, University of Calgary, Dundee University, University of Leeds, Cardiff University, University of Maastricht, University Ambrosiana and AKU, bringing together global perspectives for diversity and enrichment.

A one-credit course, 'Introductory Short Course in HPE – Theory to Practice,' is mandatory for all newly recruited AKU Faculty of Health Sciences faculty members and a prerequisite for other DED courses and graduate programmes. It focuses on trends in curriculum development, teaching/learning methods and resources, and the principles of learner assessment and monitoring. Advanced Masters-level courses are offered in curriculum development, teaching/learning, assessment, programme evaluation, leadership and research in HPE to prepare teachers, educators, researchers

(continued)

> *(continued)*
> and leaders nationally and for the region. Coordinators and directors of academic programmes are encouraged to take the 'teaching/learning' and 'assessment' courses.
>
> Faculty members may take any of these components as free-standing courses to improve teaching expertise or all courses to obtain diploma/degree qualifications in HPE. Faculty members who wish to be educators or spearhead academic programmes have the opportunity to complete the requirements for the Advanced Diploma or Master of HPE degree.
>
> Evidence of excellence and/or scholarship in teaching, discovery, integration and/or application serves as the basis for university-wide teaching awards, academic promotion, appointments to academic leadership positions and nominations for national awards, including the Pride of Performance Award from the Higher Education Commission.
>
> Through its work with medical schools, accrediting and regulatory bodies, DED has brought about educational reforms and influenced national undergraduate and postgraduate curricula and policies.

Addressing needs for faculty development creates academic educator career path(s)

Faculty development for educators must be designed to meet institutional needs and be aligned to support academic career trajectories. Applying a systematic process, AKU created the DED and its programmes to enhance and reward faculty members' skills as teachers and as educational leaders and administrators.

Clear goals

The requirement that all faculty complete a basic education course establishes that education is a discipline requiring training and expertise. The multiple types and levels of programming provided by the DED allow faculty and coordinators to select the opportunities that are best suited to meet their needs and professional goals as educators.

Adequate preparation

Faculty in the DED are experienced educators who have pursued advanced professional training in diverse settings. This expertise allows them to share best practices, approaches from the literature and personal experience in their work with faculty members from national institutions to support programmatic improvement. Their knowledge and skills as educators also ensure that the educational programmes are designed to meet national health priorities and the learners' educational needs, and are aligned with institutional goals.

Appropriate methods

Multiple venues, formats and progression levels (e.g. certificate, degree) provide faculty with a flexible approach to developing educational expertise needed to meet their career goals. Over a period of 25 years, the DED has served as a catalyst in establishing and sustaining institutional recognition and reward structures for education at each stage of a faculty member's career.

Case study 23.3 Institution(alising) education in a healthcare system, Singapore

Sandy Cook, Robert Kamei and Koo Wen Hsin

Singapore Health Services (SingHealth) is the largest public health cluster in Singapore serving as a clinical service-focused healthcare system, providing clinical education supported by outstanding educational role models and numerous faculty development programmes. Educational scholarship, however, was not well integrated with clinical care and research. In 2011, SingHealth's interest in integrating educational scholarship with its clinical care and research initiatives resulted in the creation of a 'functional ecosystem in the form of an Academic Healthcare Cluster' with Duke-National University of Singapore Graduate Medical School in Singapore (Krishnan and Ng 2012). An Academic Medicine Education Institute (AM·EI) (www.academic-medicine.edu.sg/amei/) was established in 2012 to provide resources to support clinical educators' academic efforts in education; to integrate and coordinate faculty development programmes; and to develop a community of scholarly clinician educators to influence the overall education culture of the institution. Open to all healthcare professionals, from trainees to experienced teachers, AM·EI merges a teaching academy concept with comprehensive faculty development and career mentoring/advising to advance educational scholarship at all membership levels (Associate, Full, Fellow, Scholar).

The AM·EI has established three workgroups (Advocacy, Professional Development and Scholarship) that facilitate and support the institute's goals. For example, the Advocacy workgroup identifies and recognises excellence in educational efforts; defines promotion criteria for health professions educators; and supports efforts to improve education. The workgroup has developed an educator portfolio framework based on the key domains for the Academy of Medical Educators (www.medicaleducators.org)) competencies (designing and planning learning; teaching and supporting learners; assessment and feedback; educational research; educational management and leadership as core values). The portfolio is now a required component for our Appointments, Promotions and Tenure committee for all educators. An annual Golden Apple Award system has been established to recognise teaching excellence, innovation and creativity. The Professional Development Workgroup has established 17 Academy of Medical Educators domain-focused professional development workshops offered two to three times per year, a monthly Medical Education Grand Rounds series and three education fellowships (one year or more in length). AM·EI has also been charged to provide faculty development to the SingHealth Residency Program. Since AM·EI's inception in September 2012 through to June 2014, the Institute has enrolled over 1,500 interprofessional members.

Case study 23.4 Aligning academic promotion with medical school missions and faculty roles, Eastern Virginia Medical School, United States

Elza Mylona, Aaron I. Vinik and Christine C. Matson

The Eastern Virginia Medical School (EVMS) enrolled its first medical student class in 1973. EVMS aspires to be the most community-oriented medical school in the country, collaborating to meet the healthcare needs of the community by focusing on community and population health in its clinical, education and research activities. To accomplish this mission, the school aspires to attract and retain

(continued)

(continued)

exceptional faculty who are outstanding in their professional goals and accomplishments, and who will thrive and find professional satisfaction in academic culture.

All faculty members are expected to demonstrate effective teaching, ongoing participation in scholarship and active engagement in service, with a level of expertise appropriate to their rank. As a community-based medical school, EVMS depends greatly on clinical faculty to teach and mentor medical students, residents and fellows, and improve the educational mission. Historically, EVMS's promotion criteria emphasised research-based activities limiting the number of clinical 'teaching' faculty promotions. In 2012 EVMS revised its promotion criteria and created a single academic track, retaining the appropriate rigour and clarity associated with scholarly work, yet allowing faculty to create a realistic and attainable pathway for academic promotion in their area of strength.

All EVMS faculty (full-time salaried; full-time non-salaried; and community faculty) can demonstrate scholarship in any of the four faculty responsibility areas: clinical care, education, research/discovery and administration. Excellence in each area is evaluated using Glassick et al.'s (1997) criteria, elicited as part of the guidelines for each area. Thus far, 25 faculty members have gone through review for promotion under the new guidelines and reported that the concept of 'fair' expectations across all types of activities has struck a positive chord.

Resolving incongruities between teacher roles and organisational expectations and recognition

In order to be valued, educators must be able to document what they do and provide evidence of quality in a format that facilitates a consistent and efficient review by those charged with making recognition and reward decisions.

Clear goals

The Advocacy Workgroup at SingHealth and the EVMS promotion criteria provide explicit guidance to assure alignment of educator role expectations with promotion and career paths.

Appropriate methods

SingHealth utilised the international Academy of Medical Educators competencies to create a standardised template for an educator portfolio that allows faculty to document the work that they do within established domains of activity. AMEI facilitates completion of a portfolio by collecting data for use by faculty in creating their portfolios. At EVMS, the promotion criteria are derived from the Carnegie Foundation for the Advancement of Teachers seminal works on scholarship and the criteria for its assessment. Each adapted their criteria to align with organisation-specific missions and to support faculty roles with processes and resources.

Significant results

Each organisation has achieved early success in terms of numbers (e.g. AMEI membership, attendance at events, number of faculty reviewed for EVMS promotion) and perceptions of fairness of expectations. Both have plans to continue to determine long-term impact in terms of catalysing quality improvement in educational activities, advancing educational scholarship and facilitating the recognition and promotion of educators.

Effective presentation

Each organisation used workgroups to formulate their approach and included strategies to disseminate their plans and preliminary results. The ongoing communication of results will help to ensure that the resources, opportunities and criteria for success as educators are understood by all stakeholders: from individual faculty and their supervisors and mentors to the implementation agents and decision makers who have been tasked to carry out the work/apply the new criteria.

Reflective critique and summary

At the end of every journal article, authors typically review their findings, discuss the implications of their work within the larger context of related work and highlight next steps so that others may build on their work to advance the field. This reflective process allows us to improve continuously as individuals and collectively to enhance our work as a community of educators. Consistent with this process, we asked each of the case authors to reflect on how the initiative(s) described in their report contributes to valuing education in their organisation and to the institution's culture. Their reflections and those of the chapter authors reveal recommendations that can serve as guideposts for individuals and organizations who want, in the words of Eastern Virginia case study authors, 'education and teaching to be taken seriously . . . seen/accepted as an intellectual endeavour that is equally valued with research and that can provide recognition and rewards to its scholars'.

Create forums that bring teachers together

Efforts can start small within a department or on a larger scale, within a medical school, and then extend to the university, healthcare systems and/or nationally. As the case study authors from Aga Khan University reflected,

> Through its multi-level courses, DED brings together teachers and educators at different levels of their careers fostering a community of educational leaders. It provides a platform for networking and sharing best practices from different institutions, different disciplines and different health professions across the country, thus facilitating and sustaining faculty engagement and collaboration for innovative teaching and learning.

Work simultaneously at the individual and organisational levels (e.g. university, healthcare system, accreditation bodies)

Case and chapter authors alike emphasise the importance of working to develop individuals as educators, be it through journal clubs, workshops and/or formal coursework leading to a degree. At the same time, assuring that the organisation and its infrastructure support educators requires the availability of educational expertise. Organisation of this expertise within a department or academy of medical educators facilitates the coordination of efforts to develop educators and enhance educational programmes. Last, but not least, promotion guidelines and awards/recognition processes must acknowledge the activities and impact of the work of educators. As the Singapore case study authors reflected, to achieve AM.EI's goal of building a community of educators,

> AM.EI and SingHealth established two strategic activities. First, we invited key education leaders to participate in a Fellowship Program in Medical Education . . . Second was the creation of a clinical educator track and guidelines for promotion along with the centralized documentation infrastructure to help program leaders be aware of the educational contributions of their faculty to facilitate the process of promotion.

Be visible

It is vital to communicate to all levels of the organisation continuously the importance of education and of the roles and activities of teachers. As indicated by the authors of the Singapore case study, 'The mere presence of the AM.EI has raised interest and awareness of the importance of quality medical education activities and as faculty are trained . . . and being promoted, this culture will continue to grow.'

Plan for sustainability and growth through graduates

Individuals participating in the forums for educators gain expertise and they in turn must be engaged to teach/mentor the next generation of teachers. Over time, scholarly results are visible and have high impact. For example, the case study authors at AKU reported that their

> programme alumni head departments of medical education in their own institutions, are spearheading innovations using educational experimentation grounded in research theory to bring about change and continuous quality improvement in Health Professions Education.

Recognise the time and effort required

Building and sustaining a community of educators takes time and sustained effort. As the Aga Khan case study authors commented, 'it just doesn't happen . . . it has taken a quarter century to get here'.

As health profession educators, we and our sponsoring organisations are entrusted to prepare the next generation of healthcare providers who will be responsible for delivering safe and effective care for patients and populations, at the lowest possible cost (Institute for Healthcare Improvement 2014). To fulfil this public trust, educators and organisational leaders must have the courage and commitment, as evidenced in our case studies, to develop, recognise and reward our teachers and educational scholars continuously; to create forums that bring teachers together, make these efforts visible, work simultaneously at the individual and organisational levels to advance education and educators, all the while recognising that change takes time but does yield results in terms of improving our educational programmes to meet healthcare needs.

As educators we are not alone. Common language and frameworks are emerging to help us communicate and share best practices, strategies and outcomes for developing and rewarding teaching expertise and educational scholarship. The Carnegie Foundation's work on scholarship has emerged globally as a cross-cutting, systematic, criteria-based framework informing the work and case studies presented in this chapter. Application of this framework also assures that our efforts to develop, assess and value medical teachers and their work as educator scholars is rigorous, equitable and transparent. Using the scholar criteria to guide and evaluate our work will enable us to improve health profession education continuously and fulfil our entrusted roles.

Take-home messages

- A rigorous, equitable and transparent criteria-based framework is now available to develop, assess and value medical teachers and their work as educators.
- Educators should create and sustain visible forums to bring teachers together to share evidence-based best practices to facilitate and sustain innovative teaching and learning.
- Educational leaders must partner with organisational leaders to ensure that the organisation and its infrastructure support educators, including revising academic promotion and award processes.

Bibliography

Boyer, E.L. (1990) *Scholarship reconsidered. Priorities of the professoriate*. Lawrence, NJ: Princeton University Press.

Glassick, C.E., Huber, M.R. and Maeroff, G.I. (1997) *Scholarship assessed: Evaluation of the professoriate*. San Francisco, CA: Jossey-Bass.

Grammaticos, P.C. and Diamantis, A. (2008) 'Useful known and unknown views of the father of modern medicine, Hippocrates and his teacher Democritus', *Hellenic Journal of Nuclear Medicine*, 11(1): 2–4.

Gusic, M.E., Amiel, J., Baldwin, C., Chandran, L., Fincher, R., Mavis, B., O'Sullivan, P., Padmore, J., Rose, S., Simpson, D., Strobel, H., Timm, C. and Viggiano, T. (2013) *Using the AAMC toolbox for evaluating educators: You be the judge!*, MedEdPORTAL. Online. Available HTTP: www.mededportal.org/publication/9313 (accessed 6 August 2014)

Gusic, M.E., Baldwin, C.D., Chandran, L., Rose, S., Simpson, D., Strobel, H.W., Timm, C. and Fincher, R.M. (2014) 'Evaluating educators using a novel toolbox: Applying rigorous criteria flexibly across institutions', *Academic Medicine*, 89(7): 1006–11.

Hutchings, P. and Shulman, L.S. (1999) 'The scholarship of teaching: New elaborations, new developments', *Change*, 31(5): 10–15.

Institute for Healthcare Improvement (2014) *The IHI triple aim*. Online. Available HTTP: www.ihi.org/Engage/Initiatives/TripleAim/Pages/default.aspx (accessed 30 June 2014).

Irby, D.I. (1994) 'What clinical teachers in medicine need to know', *Academic Medicine*, 69(5): 333–42.

Kirkpatrick, D.L. and Kirkpatrick, J.D. (2006) *Evaluating training programs: The four levels* (3rd edn), San Francisco, CA: Berrett-Koehler Publishers.

Krishnan, R. and Ng, I. (2012) 'Academic medicine: Vision to reality', *Annals Academy of Medicine*, 42(1): 2–4.

Simpson, D., Fincher, R.M., Hafler, J.P., Irby, D.M., Richards, F.B., Rosenfeld, G.C. and Viggiano, T.R. (2007) 'Advancing educators and education by defining the components and evidence associated with educational scholarship', *Medical Education*, 41(10): 1002–9.

24
ACCREDITATION AND PROGRAMME EVALUATION
Ensuring the quality of educational programmes

Dan Hunt, Ducksun Ahn, Barbara Barzansky and Donna Waechter

> *Strategies to evaluate the curriculum and to provide continuous information to guide decisions are now available. How schools are accredited varies in different regions of the world.*

Two related processes are essential to assure the ongoing quality of a medical education programme: accreditation and programme evaluation. Accreditation is an external review system that uses pre-established regionally accepted standards of educational quality. The focus of accreditation may be an institution, such as a college or university, or an educational programme leading to a specific degree, such as the MD (medical doctor). Accreditation tends to be episodic, occurring at specified intervals and reviewing institutions or programmes as of a given time. Programme evaluation, as defined here, is an ongoing process of review that occurs internal to the medical school using school-developed process and outcome criteria. Programme evaluation, which can be both formative as well as summative, allows the identification of strengths and areas needing improvement. Thus, programme evaluation and accreditation are two tools for quality and improvement that are complementary and may utilise similar criteria. The systems ideally are designed to provide information on both the processes and outcomes of a medical education programme, although along different time lines, with one using internal reviewers and the other using external, peer, reviewers. The results of programme evaluation inform accreditation as well as supporting ongoing quality improvement. This chapter will describe the basics of accreditation and programme evaluation systems. The reader is referred to Chapter 17 for best practices in assessment of students, which supports both programme evaluation and accreditation and, therefore, is the third side of the triangle to sustain quality medical education programmes.

Definition, purpose and need for accreditation

The Council for Higher Education Accreditation in the USA defines accreditation as both a process and a status, a means to ensure and improve higher-education quality, assisting institutions and programmes using a set of standards developed by peers. The result of the process, if successful, is the awarding of accredited status. All accrediting organisations create and use specific standards to ensure that institutions and programmes meet at least threshold expectations of quality and that they improve over time. These standards address key areas such as faculty, curricula and student learning outcomes, student support services, finances and facilities. All accrediting organisations use common practices, including a self-study by the institution or programme against the standards, an on-site visit by an evaluation team of peer experts and a subsequent review and decision by the accrediting body about accreditation status. Depending on the accrediting body, this review is typically repeated every 3–10 years for the institution or programme to sustain its accreditation (Council for Higher Education Accreditation 2010: 1).

The World Federation for Medical Education (WFME) recommends that, for the accreditation of medical education, there should be four specific stages:

1. institutional self-evaluation of the medical school;
2. external evaluation based on the report of self-evaluation and a site visit;
3. final report by the review team containing recommendations regarding the decision on accreditation;
4. the decision on accreditation (World Federation for Medical Education 2005).

Programme evaluation: five case studies

Accreditation as a tool for continuous quality improvement

Accreditation can serve as a framework for comprehensive internal programme evaluation and as a tool for continuous quality improvement. The first case study below, from the University of California, Davis (UCD), describes how one medical school in the USA used accreditation standards related to student mistreatment to improve its clinical learning environment and by extension the general culture of the institution.

Case study 24.1   Accreditation standards as a tool to drive organisational culture change, The University of California, Davis, United States

Mark Servis and Claire Pomeroy

UCD is a public school of medicine in Northern California, USA, founded in 1966 with a mission to train the next generation of physicians to serve California. Over the past decade, the school has experienced dramatic growth in the size and scope of both its clinical operations and its research enterprise. The transition of this school from a small, local, training programme to a major academic health system providing the full breadth of academic experiences engendered exciting and

(continued)

(continued)

sometimes stressful changes. Our experience highlights the key role that the Liaison Committee on Medical Education (LCME) accreditation standards can play in achieving a high-quality training environment and supporting, and even driving, important organisational culture change.

After an LCME accreditation visit in 2006 identified multiple areas of non-compliance with standards, the faculty undertook a series of quality improvement initiatives in collaboration with the recently appointed Dean. Compliance with LCME standards necessitated acceleration of curriculum reform, improved career counselling and updating physical plant facilities, as well as ongoing attention to the learning environment and prevention of student mistreatment. While many faculty and school administrators had been working on these areas, the results of the LCME review focused attention on the urgency to address these critical issues and served to catalyse real change. Delineation of optimal approaches was facilitated by a consultation from the LCME Secretariat later in 2006, and by the requirement for ongoing monitoring, including status reports and a follow-up limited site survey. As a result, significant changes were made in administrative leadership, curriculum integration, centralised oversight of education programmes, timely reporting of grades, student wellness and career advising. Policies and education programmes to reduce student mistreatment were strengthened and highlighted throughout the organisation. By 2007, the LCME deemed that substantial improvements had been made in compliance with the standards.

In 2010, however, LCME highlighted renewed concern about non-compliance with standards focusing on student mistreatment and the learning environment. Rates of mistreatment reported by UCD fourth-year medical students in the annual Association of American Medical Colleges (AAMC) graduation questionnaire were much higher than the national average. These results were obviously alarming to the faculty and administrative leadership, and discordant with the historical perception of the school as a supportive and friendly institution.

Clearly, the LCME standards were shining light on aspects of the school's organisational culture which needed to be addressed explicitly. Prompted by the 2010 findings, the school undertook a comprehensive review of compliance with all of the LCME accreditation standards, assigning letter grades for each standard and creating implementation teams to develop recommendations for any standard deemed by the teams to have a 'non-passing' grade. For example, for standards regarding student mistreatment and the learning environment, the Dean appointed a Learning Environment Task Force with representation from faculty, administration, nursing, residents, students and staff to understand the student mistreatment problem and create an action plan to improve compliance and, most importantly, the student experience. Based on the positive experience with the LCME Secretary's consultation in 2006, the Dean requested another LCME consultation visit specifically to solicit advice on best practices in creating a positive learning environment. In addition, the status reports and action plans required by the LCME to monitor progress served as useful prompts to keep planned corrective actions moving forward.

The school identified several factors contributing to the student mistreatment problem:

- The school had not recognised or addressed its evolution from a smaller programme with a 'family' atmosphere into a larger, and often less personal, academic enterprise.
- Students were not adequately prepared for the more autonomous and self-directed learning environment of the third year which was focused in very fast-paced clinical settings, having been conditioned to a more nurturing pre-clinical experience in the first 2 years.
- Increasingly busy and stressed clinical care providers often viewed students as peripheral to the clinical teams.
- Students were insufficiently involved with the school's early efforts to address mistreatment, being identified as victims and not the source of important input into solutions.

Indeed, students were seen as the 'canary in the coal mine' in identifying environmental problems experienced by other members of the clinical teams, from overworked trainees to stressed staff, to clinical faculty trying to juggle multiple mission expectations. In fact, student mistreatment was considered to reflect cultural issues which were also likely to be linked to patient satisfaction with their care experience. Consideration of the LCME standards focused attention on the importance of respect and inclusion at all levels of the organisation.

An action plan to achieve excellence in the learning environment for students and to ensure that the organisation's humanistic values, as articulated in the school's Principles of Community (University of California, Davis 2014), were reflected in clinical settings, included:

- revision of the mistreatment policy to improve transparency and enforcement;
- creation of a Learning Climate Committee with empowered medical student representation to monitor, develop and implement interventions, such as required educational sessions on the learning environment for clinical departments, and to measure outcomes;
- tracking the learning environment, including identifying both positive and negative experiences through anonymous student surveys every 8 weeks in the third and fourth years, and sharing anonymised results across the organisation as a form of appreciative inquiry and emergent design to promote culture change;
- development of a comprehensive professionalism curriculum for students in order to address the 'hidden curriculum';
- creation of new professionalism awards for residents and faculty to promote a positive learning environment and funding for a Clinical Educator's Masters programme to reward excellent faculty teaching in clinical settings.

To date, the impact of these interventions has been positive, with rates of student mistreatment declining to the national average, as measured in the 2012 AAMC graduation questionnaire, and falling further in 2013, as measured by the school's recent student survey.

The LCME accreditation process and the requirements for compliance with LCME standards facilitated identification of needed changes at the UCD School of Medicine and galvanised institutional efforts to implement quality improvements. As one example, the requirement to provide a positive learning environment focused attention on this key issue, necessitated that we overcome denial and minimisation and lent urgency to the implementation of myriad and far-reaching interventions to drive fundamental cultural change. The consensus agreement about the importance of accreditation helped overcome resistance to change and accelerate implementation and acceptance of new pedagogy, administrative policies and investment in education faculty, programmes and facilities. LCME standards are an effective tool to catalyse organisational culture change in schools of medicine and academic health centres.

Accreditation as a tool for change and guide for new school development

In addition to quality improvement, accreditation can serve as an agent of social change. New peer-developed standards can be designed to move educational programmes into areas, such as diversity and social accountability, that they might not otherwise pursue. A third value added through accreditation is its regulatory function in that it establishes minimum levels of resources and systems that must be in place for a specific certification of degree programmes. The prospective specification and review of resources and processes serve to protect students as they invest their time and money; aid institutions in planning; and provide the stimulus for the acquisition of the needed resources, at the same time that protecting the public from poorly trained healthcare personnel. The Northern Ontario School of Medicine case study describes how Canada's first new medical school in 30 years used accreditation standards to guide it in securing the resources and establishing the systems needed to admit its first class of students.

Case study 24.2   Using medical education accreditation standards as the foundation for creating Canada's first new medical school in 30 years, Northern Ontario School of Medicine, Canada

Joel H. Lanphear and Marie Matte

The Northern Ontario School of Medicine (NOSM) was established in 2003 with an explicit social accountability mandate to:

> address the healthcare needs of underserved populations of First Nations, Francophone, and Anglophone peoples across the province. The school embarked on an innovative distributed community-engaged education model ... to address the shortage of healthcare providers in rural and remote communities, especially across Northern Ontario.
>
> *(Strasser et al. 2009: 1459)*

Creating a new medical school is a complex task requiring attention to governance, admissions, curriculum, faculty appointments, faculty development and finance. The LCME accreditation standards for medical schools in the USA and Canada provided the framework for the creation of these programme initiatives.

The LCME standards are not prescriptive and, while they do not provide specific details on 'how' a particular issue needs to be addressed, they do provide the guidance on what needs to be in place to ensure a quality medical education programme. The structures and processes required to meet the standards are left to the faculty.

The development of the school's governance, financial, and faculty appointment and tenure processes were all guided by the LCME accreditation standards.

While the curriculum design and the admission system at NOSM were based on medical education research, the actual development and implementation processes were all guided by the LCME standards. The medical education research supported three principles that were used as the foundation of the NOSM curriculum and admission systems. These principles pertained to a programme's success in meeting its goal of producing graduates who ultimately decide to practise in smaller rural and remote communities. These principles are:

1. an admissions system minimising the barrier(s) to applicants from smaller communities;
2. a curriculum designed to provide students with the capabilities needed to practise in smaller communities;
3. a curriculum design that placed students in context – i.e. smaller communities to be taught and mentored by physicians who themselves had chosen to practise in small communities.

The admission standards and criteria, although guided by the LCME accreditation standards, were set by the faculty. They stipulated that the decision to admit a student must be made by the school's admission committee so that no outside influence or favouritism can be exercised. The accreditation standards do not prescribe what those criteria must be. At NOSM, the faculty chose not to use the Medical College Admission Test (MCAT) commonly used by schools in Canada and the USA because of concern that it could be perceived as a barrier for students from smaller communities and/or from different cultural or language backgrounds. The faculty chose to use the combination of objective structured mini-interviews and the college grade point average as the key criteria for decision making. Pre-med requirements were minimised based on the premise that courses like organic chemistry are not essential for the practice of medicine, and worse, might be a barrier for students who had their high school education in smaller communities without the rich science options of a large urban high school. In addition, the faculty decided to give extra weight to students who grew up in smaller communities, given that students from smaller communities are more likely to return to similar communities.

The LCME again served as a benchmark for development of learning opportunities outside the urban, specialty-based environment where students could learn from and be mentored by the non-specialty physicians in non-urban, smaller communities. This allowed the school to design a curriculum that placed students in remote First Nation communities and Reserves for a month while continuing the first-year curriculum. Many of these communities were not accessible by road and were as small as 350 people. In the second year, students spent 2 months distributed across Northern Ontario in communities of approximately 5,000 people. By developing specific objectives as the basis for student assessment and tracking systems, the faculty were able to document that, regardless of location, students had comparable educational experiences with comparable assessment results.

While requiring active learning, varied forms of student assessment and narrative feedback, the LCME standards do not prescribe specific content from any particular discipline, nor do they prescribe how teaching should be conducted. This allowed the faculty to develop a case-based curriculum with a minimal number of lectures (generally 3 hours a week) that emphasised active learning in small-group settings. In this way, students were able to refine their problem-solving skills while learning clinical skills from the physicians in the smaller communities. The need for large departments of basic scientists and clinical specialists was therefore minimised.

The LCME standards do not prescribe department or discipline-based clinical training. This allowed the medical educators at NOSM to design a clerkship programme that required all students to complete their clinical year (Year 3) in a longitudinal integrated clerkship model for 8 months. These clinical experiences were carried out in more than ten communities (each approximately 20,000 people) across Northern Ontario. In the fourth year, students trained with specialists in the two larger cities in Northern Ontario. Thus, the LCME standards support the development of a community-engaged education continuum ranging from First Nations and Reserve communities in Year 1, small rural communities in Year 2 and small urban communities in Year 3.

The early results are in. At the time of writing, four classes have graduated since the school's first class entered in 2005. Sixty-one per cent of all MD graduates have chosen family practice (primarily rural) and 65 per cent of these are practising in Northern Ontario (Strasser et al. 2013).

National accreditation systems evolve and improve over time

In the context of medical school expansion and desire for the assurance of quality educational programmes, more and more countries around the world are developing their own accreditation systems for medical education programmes. The case study from Taiwan below illustrates how this country's medical education leadership revised its accreditation standards to fit the country's needs better.

Case study 24.3 Overhauling the accreditation standards of the Taiwan Medical Accreditation Council

Chi-Wan Lai, Keh-Min Liu, Yan-Di Chang and Chyi-Her Lin

The Taiwan Medical Accreditation Council (TMAC) was established in 1999 and began accreditation of medical schools in 2001. However, over time, TMAC found that the narrative format of the original TMAC accreditation standards did not lend itself to ensuring consistent decisions about schools. In addition, it made it difficult for medical schools to understand easily the areas that needed improvement. At the same time, TMAC had been very impressed by the reformatting of the LCME standards in 2002, which enhanced the clarity and meaning of the standards and facilitated the ability to recognise chronic noncompliance.

The TMAC consulted with the LCME in 2008, expressing an interest in overhauling its accreditation standards. Five specific steps were taken:

1. In July 2009, two secretaries and an assistant secretary of the LCME and the President of the Foundation for Advancement of International Medical Education and Research (FAIMER) travelled to Taiwan to conduct a 3-day workshop on global medical education and the development of the accreditation system in the USA. The issues discussed included the content and revision of accreditation standards, the selection and training of surveyors, the accreditation process and determination of the accreditation results. The conference was attended by TMAC members and experienced surveyors and ample time for discussion was provided. The visitors formulated a set of proposals which included 39 essential standards considered to be important and relevant to medical education in Taiwan.
2. In March 2010, the ex-chair of the LCME Subcommittee on Standards (SOS) spent 2 weeks in Taiwan to help the TMAC-SOS overhaul its accreditation standards. Members of TMAC-SOS, consisting of five TMAC members and two external members with a medical education background, were first introduced to the ways in which the LCME standards had been reformatted from prose to numbered standards that allowed the use of explanatory annotations. The differences in culture across the two countries were taken into account and the existing TMAC standards were reformulated into clearer direct statements.
3. The first draft of the new standards was translated from English into Chinese and disseminated to all medical schools in Taiwan during the following 2 years. The TMAC then held several meetings with school representatives for the purpose of further revision and clarification. It also explained the process and introduced the new standards at the biannual Deans' Conference on two occasions.

4   In 2012, five medical schools in Taiwan were due for 'full review' in the second cycle of the TMAC accreditations, and TMAC members of the TMAC-SOS each participated in the visit of a particular school to perform a 'test run' on the newly drafted standards.
5   In 2013, TMAC-SOS held several meetings to discuss findings from the 'test run' and the feedback from schools. It also took into consideration standards used by other international organisations. The new TMAC-SOS standards were presented to the Deans' Conference in September 2013, and were ready for implementation in 2014.

With the assistance of the LCME, the accreditation standards of the TMAC have been extensively overhauled, and members of the Council are currently revising the TMAC Institutional Self-Analysis. The Council has especially come to appreciate the following areas of relevance in the process:

1   The value of learning from others' experiences, particularly the process by which LCME established the American accreditation system and carried out the development, application and revision of standards. The TMAC also learned through the participation of its members as international observers in two LCME accreditation visits in 2009 and, since then, has maintained regular updates by attending the LCME sessions at the annual AAMC meeting.
2   The impact on accreditation standards in diverse countries of differences in the structure and history of the medical education system and of differences in language and culture.
3   The process of overhauling the accreditation standards, which includes maximising communication between accreditation organisations, the deans and other representatives of medical schools, and the value of carrying out a 'test run'.
4   The importance of involving key persons in the process, including surveyors and schools, to increase the precision of the standards, and to help schools identify areas for improvement as well as achieve the standardisation of medical education at a national level.

Institutional versus programme accreditation

When examining a country's use of accreditation, it is important to distinguish between systems that accredit institutions and those that accredit educational programmes. Almost all countries have some form of institutional accreditation, whereas a separate and independent system to accredit medical education programmes is less common. Institutional accreditation provides a broad level of oversight across many different levels of learners and many different types of degrees or certifications. Institutional accreditation systems can often include programmes ranging from early primary school to advanced degrees in medicine, law and nursing. Such broad coverage of diverse educational offerings means that the standards for institutional accreditation cannot include the specificity and granularity needed for advanced and technical degree programmes such as medicine, nursing and other healthcare education programmes. Thus, more and more countries around the world are developing specialised programme accreditation for the healthcare fields. This is happening at the same time there has been a dramatic increase in the number of new medical schools emerging around the world. It becomes important to create systems of oversight that will ensure that all schools and their graduates meet quality standards. In simplistic terms, institutional accreditation is necessary but not sufficient for the complexities of assuring quality of medical education programmes. The description below of the relatively new medical education accreditation system for South Korea is a good example of a country taking on this challenge to provide this important level of quality assurance.

Case study 24.4   Developing an accreditation system from South Korea

Ducksun Ahn

In 1996, the Ministry of Education in Korea conducted institutional evaluation of all medical schools and published their ranking. The medical professional community criticised the validity of this evaluation as it was performed by non-medical faculty members, and further rejected the idea of creating a hierarchy among schools as it only assessed relative excellence. The institutional evaluation was not well suited for medical education and did not mitigate the problems resulting from the rapid expansion of medical schools (six schools with 805 students in 1950, increased to 41 with 3,072 students in 1997).

This was the impetus for the research and development of a national programme evaluation system for quality control of basic medical education. In 1997 the Accreditation Board for Medical Education in Korea (ABMEK) was established to do this; and in 1999, ten newly established medical schools were evaluated against the standards developed by this group.

After this successful pilot study, ABMEK expanded and became the Korean Institute of Medical Education and Evaluation (KIMEE) and officially launched its first accreditation in 2003. All 41 medical schools in the country voluntarily agreed to participate in the first cycle, which started in 2000 and ended in 2005. One medical school refused to participate after two consecutive follow-up visits due to poor evaluation results. It was only in 2011 that KIMEE, with the help of the National Assembly, passed a new health act preventing graduates of non-accredited medical schools from sitting for the national licensure examination.

Initially standards were developed by benchmarking other international organisations. The main objective of the first accreditation was to obtain full voluntary support from all 41 medical schools, and therefore special attention had to be paid to avoid burdening schools with excessive preparatory activities while still pushing newly established medical schools to meet the minimum standards. The first standards were related to resources, entry-level student characteristics and other input-driven issues, and were relatively easy for the established and long-standing medical schools. Over time, the standards became more stringent, increasing from approximately 50 to the current 97 items.

After the KIMEE completed its first accreditation in 2003, the overall satisfaction rate with KIMEE was a little over 70 per cent, and the most recent survey in 2011 showed it to be currently over 90 per cent. All medical schools, with one exception, acknowledged the necessity of a quality assurance system and supported the current accreditation programme. Annually, all medical schools pay fixed annual dues to the KIMEE for its accreditation work. In addition, the Korean Medical Association (KMA) subsidises approximately half of the remaining budget to the KIMEE, with the Korean Hospital Association (KHA) sponsoring the rest.

Accreditation in itself is a relatively new concept for East Asian countries. The South Korean government is still very much in a state of confusion in this area, and the Ministry of Education attempts to exert control over this voluntary programme through an official recognition process create tension between the Ministry of Education and the professional accrediting agencies. However, overall, the quality assurance systems that have been put in place show continued improvement and the consistent exchange with other international agencies (e.g. LCME, WFME, UK General Medical Council (GMC), Australian Medical Council (AMC) and the Royal College of Physicians and Surgeons of Canada (RCPSC)) continues to bear positive synergistic effects.

International recognition of accreditation

To stimulate further the global movement for accreditation, on 21 September 2011 the Educational Commission for Foreign Medical Graduates (ECFMG), in the USA, announced that, beginning in 2023, physicians receiving medical degrees outside of the USA and Canada who apply for residency or fellowship training in the USA must graduate from a school,

> that has been appropriately accredited. To satisfy this requirement, the physician's medical school must be accredited through a formal process that uses criteria comparable to those established for US and Canadian medical schools by the Liaison Committee on Medical Education (LCME) or that use other globally accepted criteria such as those put forth by the WFME.
>
> (ECFMG 2010: 1)

The reasoning for this requirement not being scheduled to take effect until 2023 is that there is no existing universally accepted accreditation process for medical schools. The ECFMG stated the hope that this requirement would stimulate development of such a system. The WFME philosophy, while supportive of the ECFMG decision and partnering with this effort, has a different perspective on whether there should be a universally accepted system for accreditation. Instead, WFME asserts that each region or country should develop its own accreditation system. To facilitate this approach, the WFME offers examples of accreditation standards and supports a process to recognise accrediting bodies. This recognition process allows countries or regions to have their accreditation systems reviewed through a peer review process. Schools that are accredited by a WFME-recognised accreditor satisfy the ECFMG requirement. The recognition process requires the submission of documents describing policies, standards and governance. A team of three international medical educators then observes a team conducting a survey visit, and this same team from the WFME then attends the accreditation meeting where that school is discussed. This recognition process was first applied to the Caribbean Accreditation Authority for Education in Medicine and other Health Professions (CAAM-HP), which received WFME recognition status on 10 May 2012. The Association for Evaluation and Accreditation of Medical Education Programs, Turkey (TEPDAD) received its recognition on 31 July 2013. The LCME was similarly reviewed and received its recognition on 28 January 2014.

Ensuring that new medical schools meet quality standards

One of the urgent issues that countries must consider when deciding whether to adopt a programme-level accreditation for their medical schools is the dramatic and relatively unregulated growth of new medical schools around the world. It should come as no surprise that many of these new schools are emerging in countries without medical education programme accreditation systems in place. The countries most vulnerable for unregulated growth and, therefore, students and the public most at risk, are those that have neither programme accreditation nor national licensing examinations. Brazil is one such country that is without programme accreditation or a national examination system and has seen the number of medical schools increase from a little over 120 in 2005 to over 180 by 2007, with that number holding steady as of 2013. Many or most of these new schools are private, for-profit entities, and the types of resources available for the students and the quality of the programmes themselves are unknown. The number of graduates of these new schools has exceeded this country's ability to provide postgraduate training and, since postgraduate training is not a requirement, many of these graduates will simply go directly into practice. With the absence of an accreditation system, no one knows the quality or the resources of these new programmes and, with no national licensing examination, the knowledge and skills levels of the individual graduates are also unknown. For example, there are many key questions that cannot be answered:

- How much direct patient care experience do these graduates have?
- How much of the sciences basic to medicine have they learned, and to what extent do they know how to apply this knowledge in the care of patients?
- To what extent were there opportunities for active learning to ensure that these graduates will know how to be, and be willing to be, lifelong learners?

There are many challenges for a country that seeks to set up programme-level accreditation for the first time. As difficult as it is in deciding what standards to use, how to create the supporting documents or train team members, the hardest part is establishing the governance system that grants authority to a peer group. This is most difficult in countries that have strong central government control and don't have as much experience in delegating authority to non-governmental groups. Then the issues of how the accreditation system is funded and how you manage the potential conflicts of interest with the funding source are both barriers to overcome. Indonesia is a country that is in the process of establishing a new programme accreditation system for several healthcare disciplines while at the same time creating a national examination for all medical school graduates.

Case study 24.5 Establishing a quality assurance system of medical education in Indonesia

Puti Marzoeki

Concern about the quality of Indonesia's medical doctors has been growing in the country for the last two decades. Frequent reports of malpractice and cases of neglect have triggered public debate, and at the same time raised people's awareness and expectations about the quality of available care. Increasingly, individuals who can afford it prefer to go overseas for their healthcare needs. Meanwhile, the number of medical schools has expanded by 80 per cent during the last 10 years, from 40 schools in 2003 to 72 schools in 2013; and of those 72, about 60 per cent are private medical schools. The tuition fees, particularly in private medical schools, have more than tripled during the same period of time. Concerned about the quality and increasing costs to students, the Directorate General of Higher Education suspended the licensing of new medical schools in 2011 until a more effective regulatory framework for medical education is in place. The urgency on the part of the government for this regulatory and quality assurance system is partly driven by the increased globalisation of the labour market under the Association of South East Asian Nations (ASEAN) and the Asia Free Trade Area (AFTA).

Support for medical education reform in Indonesia began in 2005 with the introduction of a competency-based curriculum that included a student-oriented approach that utilised problem-based learning, the integration of disciplines, community orientation and early exposure to clinical settings. The period of study was shortened by 1 year to accelerate production in response to the need for more doctors. A 12-month internship was added in 2012 that provided enhanced clinical supervision. The Indonesia Medical Council, as part of the reform, facilitated the development and publishing in 2006 of standards of competencies for medical doctors and standards of basic medical education. This effort was the foundation for subsequent accreditation work as it effectively engaged multiple stakeholders. The stakeholders involved in developing and adopting these documents and standards were the Indonesia Medical Association and the Association of Indonesia Medical Association Institutions, the College of Indonesian Doctors, the Ministry of Health and the Ministry of National Education. The Indonesia Medical Council also commissioned a consortium to develop the National Competency-Based Examination at the same time that the accreditation system was being developed. This national examination was administered for the first time in June 2007.

These efforts continued under the Health Professional Education Quality (HPEQ) programme launched in 2010 that involved both government and non-government stakeholders through task forces specially formed to support the reform process. The main reform agenda included strengthening the methodology of the National Examination, and establishing a specific accreditation system for health professional education, including medical education. The reform included the establishment of two independent bodies: an independent accreditation agency for health professional education (Lembaga Akreditasi Mandiri Perguruan Tinggi Kesehatan: LAM-PTKes), and an independent agency for developing the methodology and quality assurance system of the national examination (Lembaga Pengembangan Uji Kompetensi: LPUK).

Like many other countries, Indonesia has for the past 20 years had an agency that provided institutional accreditation, but this covers some 3,100 higher-education institutions and 16,200 study programmes in Indonesia. The standards for this institutional accreditation are far too broad to provide detailed focus on healthcare programmes, and that is why this next level of accreditation for medical schools and other health professional schools has been instituted. Even before the launch of the HPEQ programme in 2010, the Indonesia Medical Council engaged the institutional accreditor with a memorandum of understanding to collaborate in strengthening the accreditation of medical schools. This memorandum allowed the development of specific accreditation instruments for assessing medical education. The HPEQ played a strategic role in accelerating the establishment of an accreditation system specific to seven disciplines: medicine, dentistry, nursing, midwifery, pharmacy, nutrition and public health. Consultations were carried out with international and national experts and teams of Indonesians were sent overseas to learn from different more established accrediting organisations. The design of the system called for accreditation by an independent accreditation body established specifically for accrediting health professional education (LAM-PTKes). The inclusion of the seven disciplines opened up the opportunity for interprofessional communication, although accreditation of all seven disciplines by a single accreditation agency is challenging. The system is formative, aiming for continuous quality improvement, with financing independent from the government.

The process of establishing the accreditation system for Indonesia continues. While the blueprint of the accreditation system, the accreditation instruments and the accreditation business process are ready, ensuring synergy with existing government regulation and building consensus through broad-based participation of all stakeholders, including government and non-government entities, have required more time than expected. After lengthy debate and arduous legal process, the Minister of Education and Culture released a decree in October 2014 recognising LAM-PTKes as an independent accreditation body for health professional education.

(continued)

> *(continued)*
>
> Several lessons from the Indonesia medical education reform process are:
>
> - Existing government regulations are often not ready to support a professional community-led, peer review, quality assurance system. Transferring the authority from the government to non-government entities is difficult.
> - Strong collaboration between government and non-government entities is essential in conducting the reform process.
> - Building the capacity of professional associations is an important investment in developing the capacity for medical education quality assurance.

The efforts being made by Indonesia to institute a country-wide accreditation system are notable for the decision to move forward to address the relatively unregulated growth of new medical schools. Also important to draw from this case study is the essential but challenging need for consensus among the many stakeholders to create a decision-making body that can function independently to peer review programmes according to the standards. For countries that are used to centralised government appointees having the authority for decision making, it takes time and consensus building to establish the trust of independent decision makers that are comprised of practitioners and academics.

External evaluation: accreditation

Governance, financing and authority

There are different types of governance models for programme accreditation around the world. When evaluating the pros and cons of different models, the basic questions are: 'Who is underwriting or funding the programme?' and 'How independent are the accreditation decisions from the influences of this funding?' Many accreditation systems are fee-based, independent, free-standing entities. Often, a fixed annual fee is levied by the accrediting agency and/or individual fees for specific services are charged. This free-standing governance model raises a potential conflict of interest when the accreditation agency that charges fees for a service is the agency that prescribes the service itself. This ethical dilemma is not unlike the role of the physician who both treats the patient and prescribes a service (procedure or revisit) that financially benefits the prescriber. It is an issue that must be acknowledged and openly discussed.

Other governance models entail partnerships with professional associations and/or government agencies. These sponsoring partners often play a role in the financing of the accrediting agency, which lessens the cost burden to the schools. In this case, care must be taken to ensure that potential conflicts of interest do not arise, and that the decisions made by the accreditation committee are free of any interference from these stakeholders. One model of managing the potential conflict is that the group that makes the accreditation decisions is left to make and carry out those actions independently. The sponsoring associations or governmental agencies that are participating in the funding are blinded to these decisions but they can participate in policy deliberations that expand the scope of the work or have major budgetary implications.

Standards are the lens through which accreditation views the world

Standards are the statements that unify the examination system of accreditation. An important first step in developing a regional or national medical education programme accreditation system is the creation of a set of national standards. Ideally, this process includes a variety of stakeholder groups. There are many good examples of standards for medical education programmes, including standards developed by the WFME, the GMC for the UK, the AMC for Australia and New Zealand and the LCME for the USA/Canada. However, it is important to emphasise that, while existing standards can be good models for a specific region or country, it would be a mistake simply to adopt a set of pre-existing standards. Failing to go through the process of creating country-specific standards would miss the important process of gathering medical school faculty, practising physicians, students and representatives of the public to debate what is best for that specific country. The example described earlier related to Taiwan's reformulation of its existing standards is an excellent model for others to follow. This process is more likely to lead to standards that are more widely accepted and understood, which is vital to the implementation of any accreditation system. In the end, the standards throughout the world may look far more similar than different; however, the process of reaching consensus for a given country or region is crucial.

The standards inform the documentation that needs to be collected by the survey team and included in the survey report. They also create the framework that facilitates objective decision making about accreditation status and consistent review across programmes. A brief review of how the WFME standards are formatted can assist in understanding the layers of meaning that are inherent in well-written accreditation standards.

International standards

The WFME standards were first published in 2003, modelled in part on the LCME standards, and were revised in 2012 (WFME 2012). The standards are structured according to the following nine areas: mission and outcomes, educational programme, assessment of students, students, academic staff/faculty, educational resources, programme evaluation, governance and administration, and continuous renewal.

The nine areas are defined as 'broad components in the structure, process, and outcome of medical education' (WFME 2012). Under these nine areas of standards are a total of 36 more specific sub-areas which correspond to performance indicators. In the case of the WFME, the standards are specified for each sub-area using two levels of attainment:

1. a *basic standard* is an area that must be met by every medical school;
2. a standard *for quality development* indicates a level that would be expected as a best practice for a medical school.

Annotations supplement the standards by providing examples or clarification of language of the standards. Listed on the WFME website (World Federation for Medical Education 2014) are 100 basic standards, 91 quality development standards and 121 annotations.

As an example, consider the WFME *basic* standard related to educational outcomes (1.4):

> The medical school *must* define the intended educational outcomes that students should exhibit upon graduation in relation to:

- their achievements at a basic level regarding knowledge, skills, and attitudes (B 1.4.1);
- appropriate foundation for future career in any branch of medicine (B 1.4.2);
- their future roles in the health sector (B 1.4.3);
- their subsequent postgraduate training (B 1.4.4);
- commitment to and skills in lifelong learning (B 1.4.5);
- the health needs of the community, the needs of the healthcare system; and
- other aspects of social accountability (B 1.4.6).

(WFME 2012: 20)

The WFME *quality development* standard for that educational outcome area is:

The medical school should:

- specify and coordinate the linkage of outcomes to be acquired by graduation with that to be acquired in postgraduate training (Q 1.4.1);
- specify outcomes of student engagement in medical research (Q 1.4.2); and
- draw attention to global health related outcomes (Q 1.4.3).

(WFME 2012: 20)

These standards are 'non-prescriptive'. This means that they do not specify exactly what or how something must be done, but instead they indicate the areas that must be addressed. It is up to the faculty of the medical school to determine how to ensure that students develop the skills of lifelong learning and the commitment to apply them. It is up to an accreditation survey team to determine if that is taking place appropriately at that school.

In contrast, 'prescriptive' standards are much more specific. As an example, the accreditation standards for postgraduate or residency training in the USA are prescriptive in nature. They indicate, based on how many new residents enter the programme each year, exactly how much time must be allocated for the programme director and how many assistant directors must be in place. There are pros and cons for both types of standards. Prescriptive standards are much easier to measure, verify and document. A disadvantage of prescriptive standards is that they do not allow variations based on unique missions of a school and they restrict mission-based innovation. Prescriptive standards tend to be more common when there are many (hundreds and hundreds) of programmes to be accredited. Non-prescriptive standards are more difficult to measure and require assessment by experts familiar with that type of programme. On the other hand, they allow faculty to adjust their educational programme and the resources to address specific needs and missions of the school. Non-prescriptive standards can be frustrating to a university president who wants to know how many faculty she will need to establish a medical school. The answer, with non-prescriptive standards, is that it depends on the mission of the school, the nature of the curriculum, whether it was based in the community or in a research institution, etc. However, what a university president sometimes understands from that response is 'we can't tell you, but we will know it when we see it.' Non-prescriptive standards, while fostering creativity, require thorough guidelines for schools that are preparing for a review and careful training of the survey team and the committee in order to reduce subjectivity and support consistency in the decision-making process.

Survey teams and decision-making committees

The survey teams are primarily peer based and composed of different combinations of faculty from basic sciences, clinical sciences, medical school administration and, in a number of countries, students. The size of a team varies in different countries, with as many as ten in Taiwan to three or six in other countries. Teams should include 'peers' who are either physician practitioners or faculty involved in a medical school, but team characteristics vary based on the members' areas of expertise and the types of settings in which they practise or the nature of the schools in which they teach. Teams should be created based on the type of school that is about to be surveyed. For example, an intense research-based medical school will often have at least one team member (but not all) from another research-intense medical school. In the construction of a team, careful attention must be paid to conflicts of interest, so as to manage real and perceived challenges to objectivity. In the USA, teams will occasionally have observers who are there from other countries to afford them an opportunity to experience an accreditation survey visit. One unique aspect of team composition in the USA and Canada is the role of the fellow. A fellow is an individual who has been nominated by the dean of a medical school that will undergo its own accreditation survey visit in the next 2 or 3 years. Fellows are nominated to a team because they are designated to manage their own school's self-study in the future. This allows them the opportunity to see how to prepare for their own school's accreditation visit.

Team training is essential and particularly important when the standards are non-prescriptive. Cases using school information (in an anonymous fashion) that highlight the complexities inherent in some standards are very effective in assisting team surveyors to understand their meaning and application. Webinars and online asynchronous modules greatly improve the ability to ensure that all team members are prepared for their responsibilities. Also essential is a process to gather evaluation information after each visit about the quality of each team member. Evaluations from the school that was visited can be helpful; however, more useful are evaluations completed by team members about other team members. Assessing the quality of team members' knowledge of the standards, the quality of their preparation, the conduct during the survey visit and the quality of their written contributions are important evaluation benchmarks.

The level of detail in a survey team report varies among accreditation agencies. Some use reports that document only the areas that have been judged to be out of compliance. Others require teams to write more extensive reports providing evidence as to the status of all standards. The committee or council that will receive the report from the survey team and make the accreditation status decision is again comprised of peers, but in some countries, may also include students and members of the public who have no connection to medical education except as recipients of healthcare services. This committee is often staffed and managed by individuals either experienced in accreditation or familiar with medical education, or both.

The number of staff needed to manage an accreditation system depends on the number of schools in the country/region, the length of the accreditation term (and the corresponding number of survey visits per year), the information technology and other resources available for this activity and the nature of the standards. As an example, the LCME, which utilises an 8-year accreditation term, makes decisions for 141 medical schools in the USA and 17 medical schools in Canada, and is in the process of overseeing the development of 18 new medical schools, some of which are included in the total numbers of schools for both countries and some that are still in the very early stages of accreditation. To support this effort, the LCME has four full-time professional staff who, prior to joining the accreditation team, had extensive experience as faculty members and held various administrative roles in medical school dean offices. Supporting them are six administrative staff. The LCME meets three times annually and each meeting is approximately 3 days in length. The agenda for each meeting includes the reports from approximately six to seven full surveys, 30–40 status (follow-up) reports, and four to ten proposals for class size expansion and new branch campuses. Each of the 19 members of the LCME serves as a primary or secondary reviewer for a number of these reports. For each report, the reviewer makes a general recommendation for accreditation status and follow-up to the entire committee, with ample time for discussion. Having web-based documents with efficient reviewer reporting worksheets so that all members can preview the reviewer's recommendations is essential in order to get this volume of decision making accomplished in the allotted time frame. This process, while supporting efficient decision making, has implications for information technology and staffing needs.

Follow-up of findings

The decision-making committee reviews the team report and then comes to a decision related to the accreditation status of a given medical education programme. There are a number of choices that a committee may have when determining accreditation status. Withdrawal or denial of accreditation is always an option; however, it is generally exercised only in egregious situations and after all other remedial options have been exhausted. The safety of the public must be paramount at all times, and the welfare of the students at the institution being judged must also be considered. Removal of accreditation strands the students who are currently enrolled. When the situation is not serious enough to warrant withdrawal of accreditation, decisions are more focused on quality improvement. It is often said that an ideal outcome of an accreditation survey visit is that the medical school's internal self-study preceding the team visit identified areas in need of improvement that are consistent with the survey team's findings. This allows schools to begin to correct problem areas before the survey team arrives. For example, schools may have identified the need for renovations to certain facilities and have begun that work. However, at the time of the visit, the work is not complete. The LCME uses the term 'in compliance requiring monitoring' to indicate that a school, having identified the problem during its self-study, has already started but not yet completed the corrective action. This, and any areas that have been found to be non-compliant (i.e. not meeting one or more of the requirements of a standard), requires some form of follow-up. In most cases, when there are only a few areas needing follow-up or there is no immediate threat to the integrity of the medical education programme, the follow-up consists of a written report within 1–2 years with documentation that the issue has been resolved. In cases where the problems are more extensive or systemic, or if the situation threatens the quality of the medical education programme and student outcomes, another team may need to be sent to the school to provide a more thorough review of the corrections that have been put into place.

Confidentiality versus transparency

Just how transparent accreditation decisions should be is a frequent topic of conversation when directors of accreditation units gather for discussion. Those who argue for full disclosure of the team report and all decisions made by the accrediting committee make the point that the public – and especially the students – have the need and the right to know the strengths and weaknesses of a given educational programme. Some suggest that increased transparency would facilitate the quality improvement aspect of accreditation in that potentially more people would have access to problems that were identified, and thus, they could play a more effective role contributing to solutions.

Others argue that publicly publishing the survey report could hamper the directness that is used in describing problem areas and lead to less rigorous review. At the very least, all accreditation agencies should publish the accreditation status of each school and the date of its next scheduled visit. Accreditation agencies should also periodically publish reports that provide an overview of the actions taken, the standards that are most likely to give schools challenges and examples of best practices in meeting standards.

Accreditation summary

Accreditation of medical education programmes and other healthcare provider degrees is gaining more and more attention around the world. As movement of healthcare providers from one country to the next becomes commonplace, so grows the need to have systems in place to assure that the schools from which they graduate have provided their students with the basic medical knowledge, skills and attitudes. The WFME asserts that medical education accreditation should be a local phenomenon and provides both examples of standards and a recognition process for existing accrediting bodies. As described in the case studies from Taiwan and Korea, international consultation can be useful but ultimately, the standards and the procedures must be specific to that country or region. The Indonesian case study provides an example of an accreditation process in the middle of development and shows us that writing the standards and procedures is the easy part; the hard part is establishing the governance and the authority across the diverse schools within that country. Quality improvement and assurance are, at the end of the day, the most important aspects of accreditation. The case study from the USA shows us how standards and external peer review can lead to improvements in the learning environment, and the Canadian case study demonstrates how the standards can be used to create the blueprint for a new medical school.

Each school, in order to prepare for external peer review accreditation, must have in place its own systems that collect information to answer its own questions about how well the school's missions, goals and learning objectives are being met. This is where systems for programme evaluation become paramount.

Programme evaluation to support accreditation and quality assurance

While accreditation is a process that occurs at specified intervals, internal programme evaluation should be ongoing. Medical schools should have systems and processes in place to collect and interpret quantitative and qualitative data about educational programme quality. Which data are collected, and the timing of data collection, should be based on a set of overarching questions that administrators and other stakeholders have identified about the educational processes and outcomes. For example, is the programme meeting its missions, delivering a quality educational programme, appropriately supporting its students and faculty, and mobilising its resource in the most efficient and effective ways? The questions that guide programme evaluation, and the data collected to answer them, may be derived, in part, from accreditation standards. However, medical schools should create their own internal set of process and outcome questions that specifically focus on institutional priority areas.

Medical school programme evaluation systems for external and internal purposes should be designed with the following elements in mind:

1. what and when to evaluate;
2. what methods can be used in the evaluation;
3. what resources are needed to implement the evaluation system;
4. what evaluation data support decision making;
5. how the school will ensure that the changes needed to support quality improvement are implemented.

What to evaluate

Accreditors typically expect that schools evaluate both the outcomes and processes of the medical education programme and such a framework is useful for internal quality assurance purposes as well. Operationally, outcomes evaluation means determining the graduates' success in achieving the objectives of the medical education programme which, in turn, should be derived from the mission and goals of the medical school. Making such a judgement requires schools to define the educational programme objectives in outcome-based terms and to identify the measures that will be used to determine students' attainment of these objectives. Such outcomes typically include student knowledge, skills and professionalism, and could include mission-based outcomes such as specialty and practice choices and practice locations. Identifying how well the educational programme is working (i.e. the process dimension) includes evaluating student satisfaction with various areas, such as individual courses and clerkships and the curriculum as a whole, student support and counselling services, access to faculty, teaching facilities, and information and library resources. To identify if the educational programme is working well, faculty satisfaction may also be evaluated. The timing of such evaluations may vary. For example, schools typically evaluate performance in and satisfaction with courses and clerkships and with student services on an annual basis, while students' attainment of the educational programme objectives need to be evaluated when a cohort completes the curriculum.

In new schools, and schools implementing a new curriculum, the approach to evaluation should be structured to provide incremental information that can be used for formative purposes. For example, the quality of first-year courses would be evaluated to see what, if any, changes are needed (for example, in the organisation or density of content), and that changes could be made immediately. Then evaluation could be done to determine satisfaction with and performance in the second-year courses and to decide whether the first year provided adequate preparation for the second year. This incremental approach allows ongoing evaluation of the segments of the curriculum in themselves and in their relationship to segments prior and succeeding. As a new curriculum reaches its conclusion, a summative evaluation of both process and outcomes can be conducted.

How to evaluate

To evaluate the extent of success in meeting educational programme objectives, schools typically use the results of a variety of internal assessments of student performance, such as written examinations in courses and clerkships; observations of hands-on clinical skills; observations of cognitive skills, such as clinical reasoning; and observations of professionalism. The assessment tools, including examinations, checklists and rating scales, should provide, as far as possible, valid and reliable information. The school should have considered how each of the assessments contributes to a summative judgement about whether the individual student and the student body as a whole meet the educational programme objectives. This means that, ideally, the content of the items in the assessment instruments should be linked to the relevant objectives of the medical education programme. In addition to internal assessments, some countries have national examinations that allow normative comparisons of the school's students and graduates with a national cohort. For more information on assessment methods, consult Chapters 17, 18 and 19 in this volume.

Student satisfaction can be assessed through internal questionnaires to an entire cohort of students or to a selected group. There are several issues that schools should consider in utilising such measures. Schools should develop mechanisms to assure that response rates are high enough to provide a reliable evaluation. Strategies used include requiring students to complete the evaluation or providing incentives for students to comply. Providing information to students that the results of the evaluations are used to bring about change is also useful in motivating students to respond. The frequency and timing of evaluations are also important. Too frequent, too many, or too large questionnaires to a given group of students may decrease response rates, but too long an interval after a course has concluded can make the results less certain. To decrease the response burden on any given student, schools sometimes use a subset of students to evaluate a course, dividing the class randomly so that all courses are covered. Students typically desire confidentiality when evaluating courses or teachers, so any groups should be large enough or the process should be structured so an individual respondent cannot be identified. Finally, questionnaires often provide limited opportunities for students to explain their ratings. Focus groups can provide additional indepth information about areas that seem to require follow-up.

Resources to support programme evaluation

Accreditation standards often require that the medical school has sufficient resources to support the management and evaluation of a medical education programme. While such standards may specify only some needed resources, the internal quality assurance system should identify all the resources that the school believes to be important in educational programme planning, implementation and evaluation. Even in the absence of an accreditation mandate, a medical school should make resources available to support its internal quality assurance activities. There should be personnel, either located in a quality assurance office or as part of the medical school administration, who can develop and maintain the data collection system needed to determine if the educational process is working smoothly and educational programme outcomes are being met. This includes expertise in test development; questionnaire development; and other evaluation strategies, such as focus groups. In addition, information technology staff can support the online delivery of formative and summative assessments and course and clerkship evaluation questionnaires, as well as in ensuring data security. Information technology expertise is also needed in the implementation of a curriculum database that allows schools to identify where in the curriculum subjects related to the educational programme objectives are taught, and to determine the degree of content coverage related to each educational programme objective. The quality assurance staff should have appropriate administrative support and should have direct access to individuals and groups charged to make decisions about educational programme quality, such as the curriculum committee, and to relevant administrators.

Evaluation data that support decision making related to programme quality

Accreditation standards typically require that data about programme quality, including process and outcomes, be used for programme improvement. This should be the case for internal quality assurance activities as well. Decisions about quality should be made taking into account the following four categories of data.

Clear policies and processes

There should be clear policies and processes related to student assessment, advancement and graduation and these should be applied in a consistent way for individual students. This will result in data such as course passing and graduation rates, useful in the evaluation of such things as admission requirements.

Evaluating the curriculum as a whole

The committee responsible for the curriculum (i.e. curriculum committee) should periodically conduct a review of the outcomes of the curriculum. The review should be structured to answer several questions related to assuring that the curriculum is a coherent whole:

- To what extent does student performance indicate that the curriculum is achieving its objectives? How effective are the systems to address areas where performance is not optimal? What is the basis for any gaps in performance?
- To what extent is the content of the curriculum coordinated and integrated so that educational programme objectives are sufficiently addressed? To what extent are relevant content areas or skills taught sufficiently and appropriately sequenced across the curriculum?

Evaluating the individual segments of the curriculum (courses and clerkships)

Data should be collected about student performance in, and satisfaction with, individual courses and clerkships and as well as in curriculum segments. These data include the process as well as the outcomes of teaching. For example, it is useful to know to what extent the students think a course was well organised and addressed the stated objectives, as well as the extent to which teachers were prepared, available and organised. Students also can comment on the organisation of content and learning activities within a given year (horizontal integration) and across years (vertical integration).

Non-curricular outcomes

Based on their missions or the mandates of the country, province or state that regulates them, medical schools may have expected outcomes related to such things as the specialty choice or practice location of graduates. In order to determine whether these outcomes have been met, schools will need to collect data from students and graduates and/or from external agencies within the region. If the school finds that these outcomes are not being met, for example, the graduates are not choosing primary care practice or are not practising in the region, the school will need to determine the steps to take, and those that must be taken externally, to improve the outcome.

Decision making and programme improvement

Information about the process and outcomes of courses and curriculum segments should be reviewed by course directors, leaders of relevant departments and the committee responsible for the curriculum. A remediation plan for any identified deficiencies should be developed and there should be follow-up on the outcomes of the changes that are made. These should be reported as well, to ensure that the remediation plan has been implemented appropriately and is effective.

Decisions about the curriculum as a whole should include a determination of whether each of the educational programme objectives has been attained. This requires the curriculum committee and responsible administrators to collate the data from across the curriculum that relates to each objective. For example, for an objective related to professionalism there may be information from student performance during small groups in one year, from preceptor assessments in another year, from Objective Structured Clinical Examinations (OSCEs) and from physician evaluations during the clerkships. There should also be a review of the content associated with the professionalism taught across years so as to determine if there are gaps or redundancies and a review of student satisfaction with the teaching. All these bits of data are assembled to determine if the outcomes related to professionalism have been achieved and if the process to support professionalism teaching is working well.

To accomplish this comprehensive review of curriculum outcomes and process, the curriculum committee should have the logistical support to gather and analyse the appropriate data. Once a determination of success in meeting objectives has been made, a plan to address any gaps can be developed and implemented. For example, if the evaluation of the professionalism objective identifies that clinical ethics is not being taught, the curriculum committee should have the authority to mandate that this subject be added in an appropriate location.

Take-home messages

- Both accreditation and internal quality assurance require and depend on a robust process of ongoing programme evaluation.
- This requires planning to develop the system, resources to implement the system and appropriate authority delegated to the responsible individuals and groups to ensure that needed changes are made.
- As the WFME emphasises, medical education accreditation should be a local phenomenon. Countries establishing their own accreditation systems should draw from the experience of established programmes but they should write their own standards based on their regional healthcare issues, cultural factors and resources.
- As countries see medical education accreditation as a way to improve the healthcare workforce, attention to the potential conflicts of interest inherent in any funding scheme need to be managed carefully.
- Countries that write their own standards often initially create prescriptive standards such as expectations of square-foot formulas per student. As experience grows and training of site visitors improves, it is recommended that standards be developed that draw more upon peer judgement and focus on educational outcomes.

Bibliography

Council for Higher Education Accreditation (2010) *The value of accreditation*. Online. Available HTTP: http://cihe.neasc.org/downloads/ValueofAccreditationCHEA.pdf (accessed 20 March 2014).

Educational Commission for Foreign Medical Graduates (2010) *EFMG to require medical school accreditation for international medical school graduates seeking certification beginning in 2023*. Online. Available HTTP: http://www.ecfmg.org/forms/9212010.press.release.pdf (accessed 11 August 2014).

Strasser, R.P., Lanphear, J.H., McCready, W.G., Topps, M.H., Hunt, D.D. and Matte, M.C. (2009) 'Canada's new medical school: The Northern Ontario School of Medicine: Social accountability through distributed community engaged learning', *Academic Medicine*, 84(10): 1459–64.

Strasser, R.P., Hogenbirk, J.C., Minore, B., Marsh, D.C., Berry, S., McCready, W.G. and Graves, L. (2013) 'Transforming health professional education through social accountability: Canada's Northern Ontario School of Medicine', *Medical Teacher*, 35(6): 490–6.

University of California, Davis (2014) *Principles of community*. Online. Available HTTP: http://catalog.ucdavis.edu/community.html (accessed 23 September 2014).

World Federation for Medical Education (2005) *Promotion of accreditation of basic medical education*. Online. Available HTTP: www.wfme.org/accreditation/whowfme-policy (accessed 20 March 2014).

Accreditation and programme evaluation

World Federation for Medical Education (2012) *Basic medical education: WFME global standards for quality improvement: The 2012 revision*. Online. Available HTTP: www.wfme.org/news/general-news/263-standards-for-basic-medical-education-the-2012-revision (accessed 20 March 2014).
World Federation for Medical Education (2014) *Basic medical education*. Online. Available HTTP: www.wfme.org/standards/bme (accessed 23 September 2014).

PART 7

The future of medical education

25
LOOKING TOWARD THE FUTURE OF MEDICAL EDUCATION
Fit for purpose

Stewart Mennin

A reflection on and analysis of the practices in medical education around the world with regard to the roles of teachers and students and what students should learn, how they should learn, how we know they have learned, and how a curriculum should be developed, organised, and evaluated; an outline of key potential changes in medical education over the next decade.

You walk into the future with your back because the only thing you can see is the past.

Traditional Māori proverb

The long history of healing, medicine and science woven together with the more recent history of contemporary healthcare practices and health systems in local cultural contexts has produced the pattern of medical education observed around the world. *The Routledge International Handbook of Medical Education* explores contemporary patterns of what is working in a wide variety of settings and conditions. We turn now briefly to explore possible futures of medical education based on what we understand today and to consider conditions that could promote the emergence of future practices and theories in medical education. Looking to the future of medical education, one becomes acutely aware that the present and future can co-exist only in our shared imaginations and that the further into the future one looks, the less predictable it becomes. The gap between the present and the future of medical education is influenced and shaped by existing local and regional conditions. Questions and adaptive actions disturb those conditions such that resilience and innovation continuously emerge as fit for the function of medical education in the future.

Inquiry in the present tense (tension)

Questioning and inquiry based on present tensions and gaps between what is and what could be will create the future of the field of medical education. Medical education will continue to mature, becoming flexible enough to accommodate new and varied contexts and also capable of adapting to a strong grounding in established and proven practice (Hamilton and Yasin,

Chapter 20, this volume). It is critical that medical education emerges as a valued and essential professional career in the education and health systems of the future. Future practices of medical education will be more closely linked to the underlying assumptions and theories that inform and explain them. At the same time, theories of medical education will be played out and tested in action research and practice. Together practice and theory will continue to be a productive interdependent pair of activities promoting learning, understanding in and on action through, rich, relational, recursive and robust study, scholarship and research (Doll 1993). A few questions may serve to illustrate this point:

- How can teachers and students best work together to learn across and within the full range of conditions and settings in health practices and in health professions education?
- Who decides, and how, who goes to medical school?
- How is it decided what needs to be learned, where and when?
- How can we know learning for students, teachers, practitioners and researchers is happening, has happened and will continue to happen?
- How best can we use current resources to plan, develop, organise and evaluate medical education?
- How can advances in science and technology best serve the process of preparing present and future physicians?
- Who can be a teacher of medical students and how can the teacher best be prepared for this social responsibility?
- How do we explore and understand change?
- How do we deal with inequities in access to health and education at local, regional and global levels?
- How best can we sustain the relevance of the relationship between medical education and the health of the public?

And there are many more questions.

Students are the future: whose future? When?

Medical students are the future of medical education. Yet for most of them, their projection into the future may be focused on relatively short-term goals, and specific competencies and outcomes necessary to qualify and become a practising physician. How well prepared and how comfortable will they be as individuals and in collaborative groups to recognise and work with uncertainty? The part of the future that for them begins now can increase their experience recognising, working and learning with and from uncertainty. This is especially important early in their medical education experience as it fits seamlessly with the sciences basic to medicine and basic clinical skills (Mennin, Chapter 13, this volume). Traditionally medical education has reserved learning in authentic scenarios, i.e. those scenarios characterised as having high degrees of uncertainty, for students in the latter part of their education. This educational strategy is based on the assumption that learning, teaching, assessing and curriculum structure are additive, i.e. a step-by-step series of phases that build a foundation piece by piece over time (Bloom et al. 1954; Miller 1990). Some of medical education fits this concept; however, most of it does not (Mennin 2013). The growing importance of early authentic clinical and community experiences and assessment in the workplace has introduced higher dimensions of uncertainty earlier into the landscape of medical education. In addition, longitudinal clerkships rather than the traditional 2- or 3-month rotations have moved in this direction. This is a trend we believe will continue to grow in the future.

Another related key change occurring now and continuing into the future of medical education is the co-evolution of the relationship between students and teachers working and learning together in all levels of public health and healthcare services, promoting collaborative interdisciplinary educational experience that addresses contemporary health challenges. As we experiment with and learn more about entrustable professional activities (EPAs) (ten Cate 2005), we should be able to develop EPAs to fit all levels of student responsibility, including those early in the curriculum. There is a practical aspect to this idea as well; students can make more of a contribution to the health system earlier in their professional education at the same time as they are learning to become health professionals.

There are presently many programmes in place to reduce the gap between the profile of the local and regional populations being served by the health system and the socio-economic profile of students entering the medical professions. The assumption is that promoting equity of access to medical education among capable and qualified people around the world will decrease elitism in the selection of people who have the means to enter the present healthcare system and will foster more collaboration. Another way medical education can reach toward the future now is to focus on and select medical classes and students who are interested in working in areas of greatest need. Governments and their Ministries of Education and Health are challenged to allocate resources for health and the development of the health workforce necessary to meet the demands of the health of the public. In the near future, socially responsive admissions processes and committees will have found effective ways to collaborate to move future student and medical class profiles in this direction.

The future of medical education and technology

In the future, technology and its application will accelerate the rate at which the future appears to arrive. Some of this is already happening. It takes much longer to figure out the best application and fit for function of new technology than it does to develop the new technology itself. Medical students today are more comfortable, familiar and fluent with technology and social media than are their teachers and mentors, who are predominantly one or two generations older. Students and young teachers are more likely to be sensitive to the demands for the development and application of new technology in medical education, for example, different types of virtual classrooms, distributed learning, low- to high-tech simulation, social networking. Many forms of technology will get smaller, less costly and more accessible and as yet unimagined applications will appear. How we use them for the common good will be a continuing imperative for medical education in the 21st century.

Teaching, assessing and curriculum in, of and for the future of medical education

Medical education has moved from the large lecture hall, where communication was from one person to many, to small groups, where communication is many to many. Distributed knowledge will continue to grow and be more accessible. Fragmented curricula and isolated disciplines will be less prominent, while integration and interprofessional education will continue to grow. There is much discussion about and attention to social responsibility in medical education. What kind of social responsibilities will medical students and medical education be facing 10–20 years from now? Curriculum structure will become more fluid and capable of fitting both the learners' needs and the needs of the local population/health system. The capability to be sensitive to and act adaptively to changing circumstances will be necessary for graduates of the future. The scenarios and places in which learning experiences take place are moving toward primary integrated healthcare featuring more early clinical and community authentic learning and working experiences.

The recent recognition of the interdependence of student assessment and learning has made, and will continue to make, a significant difference for students, teachers and the field of medical education (Schuwirth and van der Vleuten 2004). This change has successfully challenged the status quo of assessment as predominantly a summative measurement problem (Schuwirth and van der Vleuten 2006). It has also raised the challenge for institutions to design assessment programmes that are fit for purpose. As assessment in the workplace and authentic practice increases, the reliance by medical educators on reductionist approaches to assessment fails to deliver data sufficient to make the inferences necessary for medical education to assure society that it is fulfilling its social contract with trust and integrity. The ability of the faculty/staff of a medical school to design and conduct a meaningful institution-wide assessment programme will be one of the more immediate future challenges in practice and research (Schuwirth and Ash 2013). Continued innovation in assessment thinking together with teaching, learning, curriculum planning and programme evaluation are and will continue to be important, especially as new medical schools are being created; hopefully walking into the future rather than running into the safety of the past.

Collaboration and the sustainability of medical education

Medical education and the practising health professions are social and collaborative by nature. Collaboration is the RNA of medical education. In the future of medical education, the tension between general practice and special interests and between autonomy and group collaborative work will be a productive and useful resource contributing to the well-being of society. The ability of medical education to study and promote a healthy workforce capable of meeting the needs of society in a rapidly changing future world is and will continue to be challenging and compelling. Well-defined outcomes for graduates of medical schools must continue to be relevant to regional health issues and vigorous in pursuit of high standards and quality. There will continue to be tension between those who hold conservative and traditional ideas and practices in medical education and those interested and willing to explore new ideas and their expression as methods and approaches that may be more fit for the future functions of a medical school. Collaboration and the recognition of the significance of cultural history are (Bleakley et al. 2008, 2011) and will be more important as international or transnational medical education evolves.

Leadership for and in the future

The formal and informal leadership (Heifetz 1994) of medical education and among health practitioners will be more and more challenging as responsibilities and duties continue to grow faster than the resources to support them. It will become essential for leadership to learn that not all problems can be solved with quick-fix, technical solutions. Working well in groups, leadership that is fit for purpose together with an enhanced sensitivity to and ability to work with both bottom-up local agents around issues and challenges and system-wide top-down influences will be a useful measure (metric) of the future of medical education and its leadership. The viability and sustainability of medical education in the future will most likely depend on how well collaboration that meets the needs of all concerned occurs. Furthermore, how medical schools, hospitals, clinics, laboratories and communities of all kinds identify, create and adapt what works and what sustainability looks like in medical education will be a useful topic of scholarship and research.

External standards and accreditation

The importance of and the role for external standards and accreditation will continue to grow in the future. Challenges will be related to the coherence of the dynamics of interactions among local needs for medical education and healthcare services and those of the greater whole of medical education in the national and international context. Whether the trend for schools in the future will be to specialise as an institution or to remain more general is not yet clear. The evaluation of institutional programs over time and of innovations in progress will become more and more important in the future as a vital source of data in decision making and resource allocation.

Collaboration

Collaboration in the future will occur among many interdependent pairs (Kelso and Engestrom 2006) co-embedded in many systems. For example:

- undergraduate–postgraduate;
- postgraduate–continuing medical education;
- continuing medical education–permanent education (Otero Ribeiro and Mennin 2010);
- personal responsibility–social responsibility;
- stability–innovation;
- familiarity–novelty;
- curative care–preventive care;
- individual–group/team;
- learning–assessment;
- urban–rural;
- primary care–tertiary care;
- hospital–ambulatory;
- local community needs–greater urban centre needs;
- and many more.

The challenge in the future will be how well individuals, departments and institutions, originally formed as independent, autonomous agents, are able to collaborate. To what extent will they be able to mobilise and value collaboration and semi-autonomy to address shared and significant problems, without feeling threatened by the fear of loss of their identity and status? This is a fundamental challenge that reaches well beyond medical education to embrace all of humanity. It's about how we get along and work together for the common good.

The future may be uncertain; however, we can be fairly comfortable about some things. The pace of change in medical education lags behind global, regional and local changes. Global conflicts, migration, displaced populations, levels of daily stress and competition for limited resources will most likely increase. Maldistribution of access to and distribution of healthcare resources by geography, economics and specialty choice will most likely continue. The need for equity of access to primary care and local healthcare workers will increase, as will the need for access to specialists. Advances in research and technology will appear more quickly than our ability to apply them most effectively. The movement toward collaboration in how we teach, learn and work together has begun and needs to grow faster and bigger. The world is becoming more, not less, complex and the challenges of cooperation, collaboration and working for the common good will require a paradigmatic change, not a programmatic change. We look forward to a future in which 'Nobody owns the truth and everyone has the right to be understood' (Doll 1993: 155).

Take-home messages

- Medical education must continue to mature and emerge as a valued and essential professional career in the education and health systems of the future.
- A closer linkage and relationship between practice and theory in medical education are a necessary interdependent pair of activities.
- Increased comfort with uncertainty across the full spectrum of medical education and practice is fit for the functioning of learning and practising in a rapidly changing world.
- Early and sustained learning experiences with authentic scenarios are important for integration, transdisciplinary and interprofessional education.
- Admission into medical school will move toward greater equity of access for all students and focus on selection of medical classes and students interested in working in areas of greatest need.
- Assessment and learning will continue to co-evolve.
- Effective collaboration and teamwork in learning, health practice and health systems will be an important measure of success.

Bibliography

Bleakley, A., Brice, J. and Bligh, J. (2008) 'Thinking the post-colonial in medical education', *Medical Education*, 42(3): 266–70.

Bleakley, A., Bligh, J. and Browne, J. (2011) *Medical education for the future: Identity, power and location*, Dordrecht: Springer.

Bloom, B.S., Engelhart, M.D., Furst, E.J., Hill, W.H. and Krathwohl, D.R. (1954) *Taxonomy of educational objectives: The classification of education goals. Handbook I: Cognitive domain*, New York, NY: Longman.

Doll Jr, W.E. (1993) *A post-modern perspective on curriculum*, New York, NY: Teachers College Press.

Heifetz, R.A. (ed.) (1994) *Leadership without easy answers*, Cambridge, MA: Belknap Press.

Kelso, S.J.A. and Engestrom, D.A. (2006) *The complementary nature*, Cambridge, MA: MIT Press.

Mennin, S. (2013) 'Health professions education: complexity, teaching and learning', In J.P. Sturmberg and C. Martin (eds) *Handbook of systems and complexity in health*, Heidelberg: Springer.

Miller, G.E. (1990) 'The assessment of clinical skills/competence/performance', *Academic Medicine*, 65(7): S63–7.

Otero Ribeiro, E.C. and Mennin, S. (2010) 'Continuing medical education: Guide supplement 35.2 – Viewpoint', *Medical Teacher*, 32(2): 172–3.

Schuwirth, L. and Ash, J. (2013) 'Assessing tomorrow's learners: In competency-based education only a radically different holistic method of assessment will work. Six things we could forget', *Medical Teacher*, 35(7): 555–9.

Schuwirth, L.W.T. and van der Vleuten, C.P.M. (2004) 'Changing education, changing assessment, changing research?', *Medical Education*, 38(8): 805–12.

Schuwirth, L.W.T. and van der Vleuten, C.P.M. (2006) 'A plea for new psychometric models and educational assessment', *Medical Education*, 40(4): 296–300.

ten Cate, O. (2005) 'Entrustability of professional activities and competency-based training', *Medical Education*, 39(12): 1176–7.

INDEX

Abbas, Farhat 308–10
Abdulghani, Hamza 274–5
Aboriginal people 5, 6, 7, 74, 192
academic ability 77–8, 80, 84
academic community 95–6
Academic Medicine Education Institute (AM.EI) 325, 326, 328
accountability 21, 24, 124, 323; *see also* social accountability
accreditation 330–47, 351; Australia 33; confidentiality versus transparency 346–7; continuous quality improvement 331–3; CPU model 14, 15; decision-making committees 346; definition of 331; evolution of systems 336–7; future of medical education 359; institutional versus programme 337–8; international recognition 51, 339; learning outcomes 32; Malaysia 48; new medical school development 297; resources 349; Saudi Arabia 51, 314, 316; South Africa 10; student involvement 89, 90; survey teams 344–6; as tool for change 333–5; transnational medical education 283, 284, 285, 287–8, 291; Tunisia 5; WFME standards 343–4
Accreditation Board for Medical Education in Korea (ABMEK) 338
Accreditation Council for Graduate Medical Education International (ACGME-I) 228
Accreditation Review Commission on the Certification of Physician Assistants (ARC-PA) 225
Accrediting Committee on Graduate Medical Education (ACGME) 28, 35–6, 38–9, 40

acquired immunodeficiency syndrome (AIDS) 49, 163, 311
Action for Global Health 45
action research 125
active learning: curriculum planning 124; new technologies 223, 234; problem-based learning 132; student engagement 86, 87, 89, 91, 93, 99
adaptive action landscape diagram 173–4, 183, 184
adaptive leadership 305, 306, 307, 313, 316
adaptive testing 257
admissions policies 12–13, 61, 65, 66, 74, 315, 334–5, 357; *see also* selection of students
adult learning theory 129
advocacy 28
affirmative action 165; *see also* positive discrimination
affordability of doctors 45
Afghanistan 44
Africa 116, 301, 311
African-Americans 3
Aga Khan University (AKU) 73–4, 308–11, 323–4, 327, 328
Ahn, Ducksun 65, 330–52
Akbarali, Laila 73–4
Al Alwan, Ibrahim A. 62–3
Al-Dubai, Sami Abdo Radman 47–50
Al-Faris, Eiad 238–9
Al Haqwi, Ali I. 62–3
Al-Hayani, Abdulmonem 39, 179
Al-Imam Mohammad Bin Saud Islamic University 313–15
Albert, M. 306

361

Index

Ali, Syeda K. 323–4
All India Institute of Medical Sciences 20–1
Allotey, P. 287
Al-Shehri, Mohammad Yahya 50–1
Alves de Lima, Alberto 268–9
American Board of Internal Medicine Foundation 4
American Society of Anesthesiologists (ASA) 273
American Society of Gastrointestinal Endoscopy (ASGE) 273
Amin, Hussain Saad 238–9
anatomy 176–7
Anderson, M. Brownell 318–29
Angoff method 242, 259
apprenticeship 151–2
apps 231
Arabian Gulf University 133, 134
Argentina 60–1, 68, 178, 267–9
Aristotle 318
Arokiasamy, John 47–50
Asia Free Trade Area (AFTA) 340
ASPIRE-to-Excellence in Medical Education 89, 99, 117, 121–2, 303
Assessing Change in Medical Education – The Road to Implementation (ACME-Tri) 172
assessment 209, 237–46, 302–3; authentic curriculum 117; authentic learning 141; case-based learning 140; clinical competence 263–77; community-based medical education 157, 161, 168; critical clinical competencies 295–6; curriculum planning 113; early clinical experience 147, 150, 153, 154; future of medical education 358, 360; integration of the sciences basic to medicine 180–5; interprofessional education 190, 198; King Abdulaziz University 179; new approaches to 29; NOSM 335; objective written tests 247–62; outcome-based education 34–6, 40; Peru 119; portfolio assessment 30, 40, 117, 172–3; problem-based learning 133, 134, 172; programme evaluation 348; progress tests 30; selection of students 82–3; social accountability 14; Social Obligation Scale 12; St George's Medical School 64; student engagement 92, 93, 97, 98; teacher's role 124; transnational medical education 285, 288, 289; Tunisia 5; Université de Sherbrooke 34; University of New Mexico 211, 212, 213; 'washback' effect 292; WFME standards 343; workplace-based 117, 173, 230–1, 238, 239, 264, 265–6, 272, 274–5; *see also* examinations
assessors 244, 265, 266

Association for Evaluation and Accreditation of Medical Education Programs, Turkey (TEPDAD) 339
Association for Medical Education in Europe (AMEE) 303
Association of American Medical Colleges (AAMC) 172, 332, 333
Association of South East Asian Nations (ASEAN) 160, 289–90, 340
Ateneo de Zamboanga University-School of Medicine (ADZU-SOM) 4, 8–9, 13, 14
attitudes 81, 102, 104
attrition rates 52; *see also* drop-out rates
Austral University 60–1
Australia: assessment 266, 275, 302; community-based medical education 158–9; distributed medical education 301–2; early clinical experience 145–6; graduate entry programmes 62, 65, 67, 68; interprofessional education 189–92; learning outcomes 32–3; new medical school development 297–8; outcome-based education 38; Parallel Rural Community Curriculum 69; positive discrimination 102; school-leaver entry 58–9, 60; selection of students 72, 74; social accountability 5–7; student employment 88; student engagement 86–7; transnational medical education 284–6, 287–8, 289, 290–1
Australian and New Zealand Association for Health Professional Educators (ANZAHPE) 190
Australian Learning and Teaching Council 32
Australian Medical Council (AMC) 283, 285, 286, 288, 291, 338, 343
Australian Survey of Student Engagement (AUSSE) 86–7
Austria 239–41
authentic curriculum 113, 114–17, 124, 126
authentic learning 128–43, 173; community-based medical education 167, 168; definition of 128; early clinical experience 151–4; theories underpinning 130–1; *see also* problem-based learning; task-based learning; team-based learning
autonomy 38, 88
Autor, D. 46
Autry, Amy 227
awards 159, 324, 325, 327–8, 333

Bahrain 133, 134
Ballweg, Ruth 225–7
Bandaranayake, Raja C. 118, 134

Index

Bangladesh 73
Baron, P. 88, 91
Barr, H. 189
Barragán, Elena I. 178
Barua, Ankur 47–50
Barzansky, Barbara 330–52
basic medical sciences 39, 104, 118, 119; assessment 180–5; authentic curriculum 117; community-based medical education 161; early clinical experience 144, 149, 150; graduate versus school-leaver entry 60, 65, 68, 69; Gulf Medical University 97; integration of the sciences basic to medicine 171–87; problem-based learning 58, 116, 132; scientific foundations of medicine 31; task-based learning 137, 138
Bateson, G. 217
Batra, Bipin 259–61
Battiola, Richard J. 321–2
Beane, J. 175
Beck, John 290
Bédard, Denis 33–4
behavioural objectives 37
behavioural theory 130, 209
belonging 88, 99
Ben-David, Miriam Friedman 180
benchmarking 47, 48
Bensimon, E.M. 87
Bernier, Frédéric 33–4
best practices 263–4, 266–73, 275, 276, 320, 324, 327, 329
Bin Abdulrahman, Khalid A. 86–100, 304–17
bio-psycho-social approach 102
Biomedical Admissions Test (BMAT) 72
Birch, S. 44–5
Bland, C.J. 306
Bleakley, A. 209, 282
blogs 123, 221, 223–4, 228, 229, 230, 233
Boelen, C. 10, 11, 14–15
Bologna Process 87
Bond University 58–9, 145–6
Bowden, J.A. 37
Bradley, Philip 283–4
'brain drain' 46
Brazil 165, 166, 167, 267, 275, 339–40
BRICS countries (Brazil, Russia, India, China and South Africa) 275
Brill, John R. 321–2
British Columbia (BC) 299–300
British Standards Institute 261
Brown University 38
Bryson, C. 88

Burch, Vanessa C. 263–77
burnout 88
Byamugisha, Josaphat 227

Canada: accreditation 334–5, 339, 343, 345, 347; assessment 275; basic medical sciences 172; as benchmark for Malaysia 47; distributed model of medical education 299–300; medical schools 3; outcome-based education 28, 33–4; productivity of nurses 44–5; selection of students 74, 78–9; social accountability 7–8; survey teams 345; transnational medical education 289
Canadian Interprofessional Health Collaborative (CIHC) 196
Canadian Physician Competency Framework (CanMEDS) 28, 38–9, 82
capabilities 190, 191
Capacity Body (Netherlands) 48
Capey, Steve 265–6
career choices 69, 75, 164–5
Caribbean Accreditation Authority for Education in Medicine and other Health Professions (CAAM-HP) 339
Carnegie Foundation for the Advancement of Teachers 326, 329
case-based discussions (CbDs) 264, 265, 274
case-based learning (CBL) 91, 129, 139–40
case repositories, online 228–9
Case, S.M. 248, 255
Case Western Reserve University 144, 172
Catholic University of Mozambique 116–17
Cayman Islands 52
Centeno, Angel 60–1
Centre for the Advancement of Interprofessional Education (CAIPE) 192
Challenge Model 199
Champin, Denisse 137
Chang, Yan-Di 336–7
change 125, 282; accreditation as tool for 333–5; adaptive leadership 313; change leaders 14, 189; climate of 263, 264
chart-stimulated recall (CsR) 264
cheating 261
CHEER collaboration 9–10, 14
Chen, H. Carrie 152–3
Chiasson, Paul 33–4
Chile 271–3
China 275
chronic diseases 44, 47, 192
class size 88, 135

363

Index

clerkships: assessment 239; British Columbia 300; critical clinical competencies 296; Faculty of Medicine of Tunis 5; Gulf Medical University 97; longitudinal 7, 158, 173, 174, 209, 335, 356; problem-based learning 133; programme evaluation 348, 349, 350; Université de Sherbrooke 33–4
climate of change 263, 264
clinical competence 263–77
clinical encounter cards (CECs) 264
clinical placements 6, 192, 198; *see also* early clinical experience; off-campus learning
clinical reasoning 28, 295; NOSM 7; Peru 119; problem-based learning 133; programme evaluation 348; script concordance testing 250; St George's Medical School 64
clinical skills 24, 31, 144, 148; anatomy 177; assessment 239, 263–77; integration 173, 181; Mozambique 116, 117; Peru 119; praxis 208; Primary Care Curriculum 172; role modelling 212; Russian doll metaphor 295; student-run clinics 152–3; Suez Canal University 150–1; Swansea College of Medicine 149; *see also* early clinical experience
clinical work sampling (CWS) 264
cloze 249, 252
coaching 153
cognitivism 129, 131, 209
coherence 209, 212, 218
collaboration: authentic learning 128; curriculum as collaborative activity 113, 117–21, 126; future of medical education 358, 359, 360; international 282, 288, 290, 292; interprofessional education 188, 189, 191, 192, 193–5, 196–7; outcome-based education 36–7; social accountability 11, 14; Université de Sherbrooke 34; University of Geneva Faculty of Medicine 28; *see also* teamwork
Collaboration for Health Equity through Education and Research (CHEER) 9–10, 14
collaborative learning 102, 131, 223
College of Medicine, Gulf Medical University 96, 97
communication skills 13, 20, 148, 173; ACGME competencies 35; Aga Khan University 311; All India Institute of Medical Sciences 21; authentic curriculum 114; early clinical experience 146–7, 150; Indonesia 31; interprofessional education 189, 195; King Abdulaziz University 39; leadership 306, 314; Mozambique 117; Peru 119; role modelling 123; selection of students 72, 73, 78, 80, 81–2; St George's Medical School 64; University of Geneva Faculty of Medicine 28
community: distributed community-engaged learning 7–8; early clinical experience 149–50; interprofessional education 193; research 14; student engagement 96; student mobility 104–5; University of New Mexico 211; *see also* community needs
community-based education (CBE) 30, 150, 198–9, 209; Canada 7–8; Mozambique 116; social accountability 11, 13; South Africa 10; student mobility 101, 104
community-based education and services (COBES) 195–6
community-based medical education (CBME) 157–70, 174, 307; benefits of 159–63; cultural competencies 166; implementation challenges 164–5
Community Health and Development Program (CHDP) 193–5
community needs 34, 39, 62, 160–4, 180, 294; authentic curriculum 114, 124; best practices 263, 264; early clinical experience 149–50; interprofessional education 198; medical school mission 301; new medical schools 297; new technologies 224–7; social accountability 11–12, 13–14, 15; WFME standards 344
community-oriented medical education (COME) 160
community-oriented primary care (COPC) 163, 164, 165
compassion 102, 103
competencies 15, 20, 23, 24, 173; assessment 237; Australia 32–3; authentic learning 130; Canada 33–4; community-based medical education 158, 160, 162; critical clinical 295–6; curriculum 114; digital 232–3, 234; Frenk on 4; Indonesia 31–2, 340, 341; mismatch with patient needs 22, 25; outcome-based education 37, 38, 41; selection of students 82, 83; United States 35–6
competency-based education (CBE) 27–8, 307; *see also* outcome-based education
complex adaptive systems (CASs) 158, 183, 209, 210, 217, 304
Comprehensive Community Clerkship (CCC) 7
computer-assisted training (CAT) 132–3, 150, 151; *see also* e-learning
computer-based testing (CBT) 259–61
Conférence Internationale des Doyens des Facultés de Médecine d'Expression Française (CIDMEF) 4–5

confidentiality 232, 346, 349
constructivism 87, 114, 129, 131, 209
consultation models 238
content production 232
context, input, process and product (CIPP) model 125
contextual assessment 80
contextualisation 288–9
continuing professional development 13, 15, 19, 20, 25; *see also* professional development
Cook, Sandy 215–16, 325
Coombs, Carmen 176–7
Corbin, L. 88, 91
core clinical problems (CCPs) 114–15
costs: assessment 256–7; authentic learning 141; graduate entry programmes 69; off-campus learning 105; problem-based learning 135; team-based learning 136
Council for Higher Education Accreditation 331
course evaluation 125
CPU model 10, 14–15
Craig, P.L. 68
creativity 20, 185
Cristobal, Fortunato L. 8–9
critical clinical competencies (CCCs) 295–6
critical thinking: authentic learning 131; interprofessional education 196; selection of students 73, 79; student engagement 87; team-based learning 136
Cuba 105–6
Cullen, W. 57
cultural competence 13, 20, 166
culture: assessment bias 265; community-based medical education 166; intercultural competence 291; non-prejudice 108; South African students in Cuba 106; transnational medical education 287, 288–9, 291; Western 282, 287
curiosity 108, 185, 212
curriculum 4, 113–27; adaptive integrated 172; Aga Khan University 308–10, 311; Al-Imam Mohammad Bin Saud Islamic University 315; All India Institute of Medical Sciences 20; assessment 239; authentic 113, 114–17, 124, 126; authentic learning methods 129; changing concept of 113–14; as collaborative activity 113, 117–21, 126; community-based medical education 157, 160, 161, 168; density 165; Duke-NUS partnership 216; early clinical experience 144–56; FMUA 31–2; forward-planning approach 27; future of medical education 357, 358; hidden 103, 104, 239, 333; Indonesia 340; integration of the sciences basic to medicine 171–87; international electives 107; interprofessional education 191; King Abdulaziz University 39; KSAU-HS 62; Namibian School of Medicine 312, 313; NOSM 7, 334, 335; outcome-based education 29–32, 36, 39–40, 41; Philippines 8; Primary Care Curriculum 172, 180, 210–13; problem-based learning 132, 297; programme evaluation 348, 349, 350; social accountability 11, 13, 15; spiral 35, 114–15, 137, 148; St George's Medical School 64; student engagement 89, 90, 92, 93, 113, 121–2, 126; teachers and the 113, 122–6; transnational medical education 282, 284, 285, 287, 288, 289, 292; Tunisia 5; Université de Sherbrooke 34; University of Geneva Faculty of Medicine 28–9

decentralised sites 225–7
Declaration of Alma-Ata (1978) 160
demand-based approach to forecasting 47, 48–9
demographic patterns 44, 52
Dennick, Reg 247–62
dental health 178
depression 88
developing countries 98, 105, 165
developmental model of student engagement 87
Dewey, J. 210
diagnosis 263, 299, 308
diagnostic reasoning 64
digital literacy 232–3
digital story telling (DST) 222–3
direct observation of procedural skills (DOPS) 264, 265, 269–73, 274
disability 75, 161
disadvantaged communities 13, 102, 106, 109
diseases 44, 192; early clinical experience 150; Malaysia 47; numbers of doctors required 52; South African students in Cuba 106
dissemination 321, 327
distance education 209
distractors 254
distributed community-engaged learning (DCEL) 7–8
distributed medical education 299–300, 301–2
distribution of doctors 45
diversity: admissions policy 12–13; community-based medical education 159–60; graduate entry programmes 69; South Africa 222; student engagement 89; student mobility 102–4

Index

doctors: demands of 298–9; forecasting supply 46–52; numbers required 43, 44–6, 52; role of 18–26; Russian doll metaphor 295; *see also* general practitioners
Doll, W.E. Jr 359
Dowell, Jon 72–85
'drag and drop' questions 253–4, 256
Dreesch, N. 43
Driessen, Erik 116–17
drop-out rates 61, 64, 67, 82
Dubowitz, Gerald 227
Duke School of Medicine 216–17

e-learning 29, 115, 307; interprofessional education 198; problem-based learning 132–3; student engagement 92; transnational medical education 285
early clinical experience (ECE) 144–56, 356, 360; authenticity 151–4; bridging the divide 147–9; community-based medical education 168; community needs 149–50; future of medical education 358; transnational medical education 289
Eastern Europe 46
Eastern Institute of Technology (EIT) 197
Eastern Virginia Medical School (EVMS) 325–7, 328
Easton, N. 46
Edinburgh Declaration (1988) 144, 160
Educational Commission for Foreign Medical Graduates (ECFMG) 339
educational policy 11, 12–13
educators *see* teachers
Egypt 132–3, 150–1, 198–9
Eire (Ireland): graduate entry programmes 63, 66; selection of students 72; student engagement 96, 98; transnational medical education 289
El Salvador 45
El-Wazir, Yasser 132–3
elderly people 44, 47
electives 30, 62, 101, 121; integrated curriculum 180; overseas 96, 98, 107–8
electronic portfolios (e-portfolios) 230, 231
elitism 3, 357
employment 88
empowerment 36, 87, 211
endoscopy training 272–3
enquiry 232
entrance examinations 21, 73
entrustable professional activities (EPAs) 35, 173, 174, 209, 210, 357
Eoyang, G.H. 217

equity 22, 25, 200; future of medical education 357, 359, 360; globalisation 25; Philippines 8; Tunisia 5
equivalence 287, 288
ethics 20, 173, 209; All India Institute of Medical Sciences 21; community-based medical education 166; ethical approval 164; interprofessional education 189; Peru 119; role modelling 123; social accountability 13; St George's Medical School 64; University of Dundee 115; University of Geneva Faculty of Medicine 29; University of Helsinki Medical Faculty 91
ethnicity: assessment bias 265; graduate entry programmes 66; selection of students 73, 74, 75
Europe: assessment 275; health managers 304; student engagement 87
European Higher Education Area (EHEA) 87
Eva, Kevin W. 78–9
evaluation: of assessment systems 243; community-based medical education 157; interprofessional education 193–5, 196–7, 198; programme evaluation 125, 330, 331, 343, 347–51, 358, 359; Social Obligation Scale 12; teachers as course evaluators 125
evidence-based medicine (EBM) 64, 214–15, 238
examinations: Aga Khan University 310; Arabian Gulf University 134; Australia 302; computer-based testing 259–61; critical clinical competencies 295–6; entrance 21, 73; examination cycle 248; Indonesia 32, 341; Japan 61; King Saud University 238; Medical University of Vienna 239–40; objective written tests 247–62; Saudi Arabia 63; selection of students 77–8; St George's Medical School 242–3; transnational medical education 285, 288, 291; *see also* assessment; Objective Structured Clinical Examination
experiential learning 101–2, 129, 131, 149
expertise 244, 245, 327
extended matching items (EMIs) 248–9, 250, 251
extracurricular activities 88, 96, 99

Facebook 123, 221, 224, 232
facilitator role 123, 137, 139
faculty development 13, 40, 154, 324–7; assessment 243, 244; case-based learning 140; community-based medical education 168; early clinical experience 150, 152, 154; student engagement 89, 90
Faculty of Medicine of Tunis (FMT) 4–5, 12, 14

Index

Faculty of Medicine Suez Canal University (FOM/SCU) 132–3
Faculty of Medicine, University of Airlangga (FMUA) 31–2, 160–2
feasibility 256–7
feedback 30; assessment 239, 243, 258, 259, 265, 270–1, 272, 274–5; clinical competence 264; coaching 153; community-based medical education 157, 168; complex adaptive systems 210; early clinical experience 147, 149, 150, 154; interprofessional education 196, 198; mini-CEX 268–9; mobile learning programme 231; peer-assisted learning 95; problem-based learning 172; selection of students 83; social theories of learning 131; student engagement 87, 93; teacher's role 124
fellows 345
'fill the gap' questions 249, 252
Finland 67, 91–2
First Nations peoples 334, 335
'fitness to practice' 82, 84
Flexner Report (1910) 3, 59, 144, 172
Flinders University 62, 63, 64, 69, 158–9
flipped classrooms 30, 121, 136–7, 233
fluid intelligence 77
Fogarty, R. 175, 178, 180, 183, 184
forecasting the supply of doctors 46–52
Forman, Dawn 188–203
formative assessment 209, 259; early clinical experience 149, 150, 153, 154; endoscopy training 272, 273; Karolinska Institute 140; King Abdulaziz University 179; King Saud University 238; problem-based learning 172; St George's Medical School 64; Université de Sherbrooke 34; University of New Mexico 211, 213
Forrest, Patrick 290
Foundation for Advancement of International Medical Education and Research (FAIMER) 336
Foundation Programme 265–6
Frambach, Janneke 116–17
France 46, 72
free open-access medical education (FOAMed) 224
Freeth, D. 192
Frenk, J. 4, 114
Frith, Gareth 230–1
funding 200, 201, 340, 342, 351

Gagné, Ève-Reine 33–4
Gallagher, Peter 197–8

Gasclass 224
Gavin, Katherine T. 98
gender: assessment bias 265; doctors 45–6; numbers of doctors required 52; selection of students 73
General Medical Council (GMC) 28, 63, 338; assessment 242; clinical skills 144; international recruitment of doctors 46; NUMed 284; standards 343; *Tomorrow's Doctors* 39, 114, 172, 242, 284; women doctors 45
general peer-assisted learning (G-PAL) 94–5
general practice 69, 82–3
general practitioners (GPs) 158, 159, 307–8; *see also* doctors
General Professional Education of the Physician (GPEP) 172
Germany 46
Ghana 45
Gibbs, Trevor 3–17, 304–17
Gillan, C. 197
Gladu, Daniel 33–4
Glassick, C.E. 326
Global Consensus for Social Accountability of Medical Schools (GCSAMS) 5, 301, 303
Global Determinants of Health and Development (GDH&D) 98
Global Minimum Essential Requirements 118
global view 22–3
globalisation 25, 37, 51, 96, 101, 292
Godfrey, R. 195
Goh, Poh Sun 228–9
Gomathi, Kadayam G. 97
Gordon, Chivaugn 101–9
Gordon, David 18–26
governance 300, 340, 342, 343
government agencies 341, 342
grade point average (GPA) 291, 335
graduate entry programmes (GEPs) 57, 59–70, 148, 297–8
Graduate Medical Schools Admissions Test (GAMSAT) 72
Graduate Outcome Study 6
Graillon, Ann 33–4
Grant, J. 37
Gray, Lesley 197–8
Greenhill, Jennene 158–9
Group Readiness Assurance Test (GRAT) 136, 137
Growing to be a Physician (GBP) 91
guided discovery 129, 136
Gulf Cooperation Council (GCC) 51
Gulf Medical University (GMU) 96, 97, 146–7
Gusic, Maryellen E. 318–29

Hamdy, Hossam 128–43
Hamilton, John 281–93
Hand, L. 88
Handy, Charles 307
Hanratty, Orla 98
Harden, Ronald M. 27–42, 113–27, 137, 175, 179, 289
Harris, R. 37
Hart, Ian 289
Harvard Medical School 123
Hatcher, Sharon 33–4
Hayes, K. 67
Hays, Richard 145–6, 265–6
health problem management 31
Health Profession Education Quality (HPEQ) 341
Health Professions Admissions Test (HPAT) 72
health promotion 22, 25, 164, 167, 168
Heifetz, R. 305–7
Heino, Anna T. 91–2
Heinonen, Kari 91–2
Henderson, Amanda 32–3
hidden curriculum 103, 104, 239, 333
High Level Task Force (HLTF) on Innovative International Financing for Health Systems 43
Higher Education Funding Council for England (HEFCE) 63
history taking 28
Hofstede, G. 282
Holladay, R. 217
horizontal integration 29, 64, 117–18; Bond University 145; King Abdulaziz University 179; Peru 119; programme evaluation 350; *see also* integration
Hosny, Somaya 132–3, 150–1, 198–9
hospitals 22, 148; Australia 6; Brazil 167; British Columbia 300; Malaysia 284, 285; South Africa 10; Tunisia 5
Houde, Sylvie 33–4
Hsin, Koo Wen 325
Hugo, Jannie 222–3
human immunodeficiency virus (HIV) 49, 50, 116, 163, 311
Human Systems Dynamics Institute 208
Hunt, Dan 330–52

Idaho State University (ISU) 225–6
image hotspots 253, 256
Imperial College Surgical Assessment Device (ICSAD) 272, 273
independence 108

India: All India Institute of Medical Sciences 20–1; computer-based testing 259–61; growing influence in medical education 275; innovative hospitals moving to developed countries 52
indigenous people: Australia 297, 302; Brazil 166; First Nations in Canada 334, 335; *see also* Aboriginal people
Individual Readiness Assurance Test (IRAT) 136, 137
individualism 165
Indonesia 31–2, 38, 160–2, 340–2, 347
infection control 198–9
inference 241, 244, 268–9
information management 31, 230
information overload 36
information provider role 122–3
innovation 20, 185, 282, 320
inquiry-based learning 216, 217
Institute for International Medical Education (IIME) 118
institutional accreditation 337–8
institutional delivery 190
Instituto Cardiovascular de Buenos Aires 268–9
integration 117–18, 120, 360; authentic learning 129; basic medical sciences 39, 118, 119, 144, 171–87; Bond University 145; future of medical education 357; interprofessional education 191; problem-based learning 133, 134; problems of 298; scholar approach in teaching 320; task-based learning 137; University of Dundee 115
integrity 20, 73; international electives 108; selection of students 76, 78, 79
intercultural competence 291
interdisciplinary practice 357; Australia 33; authentic learning 128; integrated curriculum 176; interprofessional education 193–5, 197
International Competency-Based Medical Educators (ICBME) 27–8
International Conference of Deans of French-speaking Medical Schools 4–5
international electives 96, 98, 107–8
international medical education 281–93
International Medical University (IMU) 289–90
internet 104, 225, 228–9, 232; *see also* social media
internships 52, 297–8; All India Institute of Medical Sciences 20–1; Flinders University 158; Indonesia 341; Mulago National Referral and Teaching Hospital 227

interpersonal skills: ACGME competencies 35; leadership 306; selection of students 72, 78, 79, 81–2, 83
interprofessional education (IPE) 29, 30, 148, 188–203, 307, 360; curriculum as collaborative activity 119; definition of 192; future of medical education 357; NOSM 7; outcome-based education 41; social accountability 13; Université de Sherbrooke 34; University of Geneva Faculty of Medicine 28; websites 201–2
interviews 72, 73–4, 78–9, 335
iPhones 230–1
Iran 65
Ireland (Eire): graduate entry programmes 63, 66; selection of students 72; student engagement 96, 98; transnational medical education 289

James Cook University School of Medicine (JCU-SOM) 5–7, 12, 13, 14
James, R. 88
Japan 61–2, 69
Jeffrey Cheah School of Medicine and Health Sciences (JCSMHS) 285, 286, 288
Jejcic, Kristijan 94–5
John Hopkins University School of Medicine (JHUSOM) 176
Jonas, S. 305
Jones, M. Douglas Jr 35–6
Jones, Paul Kneath 148–9

Kahu, E.R. 87
Kaila, Minna 91–2
Kamei, Robert 215–16, 325
Kane, M. 241, 244
Kark, Sidney and Emily 163
Karolinska Institute 139–40
Kelso, S.J.A. 212
Kennedy, Catherine 86–100
Kent, Athol 101–9
Kenya 195–6
Kerrin, Máire 75–7
King Abdulaziz University 39, 50, 179
King Faisel University 50
King Saud bin Abdul-Aziz University for Health Sciences (KSAU-HS) 62–3, 313
King Saud University (KSU) 50, 238–9, 274–5
Kirkpatrick, D. 125
Klamen, Debra L. 295–6
Knight, Sharon 227
Knight, Stephen 163–4

knowledge: ACGME competencies 35; assessors 244; core 303; curriculum 114; experiential learning 131; explicit and tacit 232–3; objective written tests 247; programme evaluation 348; Russian doll metaphor 295
Knowledge Test for General Practice 82
Korean Institute of Medical Education and Evaluation (KIMEE) 338
Korn, Abner 227
Kotter, John 305, 306, 307
Kozu, Tadahiko 57–71
Krajnc, Ivan 94–5

labelling questions 253–4, 256
Lafferty, Natalie 223–4
Lai, Chi-Wan 336–7
Laidlaw, J.M. 125
Lakehead University 7
Lamba, Pankaj 146–7
Lancet Commission 22
Lane, J. Lindsey 35–6
language issues 287
Lanphear, Joel H. 334–5
Larkins, Sarah 5–7
Laurentian University 7
Lave, J. 128
leaders, definition of 306
leadership 4, 20, 23, 24, 304–17; authentic learning 141; definitions of 305–6; doctor's role 299; educators 329; future of medical education 358; selection of students 73; social accountability 13
learning: assessment for 237, 259; community-based medical education 157, 158, 159, 161; as complex adaptive process 207, 209–11, 217; curriculum integration 183, 184–5; curriculum planning 113; definition of 209–10; experiential 101–2, 129, 131, 149; future of medical education 358, 360; improving effectiveness 207–20; interprofessional education 190, 196; new technologies 221–2, 231, 233; off-campus 104–5; positive learning environment 333; scholar approach in teaching 320; student diversity 102; student engagement 87, 89, 92, 93, 99; teacher as facilitator 123; transnational medical education 289; *see also* active learning; authentic learning; learning outcomes; lifelong learning; problem-based learning; self-directed learning
learning issues (LIs) 58–9
Learning Opportunities in the Clinical Setting (LOCS) 148–9

Index

learning outcomes (LOs) 29, 30, 32, 41, 173; assessment 34–6; Australia 32–3; Bond University 59; collaboration 37; community-based medical education 168; course evaluation 125; curriculum 113, 114, 121; examination cycle 248; implementation 39–40; interprofessional education 197–8; Nelson R. Mandela School of Medicine 163; Peru 118; praxis 209; programme evaluation 348; Saudi Arabia 39; task-based learning 137–8; teacher as facilitator 123; teacher autonomy 38
lectures 139, 161, 179, 192, 300
Lee, A. 190, 191
Leicester-Warwick Medical Schools 68
Lembaga Akreditasi Mandiri Perguruan Tinggi Kesehatan (LAM-PTKes) 341
Lembaga Pengembangan Uji Kompetens (LPUK) 341
Lester, Felicia 227
Liaison Committee on Medical Education (LCME) 332–3, 334–5, 336–7, 338, 339, 343, 345–6
Lieff, S.J. 306, 307
lifelong learning 13, 18, 22, 24, 25, 57; interprofessional education 196; King Abdulaziz University 39; stages of 19; Université de Sherbrooke 34; University of Geneva Faculty of Medicine 28; WFME standards 344
Lim, Victor 43–54, 289–90
Lim, William K. 135–6
Lin, Chyi-Her 336–7
Lindgren, Stefan 18–26
Linkoping University 189
Liu, Keh-Min 336–7
Liu, M. 256
Lo, Dr Lasz 321–3
Logic model 125
Lombardi, M. 128

Maastricht University 172
MacRae, Claire 114–15
Mahboob, Hina 321–2
Maherzi, Ahmed 4–5
Mak, Donna B. 191–2
Malaysia 47–8, 281; integrated curriculum 176–7; problem-based learning 135–6; transnational medical education 283–6, 287–8, 289–90; University Admissions Test 73; women doctors 45
Malaysian Medical Council (MMC) 283, 285, 286, 288

management 304, 305–6, 307, 308, 316; doctors 24–5; organisational 11, 12, 310; St George's Medical School 64; student engagement in management of medical school 89, 90, 91–2; teacher's role 124–5; Université de Sherbrooke 34; University of Geneva Faculty of Medicine 29; *see also* leadership
Manda, Venkatramana 97
Manderson, L. 287
Māori 197, 198, 355
market model of student engagement 87
marketisation 88
Martin, Stuart 75–7
Marzoeki, Puti 340–2
Massachusetts Institute of Technology (MIT) 46
Matson, Christine C. 325–7
Matte, Marie 334–5
maturity 60, 66, 67, 73, 104, 108
McCrorie, Peter 63–4
McHugh, Patrick 197–8
McKimm, Judy 148–9, 306, 307
McKinlay, Eileen 197–8
McLean, A.L. 95
McLean, Michelle 58–9
McMaster University 59–60, 78–9, 132, 172
MedBlogs 223–4
Medical College Admissions Test (MCAT) 72, 77, 291, 335
Medical Council of India 21
Medical Education in Europe (MEDINE2) 87
Medical Overseas Voluntary Electives (MOVE) 98
Medical School Council Assessment Alliance (MSC-AA) 257
medical schools 3–17, 18, 24; accreditation of new medical schools 334–5, 337, 338, 339–40; attrition rates 52; campus-based learning 104; challenges for the 21st century 294–303; graduate versus school-leaver entry 57–71; Indonesia 340; leadership and management 304–17; Malaysia 48; programme evaluation 347–51; satellite campuses 105; Saudi Arabia 50–1; social class of students 164–5; South Africa 50; student engagement 89–96; transnational medical education 283–93
Medical Teacher 27
Medical University of Vienna 239–41
Mennin, Regina Helena Petroni 157–70
Mennin, Stewart 171–87, 207–20, 355–60
mentoring 92, 93
Michaelsen, Larry 136
midwives 43

migration 4, 23, 46, 50, 51–2, 359; *see also* student mobility
milestones 34, 35, 40
Millennium Development Goals (MDGs) 43, 163
Miller's pyramid of competence 238, 239, 264
mind mobility 102, 103, 104, 109
mini-clinical evaluation exercises (Mini-CEXs) 119, 231, 238, 243–4, 264, 265, 268–9, 274
mini-peer assessment tool (Mini-PAT) 264, 265
mini-simulations (SIMs) 82, 83
Mining, Simeon 195–6
Mintzberg, H. 305, 306, 310
Mires, Gary 114–15
mission 298, 303; Al-Imam Mohammad Bin Saud Islamic University 315, 316; community needs 301; curriculum planning 113, 126; leadership and management 304, 314; programme evaluation 348; social accountability 12, 301, 302; student engagement 89, 90, 91; WFME standards 343
Mitchell, Veronica 103–4
mixed parallel-entry programmes (MEPs) 57, 59, 61, 62, 64–5, 68
mobile learning programme (MLP) 230–1
mobile technologies 221, 230–1
mobility *see* student mobility
modified essay questions (MEQs) 238
Moi University 195–6
Monash University Malaysia (MUM) 283, 284–6, 287–8, 289, 292
Montaigne, Michel 3
moral reasoning 79
motivation: assessment 239; culture of learning 212; early clinical experience 147; graduate versus school-leaver entry 67; Mozambique 117; new technologies 233; selection of students 73, 80, 82; teacher as facilitator 123
Mozambique 114, 116–17, 123
Mulago National Referral and Teaching Hospital 227
Muller, Alexandra 103–4
multi-source feedback (MSF) 264
multidisciplinary teams 159, 168, 191–2, 199, 308, 311
multimedia 132–3, 151, 232, 256
multiple-choice questions (MCQs) 21, 134, 136, 237, 238, 243, 248, 249, 254
Multiple Mini-Interview (MMI) 72, 78–9, 82, 84
multiple scenarios 154
Murray, Richard 5–7
Muyingo, Mark 227
Mylona, Elza 325–7

Naeem, Naghma 238–9
Namibia 311–13
narrative-based evidence 214
National Board of Examiners, India (NBE) 259–60
National Health Service (NHS) 45, 46, 270, 305
National Survey of Student Engagement (NSSE) 86–7
National University of Cuyo 267–8
National University of Rio Negro Dental School 178
National University of Singapore (NUS) 215–17, 228–9, 230, 233, 325
needs-based approach to forecasting 47
needs, future 190
Nelson R. Mandela School of Medicine 163–4
neo-colonialism 282
neo-liberalism 87
Netherlands: basic medical sciences 172; migration of doctors 46; selection of students 72, 82–3; workforce planning 48–9
Netherlands Institute for Health Services Research (NIVEL) 48
New Mexico 199–201, 210–13
New Zealand (NZ) 197–8, 289, 302, 343
Newcastle University (Australia) 67
Newcastle University (UK) 67–8, 283–4
Newcastle University Medicine Malaysia (NUMed) 283–4, 286, 287, 289, 292
non-linear adaptive action 215
non-prejudice 108
Nordquist, Jonas 311–12
North America 3, 86–7; *see also* Canada; United States
Northern Ontario School of Medicine (NOSM) 7–8, 12, 13, 14, 334–5
Northern Territory Clinical School (NTCS) 69
Northouse, P. 307
Nsubuga, Yosam 227
nurses 43, 44–5

Obenshain, S. Scott 211–12
Objective Structured Clinical Examination (OSCE) 40, 78–9, 117; apps 231; Brazil and Argentina 267–8; clinical competence 264; FMUA 32; graduate versus school-leaver entry 68; Gulf Medical University 147; King Abdulaziz University 179; King Saud University 238; Medical University of Vienna 240, 241; peer-assisted learning 95; Peru 119; programme evaluation 351; transnational

Index

medical education 285; Université de Sherbrooke 34
Objective Structured Long Case Examination Record (OSLER) 264
Objective Structured Practical Examination (OSPE) 134, 179
objective written tests 247–62
objectives: assessment feedback 258; behavioural 37; early clinical experience 150, 154; leadership 314; programme evaluation 348, 350–1; SMART 320, 322; Social Obligation Scale 12
Oblinger, D. 128
O'Brien Pallas, L. 47
Ochsner Health System (OHS) 289, 290–1
odontology 178
off-campus learning 104–5, 200–1; *see also* clinical placements
O'Keefe, Maree 32–3
online assessment 256, 257, 259–61
online repositories 228–9
open-ended questions 237
Opina-Tan, Louricha A. 193–5
organisational culture 332, 333
organisational management 11, 12, 310
Osaka University 61, 69
Osler, William 123, 147–8, 154
outcome-based education (OBE) 27–42; benefits of 29–37; challenges of 37–8; implementation of 38–40; importance of 27–8; *see also* learning outcomes

Pakistan 73–4, 308–11, 323–4
Pandey, Steve B. 270–1
Papa, Jared 225–7
paper-based testing (PBT) 259
paradoxical medical education 296–7
Parallel Rural Community Curriculum (PRCC) 69, 158–9
participation 232
partner medical schools (PMSs) 289–91
partnerships 20; Canada 7, 8; Community Health and Development Program 193; Duke-NUS 216; international 282; Moi University 195; social accountability 14
Paterno, Elizabeth R. 193–5
patient interaction 18, 24, 214, 281; early clinical experience 150; King Abdulaziz University 39; NOSM 7; role modelling 123; selection of students 83
Patterned Behaviour Descriptive Interview (PBDI) 82, 83

Patterson, Fiona 75–7
Patterson, L. 209–10
peer assessment 89, 92, 93, 95, 97, 238; mini-peer assessment tool 264, 265; University of New Mexico 212, 213
peer-assisted learning (PAL) 94–5, 99
peer reviews 9–10, 321
peer teaching 89, 92, 93, 94, 95, 99
peer-to-peer learning 121
Perdana University Graduate School of Medicine (PUGSOM) 176–7
personal growth 88, 101–2, 104; international electives 107; mind mobility 102, 103, 109; Peru 119
personalised learning 30, 121, 230
personality tests 80, 81
perspective taking 76
Peru 116, 118–19, 137
Peruvian University of Applied Sciences Medical School (UPC-MS) 118–19
Pete, B.M. 175
Philippines 4, 8–9, 193–5
photographs 222–3, 228, 232
physician assistants (PAs) 225–7
Pinjani, Sheilla K. 323–4
Pitkäranta, Anne 91–2
policy 11, 12–13; programme evaluation 349; student involvement 90, 91, 122; *see also* admissions policies
Pomeroy, Claire 331–3
Ponnamperuma, Gominda 274–5
Pontificia Universidad Católica de Chile Medical School (PUCMS) 271–3
population growth 25, 49, 52
portfolio assessment 30, 40, 117, 172–3
positive discrimination 102; *see also* affirmative action
positivism 144
Postgraduate Hospital Educational Environment Measure (PHEEM) 273
postgraduate training 25; assessment 271–3; Australia 6, 7; Brazil 340; British Columbia 300; Japan 61; online repositories 228–9; social accountability 14, 15; WFME standards 344; workplace-based assessment 265–6
practice: definition of 188; theory and 207, 208–9, 217, 356, 360
practice-based learning 35
praxis 154, 208, 209, 210–11, 215–17
preparation, educators 320, 322, 324
Preparation in Practice (PiP) 114–15
Preston, Robyn 5–7

prevention 22, 25, 150, 167
primary care 22, 157; career choices 164–5; community-based medical education 162, 163; Community Health and Development Program 194; Declaration of Alma-Ata 160; early clinical experience 145, 146, 149, 150, 154; equity of access to 359; Faculty of Medicine of Tunis 5; future of medical education 358; health advocate role 28; interprofessional education 199; JCU-SOM 6; Karolinska Institute 139; Malaysia 47; Mozambique 116; Namibia 311; negative stigma 165; numbers of doctors required 52; off-campus learning 104; University of Helsinki Medical Faculty 92
Primary Care Curriculum (PCC) 172, 180, 210–13
privacy 232
private sector: individualistic ideology 165; Indonesia 340; Malaysia 47; Saudi Arabia 51
problem-based learning (PBL) 29, 68, 116, 132–6, 209; Bond University 58–9, 145; constructivism 131; experiential learning 131; interprofessional education 189, 191, 200; key features 129; King Abdulaziz University 39, 179; McMaster University 172; new medical school development 297; Peru 119; Philippines 8; St George's Medical School 64; student-centred learning 121; teacher as facilitator 123; theory-practice divide 208; University of Dundee 115; University of Geneva Faculty of Medicine 28; University of Helsinki Medical Faculty 91; University of New Mexico 212; University of Sharjah 138
productivity 44–5
professional associations 342
professional development 19, 20, 25, 126; AM.EI 325; scholar approach in teaching 320; social accountability 13, 15; Université de Sherbrooke 34
professionalism 20, 23, 25, 173, 209; ACGME competencies 35; assessment 238, 239; authentic curriculum 114; community-based medical education 166; early clinical experience 147; Indonesia 31; international electives 108; programme evaluation 348, 350–1; social accountability 13
programme evaluation 125, 330, 331, 343, 347–51, 358, 359; *see also* accreditation
progress tests 30, 209
promotion criteria 326, 327–8
psychometric analysis 259, 261, 268

public expenditure 43
Pullon, Sue 197–8

quality assurance: accreditation 330, 337, 338, 347; Indonesia 340–2; outcome-based education 29–32; programme evaluation 348, 349, 351; student engagement 88, 89; transnational medical education 291
Quality Assurance Agency for Higher Education (QAA) 88–9
question banks 257

radiology 228–9
ranking questions 249, 251
real-world relevance 128–30
reflection: community-based medical education 157; early clinical experience 154; educators 318, 321, 327; interprofessional education 196; problem-based learning 172
Rehatta, Nancy Margarita 31–2, 160–2
Reid, Stephen 9–10
Reiter, Harold I. 78–9
relationship-centred care 210
reliability: assessment 239, 241, 245, 256, 261; selection of students 74, 77, 80
relocation 101
remote teaching 227
reporter, interpreter, manager, educator (RIME) model 35
reputation 88
research: CHEER collaboration 9; community-based medical education 162; future of medical education 359; medical school mission 298; social accountability 11, 13–14; student engagement 95–6; teachers as researchers 125; transnational medical education 286; Tunisia 5; WFME standards 344
resilience 80
resources 263, 264, 268; accreditation 333–4, 349; doctor's role in managing 24–5; scholar approach in teaching 320; WFME standards 343
retention 61, 88
reverse-planning model 27
Riquelme, Arnoldo 271–3
Risco de Domínguez, Graciela 118–19
Roberfroid, D. 46
Roberts, Trudie 57–71
role models 24, 123, 162, 212
Rolfe, I.E. 67
Ross, Simone 5–7
Round, Jonathan 242–3

Rowett, Emma 75–7
Royal College of Physicians and Surgeons of Canada (RCPSC) 28, 338
Royle, T. James 270–1
rules for learning 212–13, 218
rural areas: Australia 158–9, 297–8, 301–2; Canada 299–300, 334; distribution of doctors 45; interprofessional education 192; Mozambique 116; New Mexico 199–201, 211; new technologies 233; Philippines 8, 9; recruitment of students from 102; South Africa 222; student mobility 105; United States 225, 226
Rural Health Interdisciplinary Program (RHIP) 200, 201
Russia 44, 275
Russian dolls 294, 295

Sadaf, Shazia 323–4
Saleh, Farid 313–15
Sandars, John 221–34
Sansevero, Antonio 144–56
satellite campuses 101, 105
saturation of information 241
Saudi Arabia: assessment 238–9; graduate entry programmes 62–3, 67, 69; integrated curriculum 39, 179; new medical colleges 313–16; numbers of doctors 50–1; workplace-based assessment 274–5
Saudi Licensing Examination (SLE) 63
scaffolding 131, 233
Schmidts, Michael 239–40
scholar approach 318–29
school-leaver entry programmes (SEPs) 57–60, 61, 64–5, 66–9, 70, 297
Schuwirth, Lambert 237–46
Scotland 89, 114–15
Scottish Doctor 38–9, 172
script concordance testing 250, 252
security issues 261
selection of students 72–85, 357, 360; academic ability 77–8, 80, 84; community-based medical education 168; context 74–7; framework for selection 80–2; non-academic attributes 78–80, 84; ranking 83; selecting out 82–3; *see also* admissions policies
self-analysis 24
self-assessment 92, 93, 212, 213, 238, 270
self-awareness 31
self-directed learning 57, 58, 59–60; authentic learning 129; blogs 224; computer-assisted training 151; graduate entry programmes 67; interprofessional education 196; King Abdulaziz University 179; lack of student preparation for 332; problem-based learning 132, 172; St George's Medical School 64; student engagement 99; University of Dundee 115; University of Geneva Faculty of Medicine 28; University of Helsinki Medical Faculty 91; University of New Mexico 211
self-evaluation 331
self-organisation 210, 216–17
self-reflection 269
Sen Gupta, Tarun 5–7
sequential testing 239–40
Servis, Mark 331–3
sexual minorities 102, 103
sexuality 75
Shaafie, Ishtiyaq A. 97
Shehata, Mohamed H. K. 198–9
Shilkofski, Nicole 176–7
short-answer questions (SAQs) 134
Simpson, Deborah 318–29
simulation 29, 30, 36, 40, 209, 273; anatomy 176–7; Swansea College of Medicine 149; technologies 173; training workshop 270–1
Singapore 73, 215–17, 228–9, 230, 233, 288, 325, 328
Singapore Health Services (SingHealth) 325, 326, 328
single best answers (SBAs) 242–3, 249
situational judgement tests (SJTs) 75–7, 79–80, 81, 82, 84
Skinner, Margot 197–8
Skype 227
Slovenia 94–5
small communities 334–5
SMART objectives 320, 322
Snadden, David 299–300
social accountability 4–15, 23, 295, 301–2; Aga Khan University 73; assessment 303; authentic curriculum 117; global 20, 22; Nelson R. Mandela School of Medicine 163; WFME standards 344
social class 164–5; *see also* socio-economic status
social constructivism 129, 131, 136, 140
social determinants of health 8, 163, 169, 194
social justice 4, 8, 9, 12
social media 123, 136, 221, 224, 232–3, 234, 260
social norms 108
Social Obligation Scale 11, 12
social responsibility 11, 12, 24, 164, 209, 357
social responsiveness 11, 12
social theories of learning 131

societal needs 22, 25, 158, 301, 315; *see also* community needs
socio-economic status 73, 74, 77, 297
Soep, Jennifer 35–6
Sood, Rita 20–1
South Africa (SA): CHEER collaboration 9–10, 14; community-based medical education 163–4; digital story telling 222–3, 233; diversity 102–4; forecasting supply of doctors 49–50; growing influence in medical education 275; positive discrimination 102; student mobility 105–6
South Korea 64–5, 69, 337–8, 347
Southern Illinois University School of Medicine (SIUSOM) 295–6
Souza, Ruy 144–56, 166
specialist education 7, 19, 52, 157, 158
SPICES model 31, 113
spiral curriculum 35, 114–15, 137, 148
Sri Lanka 288
St George's University of London 63–4, 242–3
stakeholders: community-based medical education 157–8; curriculum planning 119–20, 124
standardised/simulated patients (SPs) 173, 176, 295
standards 32, 36, 302–3; accreditation 331–3, 335–40, 343–4, 347, 349, 351; Australia 33; future of medical education 359; Indonesia 341
Steketee, Carole 191–2
Strasser, Roger 7–8
stress 60, 66, 67
student-centred learning 87, 91, 99, 121, 136
student engagement 86–100, 121–2, 126; Aga Khan University 311; benefits of 87–8; challenges and constraints 88; community-based medical education 168; definition of 86–7; frameworks for 88–9; new technologies 233, 234; operationalisation of 89–98
student mistreatment 332–3
student mobility 101–9; challenges of 109; diversity 102–4; international electives 107–8; off-campus learning 104–5; whole-course mobility 105–6
student numbers 43–54; forecasting supply of doctors 46–52; numbers of doctors required 44–6, 52
Student Participation in Quality Scotland (SPARQS) 89
student-run clinics (SRCs) 152–3
student satisfaction 348–9
student-selected components (SSCs) 30, 114–15, 121

Stufflebeam, D.L. 34
Suez Canal University 132–3, 150–1, 198–9
Suleiman, Abu Bakar 43–54
summative assessment: endoscopy training 273; feedback 259; interprofessional education 198; King Abdulaziz University 179; King Saud University 238; Medical University of Vienna 239, 240; St George's Medical School 64, 242, 243; Université de Sherbrooke 34
supervision 20, 341
supply projection model 46
support 24, 89, 153
support staff 45, 349
Surjadhana, Adrianta 31–2, 160–2
survey teams 344–6
Swansea College of Medicine 148–9
Swanson, D.B. 248, 255
Sweden 139–40, 189
Sweeney, K. 213–15
Switzerland 28–9
symbiotic clinical education 158
systems-based practice 35
Systems in Practice (SiP) 114–15

Taiwan 65, 336–7, 343, 344, 347
Taiwan Medical Accreditation Council (TMAC) 336–7
Talford, David 225–7
Tan, Kok Leong 47–50
task-based learning (TkBL) 129, 131, 137–8
Tawfik, Mirella Youssef 150–1
Taylor, C.A. 306
teachers: case-based learning 139; community-based medical education 162, 168; curriculum planning 113; integrated curriculum 178, 179; outcome-based education 38; roles of 122–6, 137; scholar approach 318–29; transnational medical education 286–7
teaching: clinical 274–5, 287; curriculum planning 113; by doctors 23; future of medical education 358; interprofessional education 190; new technologies 223–4, 227, 233; scholar approach 318–29; student engagement 89, 92, 99, 122; transnational medical education 284, 289
team-based learning (TBL) 136–7, 209; constructivism 131; Duke-NUS partnership 216, 217; experiential learning 131; key features 129; Peru 119; student-centred learning 121; University of Dundee 115

teamwork 20, 23, 24, 25, 323; All India Institute of Medical Sciences 21; community-based medical education 164, 168; integrated curriculum 178; interprofessional education 189, 191, 199, 200; outcome-based education 41; selection of students 73, 76, 78, 83; social accountability 13; *see also* collaboration

technology 44, 221–34, 303; community needs 224–7; digital competences 232–3; flipped classrooms 136; future of medical education 357, 359; learner needs 222–4, 230; new opportunities for learning 227–30; 'new-technology doctors' 299; online assessment 256, 257, 259–61; scholar approach in teaching 320; simulation 173; *see also* e-learning; internet; social media

Tehran University of Medical Sciences 65

terminology 298

theory 207, 208–9, 217, 356, 360

'threshold concepts' 123

Tomorrow's Doctors (GMC, 2009) 39, 114, 172, 242, 284

Tope, R. 189

Topping, K.J. 94

Torres Strait Islanders 5, 6

Tosteson, D.C. 123

Training for Health Equality Network (THEnet) 6, 10, 14

transferable skills 58, 59

transnational medical education 281–93

transparency 346–7

Trinity College, Dublin 96, 98

Tromp, Fred 82–3

trust 20

tuberculosis 8, 163

Tuning Project 28

Tunisia 4–5

tutorial system (TS) 94

Twitter 123, 221, 223, 224

Uganda 227, 233

UK Foundation Programme (UKFP) 265–6

Um AlQura University 50

uncertainty 185, 213, 215, 217, 356, 360; adaptive action landscape diagram 174, 184; community-based medical education 159, 168; culture of learning 212; task-based learning 138

United Arab Emirates 96, 97, 138, 146–7

United Kingdom (UK): accreditation 343; assessment 242–3, 265–6, 275, 302; blogs 223–4; case-based discussions 264; clinical skills 144; curriculum 114–15; early clinical experience 148–9; Foundation Programme 265–6; graduate entry programmes 60, 63–4, 66, 67–8, 69; international recruitment of doctors 46; leadership 304, 305; mobile technologies 230–1; outcome-based education 28; positive discrimination 102; question banks 257; selection of students 72, 74, 75–7; simulation training workshop 270–1; student engagement 88–9; teacher as facilitator 123; transnational medical education 283–4, 286, 287, 289; women doctors 45–6

United Kingdom Clinical Aptitude Test (UKCAT) 72, 75–7

United States (US): accreditation 331–3, 336, 339, 343, 344, 345, 347; assessment 275, 302; basic medical sciences 172; chronic diseases 44; clinical skills 144; critical clinical competencies 295–6; elderly people 44; faculty development 325–7; graduate entry programmes 59; health managers 304; interprofessional education 199–201; Medical College Admissions Test 335; new technologies 224–7; outcome-based education 28, 35–6; positive discrimination 102; selection of students 72, 74, 79; student-run clinics 152–3; survey teams 345; transnational medical education 289, 290–1

United States Medical Licensing Examination (USMLE) 216, 291

universal testing 77

universe generalisation 241

Universidad Peruana de Ciencias Aplicadas Medical School (UOC-MS) 137

Université de Sherbrooke 33–4

Universiti Malaysia Sarawak (UNIMAS) 135–6

Universities and Colleges Admission Service (UCAS) 66

University Admissions Test (UAT) 73, 74

University of Airlangga 160–2

University of Auckland 197

University of Birmingham 68

University of British Columbia (UBC) 299–300

University of California Davis (UCD) 331–3

University of California San Francisco (UCSF) 152–3, 227

University of Cape Town 102–4

University of Colorado School of Medicine 35–6, 40

University of Dundee 114–15, 138, 223–4, 230, 233

University of Geneva Faculty of Medicine 28–9

University of Helsinki Medical Faculty 91–2

University of Leeds 230–1, 233
University of Limerick 63
University of Maribor 94–5
University of Melbourne 68
University of Namibia 311–13
University of New Mexico 172, 180, 210–13
University of New Mexico Health Sciences Center (UNMHSC) 199–201
University of Northern British Columbia 299–300
University of Notre Dame 189, 191–2
University of Nottingham 66, 68
University of Otago 197–8
University of Pretoria 222–3
University of Queensland School of Medicine (UQSM) 62, 67, 68, 289, 290–1
University of São Paulo 267
University of Sharjah 138
University of Sydney 62
University of the Philippines (UP) 193–5
University of Victoria 299–300
University of Washington (UW) 225, 226–7
University of Witwatersrand 50
upper gastrointestinal endoscopy basic training programme (UGIETP) 272–3

validity: assessment 239, 241, 244, 245, 255–6, 261, 266; selection of students 74, 75, 77, 80
values 34, 212, 307, 316, 323
Van der Vleuten, C.P.M. 256
VanLeit, Betsy 199–201
Venkatramana, Manda 146–7
Vermeulen, Margit I. 82–3
vertical integration 29, 64, 118, 119; Bond University 145; King Abdulaziz University 179; programme evaluation 350; *see also* integration
video technology 227; problem-based learning 132–3; video questions 254, 255, 256
Vinik, Aaron I. 325–7
virtual learning environments (VLEe) 223–4, 227
virtual patient pool (VPP) 91
voice, student 88, 89, 99

Waechter, Donna 330–52
Wagner-Menghin, Michaela 239–40
'washback' effect 292
Wasserman, M. 46
Wenger, E. 128
Western culture 282, 287
whole-course mobility 105–6
Wilkinson, David 290–1, 294–303
Wilkinson, T.J. 66, 67
Wilson, Ian 297–8
Wollard, R. 10, 14
women 3, 45–6, 66
WordPress 221, 223–4
workforce planning 45, 46–52
workplace-based assessment (WPBA) 117, 230–1, 238, 239, 264, 265–6, 272, 274–5
World Bank 43
World Federation for Medical Education (WFME) 63, 338, 351; accreditation standards 343–4, 347; Edinburgh Declaration 144, 160; international recognition of accreditation 339; social accountability 301; stages of accreditation 331
World Health Assembly 46
World Health Organization (WHO): community-based medical education 160; Declaration of Alma-Ata 160; international recruitment of doctors 46; interprofessional education 188; numbers of doctors required 43, 44, 51; social accountability 11, 301; world health days 97; *World Health Report* 43, 49, 311
written tests 247–62

Xhignesse, Marianne 33–4

Yadav, Hematram 47–50
Yasin, Shajahan 281–93
Young, Mei Ling 43–54
Yousuf, Naveed 323–4

Zdravkovic, Marko 94–5
Zuberi, Rukhsana W. 73–4, 308–10, 323–4

eBooks
from Taylor & Francis
Helping you to choose the right eBooks for your Library

Add to your library's digital collection today with Taylor & Francis eBooks. We have over 50,000 eBooks in the Humanities, Social Sciences, Behavioural Sciences, Built Environment and Law, from leading imprints, including Routledge, Focal Press and Psychology Press.

Choose from a range of subject packages or create your own!

Benefits for you
- Free MARC records
- COUNTER-compliant usage statistics
- Flexible purchase and pricing options
- All titles DRM-free.

Benefits for your user
- Off-site, anytime access via Athens or referring URL
- Print or copy pages or chapters
- Full content search
- Bookmark, highlight and annotate text
- Access to thousands of pages of quality research at the click of a button.

Free Trials Available
We offer free trials to qualifying academic, corporate and government customers.

eCollections
Choose from over 30 subject eCollections, including:

Archaeology	Language Learning
Architecture	Law
Asian Studies	Literature
Business & Management	Media & Communication
Classical Studies	Middle East Studies
Construction	Music
Creative & Media Arts	Philosophy
Criminology & Criminal Justice	Planning
Economics	Politics
Education	Psychology & Mental Health
Energy	Religion
Engineering	Security
English Language & Linguistics	Social Work
Environment & Sustainability	Sociology
Geography	Sport
Health Studies	Theatre & Performance
History	Tourism, Hospitality & Events

For more information, pricing enquiries or to order a free trial, please contact your local sales team:
www.tandfebooks.com/page/sales

www.tandfebooks.com